TOBACCO INDUSTRY AND SMOKING

LIBRARY IN A BOOK

TOBACCO INDUSTRY AND SMOKING

REVISED EDITION

Fred C. Pampel

Willow International Center Library

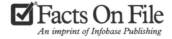

Facts On File
An imprint of Infobase Publishing

Tobacco Industry and Smoking, Revised Edition

Copyright © 2009, 2004 by Fred C. Pampel
Graphs copyright © 2009 Facts On File

Facts On File, Inc.
An imprint of Infobase Publishing
132 West 31st Street
New York NY 10001

Library of Congress Cataloging-in-Publication Data
Pampel, Fred C.
    Tobacco industry and smoking / Fred C. Pampel. — Rev. ed.
        p. cm — (Library in a book)
    Includes bibliographical references and index.
    ISBN-13: 978-0-8160-7793-9 (alk. paper)
    ISBN-10: 0-8160-7793-2 (alk. paper)
    1. Smoking—United States. 2. Tobacco industry—United States. 3. Smoking. 4. Tobacco use. I. Title.
    HV5760.P36 2009
    338.4'7679730973—dc22   2009000396

Facts On File books are available at special discounts when purchased in bulk quantities for businesses, associations, institutions, or sales promotions. Please call our Special Sales Department in New York at (212) 967-8800 or (800) 322-8755.

You can find Facts On File on the World Wide Web at http://www.factsonfile.com

Text design by Ron Monteleone
Graphs by Sholto Ainslie

Printed in the United States of America

MP Hermitage 10 9 8 7 6 5 4 3 2 1

This book is printed on acid-free paper and contains 30 percent postconsumer recycled content.

CONTENTS

PART III
APPENDICES

PART I

OVERVIEW OF THE TOPIC

CHAPTER 1

INTRODUCTION TO THE
TOBACCO INDUSTRY
AND SMOKING

Cigarette smoking is the single largest preventable cause of premature death in the United States today. Estimates of the number of yearly deaths from smoking-related causes exceed 440,000 (about one-sixth of all deaths), and smokers can expect to die 13–14 years earlier than nonsmokers. The situation has improved since the famous 1964 report of the surgeon general on the harm of cigarettes, but it remains serious. Despite falling cigarette use in past decades, 21 percent of the U.S. population in the year 2006 smoked, and roughly the same percentage used to smoke—making more than 40 percent of the population vulnerable to the risks of early death. Worse, young people today continue to adopt the habit at distressingly high levels. No wonder the U.S. surgeon general views smoking as the nation's number one public health problem.

Given that few incentives seem to remain for smoking cigarettes today, the persistence of the problem seems puzzling. Public warnings about the harm to health of smoking are so well known that people actually overestimate the risks; taxes and lawsuits against tobacco companies make the purchase of cigarettes a substantial cost; prohibitions against smoking in office buildings, public facilities, and even restaurants and bars force smokers into outside streets, alleyways, and quarantined rooms; and nonsmokers feel free to criticize smokers as a public nuisance and shame them for their inability to stop a destructive habit.

Still, about 45 million persons continue to act in ways that harm their health. Cigarette smoking is spreading across the globe and countering the decline in the United States and in European nations. China, for example, now has one of the world's highest rates of cigarette consumption. Efforts to make the United States and the world smoke-free have a long way to go.

Many suggest that the promotion and advertising efforts of the tobacco industry combined with the addictive properties of cigarette smoke explain

3

the persistence and proliferation of the habit. Private attorneys and attorneys general of many states have, in representing addicted smokers and public health programs that pay for health problems of smokers, blamed the tobacco companies for the situation. Juries appear to agree, as they have become increasingly willing to award plaintiffs large damages in suits against tobacco companies. In a major turn of events, the tobacco industry, under pressure, consented to make payments to state governments for the health costs inflicted on smokers. They now advise youth to avoid smoking and adult smokers to quit.

Yet, describing the problem seems easier than dealing with it. At one extreme, antismoking advocates, who tend to view smokers as manipulated by tobacco advertising and addicted once they want to stop, favor stringent controls and litigation. At the other extreme, defenders of smoking note that Congress has not outlawed tobacco products, and adults can reasonably decide to risk a shorter life in order to enjoy the pleasure they get from cigarettes. They worry about the threat of antismoking policies to individual rights.

Stated in less extreme but still controversial terms, the following questions have engaged the public in recent years.

- Should tobacco be regulated by the government much as other drugs are regulated?
- Is the tobacco industry, despite the mandated warnings on cigarette products, responsible for the harm of cigarettes?
- Can consumers make their own decisions about cigarette smoking, or have tobacco ads manipulated people, particularly youngsters, to adopt a harmful product?
- Does secondhand smoke from the cigarettes of others represent a serious threat to nonsmokers that requires banning smoking in all public indoor places, including restaurants and bars?
- Why do people continue a habit that so clearly harms their health? Can policies counter the attractions to smoking?

Far from obscure issues of concern only to doctors and lawyers, the debates over tobacco use and smoking policies affect most everyone in their daily lives.

THE RISE OF TOBACCO, 1870–1950

EARLY FORMS OF TOBACCO USE

A plant native to the Americas, tobacco was first cultivated in the Andes Mountains in present-day Peru and Ecuador as far back as 5000 B.C.[1] In the centuries to follow, use of the plant spread across the two continents and into the Caribbean islands. Properly prepared, tobacco could be sniffed into the nose, inserted into the mouth for chewing, or brewed like tea to make a drink. When so used, it had some medicinal properties: Tobacco's mild narcotic could ease the pain of toothache, wounds, and snakebites. And, as a powerful insecticide, it could be used for a variety of purposes. However, it had more appeal when burned and inhaled. Tobacco could be smoked after it was dried, chopped, inserted, and burned in a pipe, or after it was rolled into a leaf similar to today's cigars. When burned, tobacco seemed to have religious properties, as the smoke would rise up toward the gods in heaven.

Something more than these religious and practical purposes, however, accounts for the spread of tobacco use among diverse tribes and regions of the Americas. Inhaling the smoke into the mouth and lungs could disperse tobacco chemicals into the bloodstream and give users a mild, pleasurable experience. Smokers might find the process of inhaling to be soothing, but the chemical makeup of tobacco must have contributed to its popularity—otherwise, smoking of different plant products would have become more common. The rewards of tobacco and its main chemical stimulant, nicotine, have attracted humans for as long as the plant has been known.

Tobacco came to have social as well as physical value. Its properties made it a logical medium for youth to prove their passage into adulthood, for those relaxing and socializing to pass the time, and for competing tribes to share a common experience. Tribal shamans would blow smoke over sacred objects, warriors would smoke before battle, and the dead would be buried with their pipes. Although these activities most often involved men rather than women, they played a central part in the social life of American tribal societies.

Upon landing in the New World in 1492 and making contact with the native peoples, Christopher Columbus and his sailors received a gift of tobacco leaves, and some of the crew members later accepted the offer of the local American Indians to follow their custom by smoking the dried plant in a long pipe. Reputed to have become habitual users during their stay, the sailors were the first Europeans to try the practice.[2] Columbus returned to Spain with stories of the product but only a few seeds and leaves. Focused on obtaining gold from the New World, Columbus and other explorers did not realize at the time what influence and economic value this product would come to have.

Later brought back to Spain and Portugal in usable form during the 1550s, tobacco was first thought by Europeans to have special medicinal value, and physicians and others would plant it in palace gardens for this reason. Early on it was used mostly as snuff and mostly by health fanatics. Some claimed wondrous results from the product, recommending it as a cure for bad breath, kidney stones, and wounds from poison arrows. It soon spread from Spain and Portugal to France, Italy, and Germany. In France, Jean Nicot promoted the curative powers of tobacco to the queen, and history rewarded him: The plant was formally named *Nicotiana tabacum* and the crucial chemical in the plant was termed *nicotine*.

English explorers John Hawkins, Walter Raleigh, and Francis Drake brought the product to England starting in the 1560s, where it spread rapidly.[3] The English favored use of a pipe for their new habit. The handsome and elegant Walter Raleigh popularized the new behavior until it became something of a craze, and he even persuaded the elderly Queen Elizabeth I to try it. Smoking turned into a habit common among patrons of William Shakespeare's Globe Theatre and surrounding forums of entertainment in London, and it was the subject of an English-language book in 1595.

While many lauded the pleasurable, even narcotic properties of smoking, others found the new habit disgusting and wicked. Most famously, King James I of Great Britain published a pamphlet in 1604, soon after his coronation, criticizing the product and rebuking smokers. In harsh words he stated, "Smoking is a custom loathsome to the eye, hateful to the nose, harmful to the brain, dangerous to the lungs, and in the black, stinking fume thereof, resembling the horrible Stygian smoke of the pit that is bottomless."[4] His critical voice along with those of the emerging Puritan movement could not, however, overcome the attraction to the product and to the profits made by growers in the New World. The king soon tried to discourage its use with new taxes, but tobacco continued its growth in the English-speaking world.

The first successful American commercial crop was cultivated in Jamestown, Virginia, in 1612 by Englishman John Rolfe (who a few years later married the Wampanoag princess Pocahontas). Within seven years, tobacco had become the colony's largest export. Reflecting its Puritan background, the northern colony of Massachusetts prohibited tobacco, but such opposition did not prevent the product from becoming a central part of the American economy. Tobacco was so popular in the South that it could be used as a form of money and as a dowry in marriage. It had such a central place in the economy and the wealth of citizens that high taxes placed on the product once led Virginia planters to rebel against the colonial governor. By the time of the American Revolution, tobacco was such an important commodity that Benjamin Franklin used it as collateral in obtaining loans from France to support the war effort.

Tobacco use took various forms in the United States. During the colonial period, the pipe remained generally popular, but aristocrats tended to use snuff and those in rural areas tended to use chew. For a brief period in history, pipe smoking was also popular among women (the wife of President Andrew Jackson, first elected to the office in 1829, smoked a pipe as the first lady). Cigars were new at the time, and cigarettes were rare. Only the destitute, who rolled discarded tobacco bits, used cigarettes; that form of smoking product accordingly gained little acceptance by more respectable parts of colonial society. One exception to the disrepute of cigarettes was during a brief period in revolutionary France (1789–94) when many viewed cigarettes as a way to show solidarity with the lower class.

During the first part of the 19th century, however, tobacco use in the United States declined. The U.S. government had begun taxing tobacco in 1794, and a few leading scientists and public figures (including Benjamin Rush, a physician and signer of the Declaration of Independence) claimed that tobacco was harmful to one's health. Snuff became unfashionable, and pipe smoking and chew remained common largely in rural areas. Other tobacco products started to appear more commonly but did not yet gain widespread popularity; for example, troops during the Civil War used hand-rolled cigarettes because they were cheap, convenient, and easy to carry, yet most did not continue with the habit afterward. In fact, men tended to view cigarettes after the Civil War as effeminate and suited for dandies and Europeans in big cities. Outside rural areas, chew was increasingly viewed as unsanitary; the presence of spittoons containing spit tobacco juice and the sight of tobacco stains on floors in cities repelled many respectable people. Cigars became popular among the growing affluent business class after the Civil War, and many leaders such as President Ulysses Grant (who later died of throat cancer) and General Robert E. Lee smoked cigars regularly. Perhaps because of their expense, however, cigars did not attract widespread adoption.

THE SPREAD OF MANUFACTURED CIGARETTES

Historians mark 1870 as the starting point for widespread cigarette smoking in the United States. Prior to this year the use of tobacco seemed a curious habit that appealed to just a few groups, hardly a habit that would become an important part of society. It brought a mild form of pleasure, but the common forms of tobacco produced harshness in the smoke that made inhalation unpleasant. Moreover the process of smoking pipes and cigars was slow and tedious—suited for leisurely paced socializing but not for daily activities. Chew was unsanitary, snuff was pretentious, and cigarettes were bohemian. With the decline of tobacco use over the last 70 years, the market for greater sales seemed limited. Several new developments, however, made for changes in attitudes toward one tobacco product—cigarettes.

What led to the changes and the widespread adoption of the product over the next century? Slowly and steadily, improvements in the product itself and its suitability for modern life combined to make cigarettes widely popular. In terms of the product, manufacturers made their cigarette tobacco less harsh and more flavorful. Consisting of mild and sweet tobacco plants that were cured to make the leaves even milder and sweeter, cigarettes became easier for persons to tolerate and inhale. As discovered in 1839, bright tobacco, grown in Virginia and North Carolina, developed an unusually sweet and pleasant taste when cured in a certain way and could be smoked in greater quantities than previous forms. Another tobacco plant, white burley, first developed in Ohio in 1866, could absorb additives better than other products. Soon, sweeteners and flavors added to the tobacco also attracted new users. In addition to having a better taste, the new products had higher nicotine levels.

By itself, however, better flavor did not lead to widespread use of cigarettes. The product needed to be presented in a way that consumers would find attractive. In the past, tobacco was sold in lots that required smokers to roll their own cigarettes, which made it hard to identify a certain tobacco with a product name and identity. The creation of manufactured cigarettes that came in small boxes not only avoided the need for smokers to roll their own cigarettes but also allowed producers to display the name of the cigarette on the box. From this packaging came the emergence of tobacco brands that would attract smoker loyalty and, with the coming of advertising and promotion, the desire to buy new products. Producers could advertise their brands by name to gain new smokers and could offer picture cards that smokers liked.

Manufacturers soon realized that increasing demand for cigarettes from advertising and promotion of particular brands would do little to help the industry if they could not supply the product at an affordable price. Hiring workers to roll each cigarette by hand was expensive and kept the production costs of cigarettes high. The tobacco industry fell behind other manufacturers in its lack of a mechanized means to turn out cigarettes. A major innovation thus came with a machine invented and patented by James Bonsack in 1881. The machine dropped a small amount of granulated tobacco onto paper, shaped the paper and tobacco into a tube, and then cut the tube into equal-sized cigarettes. By 1884 the machine could produce 200 cigarettes a minute.

Combined with a helpful decrease in excise taxes on cigarettes, the ability of machines to reduce labor costs in factories made it possible to sell cigarettes to retailers at lower prices than before. Able to make larger profits themselves, the retailers did more than in the past to promote cigarettes. Cigarette manufacturers did not get a higher rate of profit with the lower prices they charged to retailers but did increase their profit through higher sales.

Cigarettes also led to a different form of smoking that seemed well suited to changing social life at the end of the 1800s. Cigars and pipes typically did not require inhaling to enjoy; rather, the pleasure came from the drawn-out process of preparing to smoke and from the aroma of the tobacco fumes. With continued effort required to keep cigars and pipes lit, they were enjoyed during leisurely talks after dinner and during periods of inactivity. Smokeless tobacco in the form of snuff or chew could be used on the go and spit on the ground by farmers and residents of rural areas, but spitting was not a habit suited for modern life in cities. In contrast to these other products, cigarettes fit the continuous, sometimes frantic activity in cities. They could be carried conveniently, lit easily, and smoked quickly. (The invention of small paper matchbooks added to the ease of use.) Clerical workers in cities, for example, could more handily smoke cigarettes than cigars or pipes while they worked. Cigarettes, more than other tobacco products, also involved social sharing: Their inexpensive cost allowed for giving them out upon request, and lighting another's cigarette signified friendship or intimacy. Although cigars remained well liked for special occasions, the smaller cigarettes became common for everyday activities.

Perhaps more important, cigarette smoking had a different and more attractive physiological effect. Smoke from cigars and pipe tobacco had properties that made inhaling unpleasant. As with chew, cigars and pipe tobacco delivered nicotine to the body through the mouth. However, cigarettes could deliver nicotine more efficiently than the other products. Cigarette tobacco had chemical properties that made inhaling easier to learn and tolerate. Because the lungs more than the mouth cavity have enormous absorbent properties, inhaling smoke effectively delivered nicotine to the body, efficiently evoked the mild narcotic pleasure, and resulted in addiction. Smokers consequently found it harder to moderate or stop their habit when they used cigarettes.

Past fashions in tobacco use had led to preferences for snuff, pipes, chew, large cigars, and small cigars, but these new trends and developments would make cigarettes the dominant product in the late 19th century and into the early 20th century. By 1924 more than 80 percent of families spent at least part of their budget on tobacco. In a study in 1935–36, about 2.23 percent of the budget of the typical American family went to tobacco products.[5] Economic downturns might produce some modest changes in cigarette use. Purchase of cheaper brands of cigarettes rather than premium brands and even use of cheap tobacco to roll one's own cigarettes became popular during periods of high unemployment and low income (particularly during the Great Depression of the 1930s). Otherwise, cigarette use spread steadily.

Some figures can describe the rise of manufactured cigarettes in the United States. In 1870 the number of cigarettes smoked per person was 0.36—in other words, less than a single cigarette a year on average. In 1879 cigars remained the most common tobacco product, followed by tobaccos for snuff, pipe, and chewing. By 1900, however, the figures for cigarettes per person had risen to 35 and by 1938 to 1,268. In the 30 years from 1870 to

1900, consumption per person had increased by 9,700 percent, and in the following 38 years from 1900 to 1938, it increased by another 3,600 percent. In 1900 tobacco for cigarettes constituted only 2.4 percent of all manufactured tobacco, and by the early 1930s it represented more than 40 percent. Smoking tobacco for pipes, the next most popular form, equaled 30 percent; cigars, 15 percent; chew, 10 percent; and snuff, 5 percent. The popularity of cigarettes would continue to rise.

COMPETITION AND MONOPOLY IN THE TOBACCO INDUSTRY

As with most industries during the late 1800s, the tobacco industry grew initially through the entrepreneurship of thousands of small businessmen. In 1864, there were no major American cigarette manufacturers, and pre-made cigarettes were imported from Europe, Turkey, and Russia. In response to concerns about the use of cigarettes by soldiers and to the desire of the government for revenue, new taxes were placed on the manufactured cigarettes, most of which were paid by importers. Domestic cigarettes made with the bright tobacco leaf were largely handrolled and used by those living outside the larger cities of the eastern United States who could not afford the high prices of the imported brands.

The growth of the American tobacco industry came with efforts to sell cigarettes made of domestic tobacco. F. S. Kinney in 1868 began to sell prerolled cigarettes largely with American bright tobacco in a store in lower Manhattan. Experimenting with various blends and even adding sugar and licorice flavor, Kinney had much success with his brands in New York City. Keeping his prices lower than the imports, he placed the cigarettes in paper rather than cardboard packages. Businesses copied his strategy in other neighborhoods, cities, and states.

Lewis Ginter, who began in the cigarette business in 1840, used his base in Richmond, Virginia, to become the first national distributor of cigarettes. Also using bright tobacco from the Virginia and North Carolina area that smokers found so appealing, he marketed his product to all parts of the country. Although not the first to use factories to roll cigarettes, Ginter began producing cigarettes in large numbers in the 1870s and contributed to the early rise of cigarette smoking. He also exploited the advantages of white burley tobacco in absorbing sweeteners and flavors by producing and marketing new flavored brands of cigarettes.

Despite Ginter's success in selling his product across much of the nation, the tobacco industry in the 1870s still consisted of hundreds of small manufacturers. In 1877, for example, government tax authorities had registered 121 cigarette brands, and local brands left uncounted by national authorities would add even more to the total.[6] The competition between small companies resulted in overproduction of cigarettes, low prices, and small profit margins. Those in the cigar business thought that the cigarette industry would collapse, and cigars would continue their traditional dominance as the tobacco product of choice. In fact, efforts to organize and monopolize the cigarette industry would put it on a sound financial basis and would lead to some of the most successful and powerful business enterprises in the United States.

James Buchanan (Buck) Duke, the man most responsible for the shape of the modern tobacco industry—and also for the spread of cigarettes—played much the same role as did John D. Rockefeller in the oil industry and J. P. Morgan in the financial industry. In 1874, he joined his father and brother to found a tobacco firm, W. Duke Sons and Company, in Durham, North Carolina. Duke's father, Washington Duke, had established a small business that produced chewing tobacco from the bright tobacco leaf. Eventually taking over the business, Buck gave up competing against more well-known brands of chewing tobacco, such as Bull Durham, and began to produce cigarettes in 1881. The competition for the product was less fierce but so was the demand from tobacco users. A wildly overwrought quote from the *New York Times* in 1883 reveals the prejudice at the time against cigarettes: "If this pernicious habit obtains among adult Americans the ruin of the Republic is close at hand."[7]

Duke showed his tremendous organizational and managerial skills in making his cigarette business successful and creating a major industrial empire. By exploiting the development of the cigarette rolling machine—he leased machines for his factories from the inventor, James Bonsack, beginning in 1884—and using his lower costs to encourage retailers to push his product, he made strong inroads on the market. With considerable expense devoted to advertising and hiring talented salespeople to further market his brand, Duke became the nation's largest cigarette manufacturer. Yet he was not satisfied. He wanted to control the industry, not just lead it.

To the dismay of his competitors, Duke intensified his advertising efforts and price-cutting strategy in the late 1880s. He bought out companies with profit margins so thin they could not invest in the machines and advertising to compete with Duke. Other, more successful companies promised to fight back, but most soon gave in and agreed to merge with Duke. In 1890 Duke, at age 33, became the first president of the American Tobacco Company. The firm produced 90 percent of domestic cigarettes and soon began trying to overtake the chewing and snuff companies in addition to cigarette companies.

Although wildly successful in creating a profitable enterprise that enriched all those involved, Duke created enemies with his strategies. No sooner had he founded the American Tobacco Company than an antitrust suit in North Carolina aimed to dissolve the company. Other suits followed, and President Theodore Roosevelt came to oppose the trust. In 1907 the circuit court found that subsidiaries of the American Tobacco Company had violated the Sherman Anti-Trust Act. With eventual support of the decision by the U.S. Supreme Court, the American Tobacco Company in 1911 had to be dissolved into four firms: Liggett and Myers, Reynolds, Lorillard, and American, all companies that would remain important forces behind cigarette production and use in years to come.

Duke's trust not only made him rich but also made cigarettes a national product with increasing acceptance and prices that a mass market of people with modest incomes could afford. Duke retired soon after the breakup of his company and devoted his wealth to expanding a small college, which was later renamed Duke University. However, his efforts to create an efficiently and rationally organized industry for growing, curing, manufacturing, marketing, and selling tobacco contributed to the spread of the product's use. Although several companies rather than one major company now existed, each one continued and even expanded the efficient generation of profits. They did so in part because of the nature of the product but also by advertising and promoting their products. Such efforts would become the key to success among these companies, and in the future several of the most famous brands—Camel, Lucky Strike, and Chesterfield—would emerge and further contribute to the growth of the industry.

ANTISMOKING MOVEMENTS

Given the enormous success of the industry, the spread of cigarettes created a backlash of resistance. During the early 1900s largely rural Protestants protested against the spreading vice of alcohol, especially among the largely immigrant Catholics and the new affluent middle classes in cities.[8] With much the same motivation the Anti-Tobacco Society was founded in 1849, publication of an antitobacco journal began in 1857, and warnings about the harm of tobacco use emerged in 1849 and 1857. The opposition to cigarettes was neither as strong nor as successful as the opposition to alcohol and did not result in national prohibition of the product, as occurred for alcohol from 1919 to 1933. While drinking became associated with debauchery, saloons, prostitution, gambling, fighting, marital discord, and drunkenness, smoking had none of these drawbacks. Cigarettes and tobacco were sold by respectable businesses, did not lead to inebriation, and were used by respectable members of society in everyday life.

Still, substantial opposition to smoking surfaced for several reasons. Because the purpose of tobacco seemed to involve little more than the search for frivolous pleasure, religious groups such as the Seventh-Day Adventists and the Women's Christian Temperance Union (WCTU) opposed its use. Although no one knew the extent of the harm smoking could cause, critics saw it as unhealthy for smokers, unpleasant for nonsmokers, and lacking social merit. Cigarettes received special criticism: Cigars and pipes seemed more dignified and less noticeable; in contrast, the tendency for people to smoke cigarettes in public and to become habituated to the daily use of cigarettes aroused the concern of crusaders. More than other tobacco products, cigarette use led to addiction and revealed weakness of character.

Antismoking groups showed particular concern about the tendency of youth to smoke, worrying that it reflected a sense of rebellion and lack of respect for authority. Young boys seemed particularly attracted to cards that were included in many packages of cigarettes. Sometimes these cards included pictures of attractive actresses in provocative poses and famous athletes whom children would want to emulate. The cards might even be used for betting games. Furthermore, smoking seemed especially common among delinquent youth and soon became associated with truancy and petty crime.

Responding to these negative characteristics of cigarette use among adults and young people, a powerful antismoking movement emerged from the temperance movement. Its leader, Lucy Page Gaston, a single schoolteacher and WCTU member, came to have much influence on the public's view of smoking. Through her tireless efforts, she significantly slowed the spread of cigarette use. In 1899 she founded the Chicago Anti-Cigarette League using the model of antialcohol groups. Two years later she founded the National Anti-Cigarette League and soon became one of the country's best-known reformers. She held rallies in schools and towns in which she decried the poisons brought into the body by cigarettes and noted cases of known murderers and criminals who smoked. She recruited converts to her organization, promoted city health clinics where smokers could go to quit the habit, and urged legislatures to ban the product. In 1920 she ran unsuccessfully for the Republican Party presidential nomination.

Her antismoking movement had some success. North Dakota, Tennessee, and Iowa first prohibited cigarette smoking in the 1890s, and 11 other states followed with prohibition in the first two decades of the new century. Other laws prevented teachers and school officials from smoking, banned passengers from smoking in railway cars and in the New York City subways, and required persons buying cigarettes to be at least 16 years old. Many famous Americans supported these antismoking efforts: Henry Ford, the successful car manufacturer, wrote a pamphlet for young people entitled "The Case Against the Little White Slaver," and Thomas Edison, the inventor, claimed that cigarettes released poisons into the body and destroyed brain cells.

In the end, however, cigarette use continued its steady upward increase. Laws to ban smoking did not stop the habit, much as Prohibition did not stop the use of alcohol. In fact the efforts to deny people the chance to use cigarettes may have intensified their appeal in some quarters. States repealed their prohibitions against smoking (except among minors) by the end of the 1920s, with Indiana being the first state to do so in 1909. Gaston continued her campaign against cigarettes into the 1920s, later focusing on limiting their adoption by women. In support of this goal the Women's Christian Temperance Union also sponsored thousands of antismoking events. The efforts failed to slow the spread of cigarettes. Gaston died in 1924, ironically of throat cancer, having had only short-term success. Not until some 50 years later would antismoking crusades have real success.

SMOKING BECOMES WIDELY FASHIONABLE

Despite its steady growth, cigarette smoking in the early 20th century remained somewhat tainted. As one historian described it, "Red blooded men smoked cigars and pipes and chewed tobacco" while the cigarette had "the taint of the dude, the sissy, and the underworld."[9] Consistent with such attitudes, cigar production reached a new record in 1917. True popularity of cigarettes would come only with their adoption by men as a symbol of rugged masculinity and by women as a symbol of freedom and independence.

Changes in the attitudes of men toward smoking began with World War I. During U.S. participation in the war from 1917 to 1918, cigarettes became popular among soldiers. Entering late into the war, American soldiers picked up the habit from British troops but were also encouraged to smoke by the free or inexpensive cigarettes supplied by the government to the armed forces; tobacco firms wisely made cigarettes available to the government for such distribution at low cost. General John Pershing, the commander of the U.S. troops, revealed the importance of cigarettes to soldiers when he stated, "You ask what we need to win this war. I answer tobacco, as much as bullets. Tobacco is as indispensable as the daily ration. We must have thousands of tons of it without delay."[10] Charitable organizations responded by sending cigarettes to soldiers overseas.

Cigarettes were easy to carry in battle and convenient to light up during breaks in fighting. Sharing them created bonds among unit members and helped pass the time during periods of inactivity. Moreover, some said that cigarette smoking helped calm the nerves when watching and waiting for the enemy. Smoking might even have given a soldier a sense of confidence and resolve when holding a cigarette between his lips in periods of danger. During the terrible battles of the war, providing a cigarette to an injured or dying soldier became a sign of compassion, an act of civility for someone suffering.

Cigarette manufacturers quickly took advantage of the popularity of cigarette smoking among soldiers. By associating the habit with patriotic fighters, advertisers could displace common views that smoking was a habit of delinquent youth, members of the underworld, and European dandies. The respectability of soldiers countered criticisms of antismoking organizations. Indeed the opposition of the American Legion and soldiers to smoking bans contributed to the repeal of state laws in the 1920s. Building on this new constituency, advertisers created patriotic copy. One such ad in 1918 depicted a muscular and determined-looking sailor standing next to a tall, sleek bomb and holding a cigarette; the ad states, "I'd shell out my last 18 cents for Murad (The Turkish Cigarette)."[11]

Along with targeting soldiers who had returned from the war, the tobacco industry knew it had to appeal to young people. Without having present-day knowledge about the addictiveness of cigarettes, the industry realized that continued growth of cigarette sales depended on the acceptance of the product by new generations. Advertisements that appealed too directly to young people would be seen as wrongly influencing children; however, testimonials by adult sports stars and celebrities could indirectly appeal to youth. A 27-year-old Charles Lindbergh, for example, lit a cigarette after his famous flight across the Atlantic.

A new market for cigarette use among women also emerged in the 1920s. Smoking by women was not unknown in the United States. In colonial times aristocratic women used snuff, and rural women smoked pipes, much like their spouses. However, with the decline in popularity of snuff and pipes, women dropped the use of tobacco and did not adopt the cigars and chew used by men later in the 1800s. Becoming largely a male activity, tobacco consumption seemed unfeminine and inappropriate for women. Men would, accordingly, segregate themselves from women after dinner in a special room to smoke cigars and would often wear special smoking jackets so regular jackets did not smell of tobacco. Women largely took the lead in antismoking movements.

The early use of cigarettes in the late 1800s thus began as a male fashion. Smoking by women in private was frowned on, and smoking in public was seen as outrageous. For example, in 1904 a New York City policeman arrested a woman for smoking in a car on Fifth Avenue, and a 1908 ordinance in New York City made public smoking for women illegal. An 18-year-old woman was expelled from Michigan State Normal College for smoking in 1922. Women nonetheless began to adopt the habit as it became popular among men but did so more in private.

Tobacco firms recognized that they could double their market if women smoked as much as men. Toward the goal of gaining more female converts, the first advertisement aimed at women occurred in 1919 for Helmar cigarettes, and by the 1920s such ads were common. The early ads were relatively tame because tobacco companies did not want to violate public taboos too severely, but they represented a new strategy in the battle to gain smokers. By 1929 women consumed about 12 percent of all cigarettes.[12]

The adoption of cigarettes by women coincided with advances toward greater freedom in other arenas of social life. Voting in elections had since the founding of the country been limited to men, but protests by women suffragists had led to ratification of the Nineteenth Amendment to the Constitution in 1920, granting women the right to vote. The right of women to smoke, in both private and public, emerged about the same time and was seen by some as, like voting, an issue of women's freedom. Other behaviors once restricted in public, such as dancing and wearing bathing suits, became acceptable for women, along with cigarette smoking. Tobacco companies aimed to exploit these new desires by challenging social conventions. Rejecting traditional views of women as protectors of moral purity, advertisers promoted images of women as stylish, autonomous, and sexually alluring.

Some figures show the rise in female smoking. In 1923, 5 percent of smokers were women, but by 1931 the figure had risen to 14 percent. Smoking levels among women lagged behind those of men but were still substantial. A 1937 survey found that 26 percent of women smoked an average of 2.4 cigarettes a day, compared to 60 percent of men who smoked an average of 7.2 cigarettes a day.[13]

With cigarette smoking viewed by youth as a behavior that helped establish their identity as adults, by men as a behavior that helped establish their masculine identity, and by women as a behavior that helped establish themselves as modern and independent, the negative perceptions that had been associated for decades with cigarettes largely disappeared. Movie stars, sports figures, adventurers, physicians, college students, beautiful women, and rugged men smoked—and tobacco advertisements did all they could to publicize such usage. The decades after the 1870s, and particularly the 1920s, thus revealed a major change in American social life: An innovative behavior that many had once viewed with suspicion as a worrisome vice and organized to protest, outlaw, and reform became not only tolerated but embraced. Overcoming the efforts of its onetime opponents, smoking became a norm that men and women followed without much thought to its long-term consequences.

THE INFLUENCE OF ADVERTISING

Cigarette manufacturers learned early that competition for sales had to involve something other than price or product distinctiveness. James Duke discovered that cutting prices destroyed the prestige of a cigarette brand, associating it with the poor and disadvantaged and thereby reducing its sales. If having the lowest prices offered no means to success, neither did differences in the product. The public liked certain types of tobacco, certain packaging, and certain kinds of flavor in their cigarettes. Makers developed new products that smokers liked, but other makers would imitate the new brands. In both price and product, different brands of cigarettes varied little.

As Duke demonstrated, the key to gaining sales was advertising and promotion. Even given similarities in price and flavor with others, a particular brand could through advertising and promotions develop brand loyalty among its users and increase its sales to new buyers. After spending nearly 20 percent of his company's gross income on advertising in his successful attempt during the 1880s to weaken rivals and create the American Tobacco Company, Duke had eliminated most competition and reduced the need for so much advertising. Yet he did not do away with it altogether. Advertising could help attract new smokers and help keep cigarette consumption rising. In contrast, advertising never emerged as important for cigars, where product differences in prices, shapes, flavor, and tobacco leaves offered the major source of appeal to customers. The markets for pipe tobacco and chew also responded less to high expenditures on advertising than the market for cigarettes did. Advertising and cigarettes became closely associated.

Upon breakup of Duke's cigarette trust into four companies, advertising competition among tobacco firms accelerated. In 1913 an advertising campaign of Richard J. Reynolds for Camel cigarettes helped make the product the nation's most popular, capturing 40 percent of the market by 1919; the R. J. Reynolds Tobacco Company subsequently grew into one of the nation's most successful. Large two-page ads that appeared in the popular *Saturday Evening Post* magazine proclaiming "The Camels Are Coming" piqued the interest of smokers. Smokers also liked the more flavorful blend of Turkish and American tobaccos in the cigarette that resembled more expensive imports. Responding to this success, other companies promoted their own products. American Tobacco introduced Lucky Strike cigarettes, and Liggett and Myers introduced Chesterfield cigarettes about the same time as Camel cigarettes. Each brand developed advertising to identify a particular image and would dominate sales in the decades to follow.

The problem for tobacco firms that gained market share through advertising was that their brands were easily displaced by advertising campaigns from other companies. The rise and fall of the major brands showed in the replacement of the top-selling Camels in the 1920s by Lucky Strikes. George Washington Hill, the president of American Tobacco, followed the precepts of his predecessor, James Duke, by using advertising to make Lucky Strike cigarettes the top seller. Chesterfields also took the lead in sales in the 1930s. Trends in sales thus followed innovations in advertising more than innovations in product and price.

Sometimes ads highlighted factual claims that one brand had superior flavor, was less irritating, and used better tobacco. Lucky Strike cigarettes claimed that physicians favored their brand, and other companies followed suit with statements that their product soothed the nerves and protected the throat. Such assertions led editors of the *Journal of the American Medical Association (JAMA)* to criticize cigarette advertisements for promising unproven benefits. However, the real appeal of ads was emotional. Much as they do today, ads in the first part of the century associated smoking with other pleasurable activities, relied on testimonies of celebrities, and depicted cigarettes as enjoyable. Camel ads, already associated by virtue of the name with the exotic Middle East, proclaimed the strong desire for their product with the slogan "I'd Walk a Mile for a Camel." Reminding smokers of the pleasant aroma of browned bread, Lucky Strike emphasized that its tobacco was toasted. Chesterfield cigarettes claimed, "They Satisfy."

Advertising also targeted specific subgroups with their images and appeals. Advertising for women often took special forms. Lucky Strike advised women in 1928 to reach for a Lucky rather than a sweet, appealing to the growing desire for young women to maintain a thin figure. A new cigarette brand from England, Marlboro, aimed to capture the female market by proclaiming that the product was as "Mild as May." Chesterfield cigarettes hired Bette Davis and Marlene Dietrich to advertise their products. Other brands emphasized that their cigarette was lighter and prettier than those smoked by men. In 1926 one Chesterfield ad reflected a new, more provocative approach: It showed a young woman asking a handsome male smoker to "blow some my way."

Did advertising contribute to the growth of cigarette use? On the surface, it would certainly appear so. Advertising of cigarettes rose at a pace similar to cigarette consumption, and advertising campaigns certainly had success in making one brand more popular than others. The tobacco companies believed in advertising and used it to increase their market share. However, it is hard to show that coinciding trends in advertising and smoking result from causal forces. The increased acceptability and fashionableness of smoking among wide segments of the U.S. population could have encouraged both more smoking and more advertising. Indeed, advertising may have followed the growth of cigarettes among various groups by appealing to those already using the product.[14]

DOCUMENTING THE HARM OF TOBACCO, 1950–1990

EARLY WARNINGS ABOUT CIGARETTES

Cigarette consumption continued its upward growth rate throughout the first half of the 20th century. Given the widespread acceptability of the practice, the number of cigarettes smoked per capita rose from 1,485 in 1930 to 1,976 in 1940. Aided by the consumption of cigarettes by U.S. soldiers in World War II (1941–45) and advertising campaigns emphasizing the war efforts of the tobacco companies, smoking rose even faster during the 1940s. By 1950 smoking per capita reached a new high of 3,552—nearly twice as high as only 10 years earlier. The major controversies came not from health concerns but from conflict over profits. Tobacco farmers had survived financial ruin during the Great Depression only by receiving government price supports, while tobacco manufacturers continued to earn high profits. A price-fixing suit against the tobacco companies in 1941 led to a fine but not to low profits. A later shortage of tobacco in the United States during the war years raised the price of cigarettes and further benefited the industry. After the war the demand for American cigarettes increased sharply in Europe, where production facilities had been destroyed.

However, growth of cigarettes slowed during the 1950s. To some degree the market had simply reached saturation: Anyone who would be prone to smoke had likely already tried and continued the habit. More important, people responded to new evidence on the damage to health caused by cigarettes. Per-person cigarette consumption actually fell after 1952 and did not return to its previous peak until 1958. Scientific evidence had accumulated for some time, but new articles about the risks of smoking in popular magazines during the years of the 1950s may have worried smokers. The change in smoking habits was not dramatic—the behavior remained common and acceptable—but it was the start of larger changes to follow.

In hindsight, one wonders why the scientific community and the population did not come sooner to the conclusion that smoking harms health. Antismoking advocates had for decades noted the potential harm of smoking. The slang term for cigarettes—*coffin nails*—certainly implied that the product was damaging. And most anyone could wonder if the large amount of smoke being inhaled into the lungs and the body would bring injury and if smoker's coughs reflected underlying problems. Perhaps the sometimes exaggerated and unscientific claims of antismoking advocates made the general public suspicious of health warnings about cigarettes, or perhaps the advertising claims, sometimes supported by physicians, that smoking brought energy and good health soothed doubts people had about smoking. Overall, however, the main reasons for the lack of attention to the risks of smoking were that the harm of smoking took several decades to emerge at a time when most people worried about diseases such as scarlet fever, influenza, and tuberculosis that killed more quickly and that scientific evidence had not yet clearly demonstrated the harm. The general medical consensus was that, when done in moderation, smoking was not dangerous.

Those looking for such evidence could by 1950 find articles published in reputable scientific journals that warned of the risk of smoking. A 1930 study by researchers in Cologne, Germany, identified a correlation between cancer and smoking, and in 1938 Dr. Raymond Pearl of Johns Hopkins University reported that smokers did not live as long as nonsmokers. Those following the trends in lung cancer noted that the death rates for men had risen from two per 100,000 in 1910 to 22 per 100,000 in 1950—an 11-fold increase. The rise in lung cancer came a few decades later than the rise in smoking, but otherwise the upward trends matched. Despite denials from cigarette companies, such evidence led scientists to suspect cigarettes as a source of the increased incidence in lung cancer. Still, proof was harder to obtain: As noted in considering the relationship between advertising expenditures and cigarette consumption, proving cause and effect from these statistical correlations is always difficult.

Other studies in the 1940s demonstrated that tobacco extract could induce cancer in laboratory animals; that cigarette smoking was associated with coronary heart disease as well as lung cancer; and that chewing tobacco led to mouth cancer. Still, defenders of the habit could dismiss the evidence as preliminary and tout the health benefits of smoking. The pleasure gained from smoking seemed for many to outweigh possible risks. Even *JAMA* was not sufficiently convinced by the evidence of the harm of smoking in the 1940s to refuse inclusion of cigarette advertisements in the publication. The American Cancer Society, clearly concerned about cigarette use, admitted that no definitive evidence at the time linked smoking to lung cancer.

The year 1950 marked a turning point in scientific evidence and attitudes about smoking. In that year, a groundbreaking study demonstrated in stark terms the association between smoking and lung cancer by examining individuals rather than statistical trends. Ernest Wynder, a medical student at Washington University in St. Louis, Missouri, persuaded his professor, Dr. Evarts A. Graham, to participate with him in a study of smoking and lung cancer. A smoker himself, Graham was not enthusiastic about the project or the ability to prove a connection between smoking and lung cancer but agreed to collaborate. With support from the American Cancer Society, the investigators surveyed 605 patients with lung cancer and then surveyed a set of patients without lung cancer yet matched in background to the lung cancer patients. The results were striking: Of the lung cancer patients, 96.5 percent smoked compared to 73.7 percent of the other patients. The 22.8 percent difference between the groups represented a huge effect in comparison to other factors known to influence lung cancer; only rarely did medical studies find differences this large.

Soon after, another study demonstrated even more strongly that cigarettes increased the risk of death. Rather than gather current lung cancer patients and ask about their past habits, a better-designed study would identify healthy smokers and nonsmokers and follow them into the future to see if deaths occurred more commonly among one group than the other. In 1952 Dr. E. Cuyler Hammond and Dr. Daniel Horn of the American Cancer Society—themselves both smokers—began a huge study of 187,000 men aged 50 to 69. After obtaining information on the current health, background, and smoking habits of the subjects, they merely kept track of deaths in their sample. After only 22 months, they found that smokers had a death rate 1.5 times higher than nonsmokers and that heavy smokers (a pack or more a day) had death rates 2.5 times higher than nonsmokers. With all causes combined, 150 smokers and 250 heavy smokers died for every 100 nonsmokers who died. For lung cancer, smokers had death rates seven times higher than nonsmokers; for every 100 nonsmokers who died of lung cancer, 700 smokers died.

A 1954 study of 40,000 physicians aged 35 and over in Britain replicated these results. Dr. Richard Doll and Dr. A. Bradford Hill found that after four and a half years, mild smokers had death rates from lung cancer that were seven times higher than nonsmokers, moderate smokers had lung cancer death rates that were 12 times higher, and heavy smokers had death rates that were 24 times higher. These figures were shockingly high. Since these findings came from a sample of physicians—a group of highly educated and affluent individuals who, other than with the habit of some to smoke, would live healthy lives—critics could not say that unhealthy lifestyles, ignorance of healthy behaviors, and poverty could account for the high death rate among smokers. That same year Wynder and Graham reported that they produced skin cancer in 44 percent of the mice they had painted with tobacco tar condensed from cigarette smoke.

The scientific evidence entered the public consciousness through a series of articles in *Reader's Digest*, whose editors and publishers took an early stand against tobacco. (The magazine had published an article in 1924 that questioned the safety of cigarettes, but without supporting scientific evidence, it did not provoke much concern.) *Reader's Digest* articles in the 1950s on "How Harmful Are Cigarettes," "Cancer by the Carton," and "The Growing Horror of Lung Cancer" alerted the public to the new evidence of the hazards of smoking. Along with similar articles in *Ladies' Home Journal*, the *New Republic*, and *Consumer Reports*, early concerns began to take shape. In 1954, for example, the American Cancer Society adopted a resolution recognizing a connection between smoking and lung cancer, and in 1958 the Consumer's Union recommended that smokers quit or cut down to avoid health risks.

THE 1964 SURGEON GENERAL'S REPORT ON SMOKING AND HEALTH

As study after study replicated the results of Wynder and Graham, Hammond and Horn, and Doll and Hill, the mounting evidence of the danger of cigarettes for health could not be ignored. Although many medical researchers criticized the studies as insufficiently rigorous in their scientific methods and defended the habit, others became increasingly vigorous in their criticism of smoking. To make a strong impression on the public, those critical of cigarettes believed that the government should make a statement on the effects of smoking—yet federal agencies worried that government support of efforts to control tobacco would harm the economy, create resistance in Congress, and make enemies of powerful tobacco companies.

With pressure from a few in Congress and organizations such as the American Cancer Society and the American Public Health Association, President John F. Kennedy referred the matter to then surgeon general Luther Terry, who agreed to supervise a comprehensive review of the evidence on smoking and health. Although part of the Public Health Service, the surgeon general was an appointed position that involved little in the way of bureaucratic administration and focused largely on informing the public and health professionals about matters relating to public health. In 1957 Surgeon General Dr. Leroy F. Burney had issued a mild statement that confirmed cigarette smoking was a cause of lung cancer and in 1959 published an article on his findings in *JAMA*. Still, his carefully qualified statements received more in the way of harsh attacks from the tobacco industry than recognition of the problem from the public.

Surgeon General Terry, on the other hand, took the approach of convening in 1962 an advisory committee of 10 biomedical experts from the nation's most prestigious universities and research institutes. The committee undertook a review of the evidence and completed a 387-page report that remained secret until its release on January 11, 1964. In the words of Terry, "The report hit the country like a bombshell. It was front page news and a lead story on every radio and television station in the United States and many abroad. The report not only carried a strong condemnation of tobacco usage, especially cigarette smoking, but conveyed its message in such clear and concise language that it could not be misunderstood."[15] More than a summary of scientific findings, the report and the recommended actions bluntly told people interested in their health and in a long life to give up or avoid smoking.

The publicity received by the report showed in the immediate reaction of the public. For the first two months after the report, cigarette consumption declined by 20 percent, and tobacco companies worried about the collapse of the industry. Although the short-term decline did not last, the overall per capita consumption in 1964 fell to 4,143 from the 1963 peak of 4,286. By itself a small decline, it nonetheless represented a major turn of events in the longtime span of the cigarette's largely uninterrupted upward climb.

Building on the reaction, the surgeon general recommended new public policies to deal with the problem. With nonsmoking the best way to reduce risks, policies would aim to have smokers give up the habit and prevent nonsmokers from starting. The recommended actions included an educational campaign on smoking and health, labels on cigarette packages to warn about the hazards, and restrictions on advertising.

After the first report on health and smoking, the surgeon general continued as an advocate against smoking, and beginning in 1967 the Office of the Surgeon General released reports nearly every year. The reports generally summarized recent research on the health consequences of smoking but eventually came to focus on specific themes. For example, a 1980 report focused on women, a 1981 report focused on changes in cigarette products, and a 1983 report focused on cardiovascular disease. A 1982 report from C. Everett Koop, the newly appointed surgeon general in the Reagan administration, on the relationship between smoking and cancer noted an encouraging decline in cigarette use from the time of the first report. It further noted in strong language that the consequences of smoking were still "the most important public issue of our time," and that cigarettes were "the chief, single, avoidable cause of death in our society."[16] The report presented evidence that 21 percent of all U.S. deaths were due to cancer, and 30 percent of those were attributable to smoking. More so than previous surgeons general, Koop became a fierce critic of smoking, approached his task with missionary zeal, and reported on the harm of smoking in several other influential reports during his tenure.

NICOTINE ADDICTION

Given the publicity of the 1964 Surgeon General's report and the desire of nearly all people to avoid dying early, it would seem that the evidence against smoking would lead to the disappearance of the habit. The percentage of the U.S. population that smoked did indeed decline, as did the overall consumption of cigarettes, but not as fast as public health advocates would have liked. In 1965, 52 percent of adult males and 34 percent of adult females smoked. Just over 20 years later, the percentages had fallen to 33 and 28, respectively—a significant decline but far from creating a smoke-free society. A substantial part of the U.S. population continued to smoke. Moreover, per-person consumption fell from its 1963 peak of 4,286 to 3,969 by 1970, but rose again to 4,112 by 1973—not an encouraging change. The number of cigarettes smoked per person fell less than the percentage of smokers because those continuing the habit consumed an increasing number of cigarettes.

The slow shift in behavior did not mean that smokers rejected the evidence about the harm of smoking and the benefits of quitting. Rather, they wanted to quit but found the process difficult. Researchers could have predicted as much. Personal experiences over the years demonstrated that cigarette smoking was at least habit forming, if not addictive. The 1964 Surgeon General's committee that authored the report recognized this fact. Some members desired to label cigarettes and the nicotine they contained as addictive, but others believed more cautiously that the evidence could not yet prove this claim. Many saw smoking as a habit, but one substantially different from addictions to drugs such as heroin and cocaine. Hard drugs required increasing amounts to satisfy the craving, but smokers of cigarettes seemed to get along on the same daily allotment. Moreover, labeling millions of smokers as addicts—akin to drug and alcohol abusers—might offend enough people to blunt the major message of the Surgeon General's report about the harm of smoking.

After the 1964 report two groups continued to research the addictiveness of nicotine—scientists employed by tobacco companies and scientists in research universities or institutes. The tobacco companies had recognized the addictive qualities of tobacco early on, but to avoid obvious negative publicity that they were enslaving smokers much as drug dealers enslaved heroin addicts, they kept the information in-house. According to documents released many years later during a civil suit, the tobacco company Brown and Williamson was informed in 1962 of research done by its parent company, British American Tobacco, that showed smokers needed continued intake of the drugging element of cigarettes to maintain physiological and emotional equilibrium. One executive wrote, in a memo that would prove damning in the suit, "We are, then, in the business of selling nicotine, an addictive drug effective in the release of stress mechanisms."[17] Cautious executives did not want to make this claim public.

Independent researchers also began to accumulate evidence of the addictive properties of cigarettes and nicotine. In one 1967 study at the University of Michigan Medical School, smokers were injected with a substance that, unknown to them, consisted of either nicotine or a placebo. Those injected with nicotine cut their consumption of cigarettes, as they received little additional lift from the cigarettes.[18] Other studies systematically described the difficulties smokers faced in stopping. Although the majority (70 percent) of smokers today state they want to quit, few can do so—only about 6 percent succeed for more than a year. The quit rate for cigarettes is lower than for many hard drugs, which reveals the powerful hold of cigarettes over smokers.

In terms of feeding an addiction, cigarettes turn out to work well as a delivery system. They allow smokers to conveniently regulate their ingestion of nicotine. After lighting up and inhaling a cigarette, nicotine reaches the brain in minutes. It stimulates electrical activity in the brain, increases metabolic activity in the body, raises the heart beat, and causes skeletal muscles to relax. Serving as both a stimulant and relaxant, nicotine mildly improves the performance of everyday tasks and moderates mood swings.[19] It can stay in the body for hours, but as it leaves, the desire to smoke grows. Lighting up and inhaling on a regular basis feeds the body's need for more nicotine. In this way, the use of cigarettes is self-reinforcing.

Viewing cigarette use as an addiction presents a different perspective on the pleasures of smoking. Smokers often state that they find smoking soothing, as the stimulant properties of nicotine for the brain can help one focus on the task at hand, and the relaxing properties for the muscles ease physical stress. Yet, the soothing nature of cigarettes may really come from the delivery of nicotine, which relieves addictive cravings and the physical discomfort caused by the cravings. In other words, cigarettes and nicotine may in the first place cause the negative feelings that more cigarettes and nicotine later remedy.

The difficulty in quitting and the evidence of addiction show in several withdrawal symptoms. Giving up smoking causes strong cravings for the product that, when not satisfied, produce irritability, restlessness, depression, anxiety, sleep disorder, and physical discomfort. Those with these symptoms often have trouble concentrating on daily tasks. The withdrawal symptoms largely disappear after three to four weeks, but the cravings remain for much longer periods, sometimes indefinitely; former smokers often say they miss the habit years after they have stopped. This continued attraction results not so much from the physical dependence but from the memory of the pleasurable feelings (stimulation of the mind and relaxation of the muscles) and behaviors (eating, drinking alcohol, socializing) associated with smoking.

In 1988 the Office of the Surgeon General released another report that this time focused on nicotine addiction. The report stated bluntly, "The processes that determine tobacco addiction are similar to those that determine addiction to other drugs, including illegal drugs."[20] Willing to go beyond statements in previous reports of the Surgeon General, the 1988 report clearly laid out its definition of addiction and how nicotine had properties similar to hard drugs. In general terms, addiction involves behavior that is controlled by a substance that causes changes in mood from its effects on the brain. Nicotine causes changes in mood through its effect on the brain (unlike, say, food that improves mood by meeting requirements for nourishment) and compels smokers to act in ways that damage themselves and society. As with addiction to hard drugs, addiction to nicotine produces uncomfortable withdrawal symptoms that require smokers to light up again. Such addiction occurs not only from cigarettes but also from smokeless tobacco (and less so, cigars and pipes), which distributes nicotine to the body through the mouth.

That many smokers quit successfully does not, according to the report, negate the claim of nicotine addiction. Spontaneous remission or unaided quitting occurs among 30 percent of hard drug users but leaves many others who face difficulties in trying to end their dependence on the addictive substances. For both drugs and cigarettes, some people are more prone to becoming addicted than others and have a more difficult time quitting. Such

25

variation occurs in most human behavior and simply means that susceptibility to cigarette addiction, if not universal, is common. Of course, cigarettes are legal and most hard drugs are not. Hard drugs more than cigarettes negatively affect the ability of addicts to participate in daily life, increase the criminal actions associated with the habit, and produce more disgust in conventional society. Still, the control of one's actions by an artificial substance and the difficulty in ending the reliance on the substance make the products similar.

Several important implications follow from these conclusions about addiction. First, smokers and those considering taking up the habit must be made aware of their addiction. By realizing that their habit comes not from a personal choice, they may be more motivated to reject or quit the habit. This would seem especially important to young people, who may begin the habit not realizing that it will addict them for decades to come. Second, education alone cannot get most smokers to quit. Many smokers fully understand the advantages of not smoking, but the addiction makes quitting difficult. For those unable to quit on their own, interventions must involve some sort of medical treatment of the addiction. Third, unlike earlier antismoking advocates, such groups today do not criticize smokers for their weakness but instead view them as victims of an addiction. More than smokers the tobacco companies that encouraged the addiction with their advertising, product marketing, and pricing strategies become the villains.

ADVERTISING TO YOUNG PEOPLE

Given the evidence of the addictiveness of smoking, public health experts turned their focus to the problem of teen smoking. Once a young person overcomes the initial unpleasant sensations and takes up smoking on a regular basis, he or she will become a long-term, perhaps even lifelong, smoker. The earlier the addiction occurs, the longer a smoker will remain a customer.

Nearly all smokers first tried cigarettes before age 20, and people who pass that age without smoking seldom ever begin. Teens might know of the harm of smoking to health but tend to think that they will have plenty of time to quit before health problems develop and underestimate the difficulty in quitting.[21] The teenage years thus prove critical in the adoption of cigarette smoking.

While recognizing the need to appeal to teenagers, the tobacco industry did not want to undermine its formally declared statement that smoking was an adult habit by appealing directly to minors. Advertising could indirectly appeal to adolescents, however, by associating traits valued by the young with smoking. Ads did not need to use teen models or students in schools but could show young adults involved in activities that youth want to enjoy. They would depict smokers as young, physically active, cool, independent, attractive to the opposite sex, and able to fully enjoy life's pleasures. Tobacco companies could, within limits, advertise in magazines and on radio and television shows that attracted the young as well as adults so they could not be accused of targeting youth alone. *Playboy*, for example, often appeals to adolescent males and includes many cigarette ads. Similarly, tobacco company sponsorship of sporting events, such as auto racing, women's tennis tournaments, and rock and jazz music concerts influence youth.

The sheer number of ads could also increase the misperception among young people that cigarettes had achieved a high level of popularity and acceptance outside their own families and schools. Until recent restriction, ads in magazines, on billboards, in sports stadiums, on racing cars, and in store displays were hard to miss. Point-of-purchase advertisements in retail outlets that sell cigarette products can easily be seen by youth. A 1992 Gallup poll found that 87 percent of surveyed adolescents could recall having seen one or more tobacco company advertisements. Even relatively young children are aware of cigarette advertising.

The most glaring and disconcerting effort of tobacco companies to attract young smokers came from the Joe Camel campaign sponsored by R. J. Reynolds for Camel cigarettes. As part of a $75 million campaign that began in 1987, the Joe Camel ads used a cartoon character along with adult models. In the ads, Joe Camel appeared as a cool party animal, with a cigarette, sporting sunglasses and a tuxedo, and with adoring young women nearby. Joe Camel also appeared on T-shirts, sweatshirts, posters, mugs, and beach sandals. The images and products appeared to be geared toward young children as well as teens—few adults would be attracted to a brand by a cartoon camel and cheap products. A study published in 1991 in *JAMA* found that a shocking 90 percent of six-year-olds could identify Joe Camel and knew his connection to cigarettes.[22]

Combined with the mounting evidence of the addictiveness of cigarette smoking, the ads directed at young children and teens encouraged the Office of the Surgeon General and antismoking organizations to further emphasize the harm of cigarette advertising. Reports by the Surgeon General's office included long chapters on the manipulation of youth by smoking advertisements and the effects of the ads on the adoption of cigarettes.[23] Controversy exists over the effectiveness of advertising, but documenting the harmful effects of tobacco had moved from medical studies of the physical harm (for both addiction and mortality) to social science studies of the social factors behind youthful adoption of cigarette smoking.

RESPONSE OF THE TOBACCO INDUSTRY

The emerging negative evidence about cigarettes in the 1950s led at least in part to a drop in sales during the middle of the decade. In an attempt to continue generating profits at past levels, tobacco companies addressed these health concerns. In 1954 they formed the Tobacco Industry Research Council (TIRC). The council aimed to counter the negative publicity about cigarettes with its own studies, press releases, and propaganda on smoking. Tobacco executives, representatives of the council, and some physicians and scientists assured the public that the harm of smoking was overstated and moderate cigarette use was safe.

The debate between critics and defenders of cigarettes often centered on the validity of the scientific evidence. The key statistical issue concerned the ability of studies to demonstrate the causal harm of cigarettes. The fact that smokers experienced premature mortality did not prove cause and effect; for example, one respected psychologist in England, Hans Eysenck, suggested that persons unable to express anger, fear, and anxiety were prone to both smoking and early death.[24] These personality traits, both inborn and learned, could account for an observed but ultimately unfounded association between smoking and lung cancer. An appropriate study would have to make sure that the personality traits of smokers and nonsmokers did not differ before concluding that smoking caused lung cancer. Scientists replied that premature death from lung cancer in societies with little cigarette smoking occurred rarely, even though the personality traits seen to cause both smoking and cancer were common in those societies. Yet, defenders of tobacco could always point to possible alternative explanations.

Other scientists with no vested interest in either the theories of the causes of cancer or the defense of tobacco companies nonetheless remained cautious about the criticisms of cigarette smoking. These scientists tended to wait for improved methodology and replication before reaching a firm conclusion about the hazards of tobacco. *JAMA* was slow, for example, to give scientific backing to claims about the perils of smoking. Ernest Wynder, one of the first researchers to identify the connection between smoking and lung cancer, faced much criticism for his work. In the 1960s, the director of research at the Sloan-Kettering Institute called Wynder's claims irresponsible but also accepted annual cash gifts from Philip Morris on behalf of the institute. Antismoking campaigns point out that the tobacco industry supported many such skeptical researchers with funding.

The battle of experts would prove futile, however—the emerging evidence against smoking was too strong. As internal industry documents released in the 1990s would show, many in the tobacco industry in the 1960s and 1970s were fully aware of the hazards of their product. The documents proposed that nicotine was addictive and smoking caused cancer. Manufacturers searched for tobacco leaves and ingredients that would most effectively deliver the chemical and limit the harm of the product, all the while publicly denying both the addictiveness and perils of smoking. This dishonesty may have kept sales from falling further but would provide grounds of fraud and misrepresentation for groups to later sue tobacco companies.

Rather than trying to convince hard-line critics of its case, the tobacco industry believed it should focus on appealing to those with more moderate views about the need to make changes in the smoking habits of the population. In trying to do so, tobacco ads in the 1950s claimed that cigarettes were safe. Philip Morris offered "A Cigarette That Takes the Fear Out of Smoking"; R. J. Reynolds said that "More Doctors Smoke Camels"; Chesterfield promised the benefits of "30 Years of Tobacco Research." However, these ads may have worsened rather than soothed the worries smokers had about cigarettes.

More effective ads took another form: They indirectly associated smoking with health. The Marlboro Country ads came to prominence in television and magazines in the 1960s in a campaign developed by the famous advertising executive Leo F. Burnett. The ads featured the Marlboro Man, a ruggedly handsome cowboy who lived and worked outdoors in open mountain country and enjoyed a life of hard work, fresh air, and scenic beauty. The ads did not have to state that the Marlboro Man did not look like he would succumb to lung cancer. Other ads also showed young, healthy, and active people smoking cigarettes while enthusiastically enjoying themselves.

Tobacco ads touting health claims drew the ire of the federal agency in charge of regulating business practices. The Federal Trade Commission (FTC) had since the 1950s expressed concerns about the claims made on behalf of cigarettes in advertising. Later, at the time of the 1964 Surgeon General's report on health and smoking, the commission began an investigation of cigarette advertising, concluding that some ads made false health claims, and others misleadingly implied that smokers gained vigor, sexual attractiveness, and virility from cigarettes. Hoping to preempt government interference, the tobacco industry promised to self-regulate its ads. It would no longer allow industry members to make claims that did not have medical or scientific proof or that misrepresented the social benefits of cigarettes. The effort could not, however, forestall proposals by the FTC and eventual legislation from Congress to include warnings on cigarette packages and advertisements, and the policy of self-regulation was dropped.

The tobacco industry financed several other efforts to discredit claims against cigarettes in the areas of politics, the law, public relations, and the media.[25] First, recognizing the importance of the political as well as the medical battle, a consortium of the major tobacco firms hired a lobbyist to represent their interests in Washington, D.C. Their lobbyist, Earl C. Clements, a retired representative and senator from Kentucky who had close ties to his former colleagues in Congress and to the Lyndon Johnson White House, testified formally and lobbied informally. He shrewdly led the discussion toward economic issues and away from health issues. Politicians worried about the economic harm new laws to restrict cigarette sales and advertising might bring to growers, factory workers, retailers, advertising outlets, and cities, such as Richmond, Virginia, and Winston-Salem, North Carolina, that depended on the industry. Clements's lobbying could not stop movements to restrict advertising and require warning messages on cigarettes but did stall more drastic measures.

Second, the tobacco firms hired a committee in 1963 of six well-known and successful lawyers to defend the legal interests of the industry. Early suits against the tobacco companies had failed, but the evidence presented by the Office of the Surgeon General might make the manufacturers liable for future suits. Worried that even one loss would open the floodgates of suits from other smokers, the industry prepared to fight expensive legal battles until the end. Hiring the best legal talent would prove crucial in this effort.

Third, to help publicize their views about cigarettes, tobacco firms funded the Tobacco Institute (TI), which opened in Washington, D.C., in 1958. Like any trade organization, the TI emphasized the economic importance of the industry and the dependence of millions of people on its fortunes. In addition, it extended the efforts of the TIRC to dispute the evidence behind claims of the dangers of smoking, highlighted the rights of smokers to enjoy their freely chosen pleasure, and emphasized the First Amendment rights of companies to free speech in commercial advertising.

Fourth, through its financial support of research organizations, writers, magazines, and publishers, the tobacco industry promoted its own views about smoking. Articles and books arguing for the safety of cigarettes appeared regularly, and copies of these articles and books received wide distribution free of charge. The publication of one 1967 book, *It Is Safe to Smoke*, turned out to have been subsidized by the tobacco industry.[26] Ads filled with one or two pages of dense text offered a detailed defense of smoking and the rights of consumers to enjoy the habit. With ads entitled "A Frank Statement to Cigarette Smokers" or "Do Cigarette Companies Want Kids to Smoke? No," the tobacco industry could purchase space in magazines when it could not publish regular articles.

In a highly praised history of cigarette use, *The Cigarette Century*, Harvard professor Allan M. Brandt describes the strategy behind the tobacco industry response.[27] Based on the vast information from 50 years of documents, he argues that the industry employed techniques of scientific disinformation to deny the harm of smoking. The researchers and public relation experts employed by tobacco companies and their trade organization managed to get widespread media coverage of the few dissenters from the scientific evidence of the harm of tobacco. The lobbyists and lawyers used political influence to effectively block or water down antitobacco legislation.

At the heart of the strategy was a change in the nature of disease in the modern world. Rather than linking a bacterium or virus to a specific disease, smoking greatly increased the risks of many diseases but did not guarantee death. The tobacco industry exploited the special nature of tobacco-related disease.

These efforts could not, however, halt the growing antismoking movement. In the years after the Surgeon General's 1964 report the industry had to respond to multiple threats to its well-being and profits. They met these threats with, from their point of view, varied degrees of success.

- In 1964 the FTC proposed requiring a warning on cigarette packages and in advertisements to counter what they viewed as deceptive advertising. After proposing self-regulation, the industry appealed to allies in Congress, many of whom represented tobacco-growing regions and states, for protection from the proposed regulations. Congress responded by preventing the FTC from taking action on the issue. In reaction to the lobbying efforts of the tobacco industry, the House and Senate in 1965 instead required a mild warning on cigarette packages but not advertisements. The warning stated, "Caution—Cigarette Smoking May Be Hazardous to Your Health."

- The Federal Communications Commission (FCC) agreed with a 1966 petition of a New York City lawyer, John F. Banzhaf III, that the fairness doctrine applied to cigarette advertising. Based on the view that the airways are a public resource, the fairness doctrine required equal time for presentation of competing views. Although typically applied to politicians and political parties, the fairness doctrine was extended by the decision of the commission to require the airing of antismoking ads to balance smoking commercials. Much to the concern of the tobacco industry, these antismoking ads proved effective.

- Continuing its efforts against tobacco advertising, the FTC proposed to ban cigarette advertisements from radio and television. The tobacco industry again appealed to Congress for protection, but antismoking legislators had grown in power. After much struggle, the tobacco industry first agreed to voluntarily remove their ads and then went along with a bill that banned the ads beginning on January 2, 1971 (after filling the airways with commercials during the New Year's Day football bowl games).

- Congress required that a stronger warning appear on cigarette packages and the same warning be included on advertisements. The warning stated, "The Surgeon General Has Determined That Cigarette Smoking Is Dangerous to Your Health."

- Joseph Califano, head of the Department of Health, Education, and Welfare under President Jimmy Carter, proposed several actions in 1978

31

to fight cigarette smoking. He wanted to raise taxes on cigarettes, use the government proceeds from the taxes for antismoking campaigns and programs, eliminate smoking on airplanes and in restaurants, and end government subsidies to tobacco growers. However, Califano received little support from the Carter administration. Opposition from tobacco growers, retail establishments, and cigarette makers was sufficient to block these proposals.

- On the legal front the tobacco industry lawyers had since the first filing in 1954 successfully defeated suits brought by smokers against them. In part due to the resources of tobacco firms in fighting them, few early suits even reached a jury. However, in 1988, Rose Cipollone won a $400,000 judgment against the Liggett Group for the failure of the cigarette manufacturer to warn her about the dangers of its product. Although the decision was later overturned and the family of the deceased Mrs. Cipollone dropped continued appeals to the Supreme Court after the costs rose beyond their means, the jury award represented a major defeat for the tobacco company against claims that it was liable for the harm of cigarettes. (More serious legal problems would come in the 1990s.)

Overall, the years after the 1964 Surgeon General's report were not good ones for the tobacco industry. Both the sales and the image of the industry suffered. In response to the troubles, however, the industry could follow past strategies by continuing its advertising, promotion expenditures, and product development.

CHANGES IN THE TOBACCO INDUSTRY

The cigarette industry had over the first part of the 20th century overcome opposition to its product and gained widespread respect and high profits. Cigars, the one-time major competitor of cigarettes, became associated with older rather than younger generations and had fallen on hard times. In 1950, having done its part in the efforts against Nazi Germany and imperial Japan in World War II and facing no opposition from antismoking crusaders, the industry could expect to benefit from the booming economy after the war. The three major cigarette brands, Camel, Lucky Strike, and Chesterfield, continued to dominate the market as they had for decades. Confident executives would not have predicted the threats to the financial condition of the companies that would soon come or recognize the new shape their business would take.

Economic problems for tobacco in the 1950s related to marketing as well as to health. With levels of smoking near the maximum, the market could not likely grow by attracting more smokers (except of course at the younger ages, when new smokers would first start). At the time, more than 50 percent of men ages 18 and over smoked. Those who did not smoke were unlikely to take up the habit, as they would have already had their chance to begin but for whatever reason did not like the habit. Fewer women smoked (between 20 and 30 percent). Without special efforts to create products that better appealed to women, it seemed unlikely that they would reach the high smoking levels of men. Thus, under current sales and production strategies, the market of smokers had reached saturation.

One way to increase sales came not from attracting more smokers but from encouraging each smoker to consume more cigarettes. Sales of cigarettes in cartons made a new package easily available to smokers when they finished an old one. Sales of cigarettes in ubiquitous vending machines similarly made it easy to find cigarettes outside the home. These changes made smoking even more than in the past an activity not reserved for special times and places, but something that one could indulge in throughout the day.

Perhaps more important, cigarette companies developed a new form of cigarettes—king size—that might lead to more smoking. Slightly longer than regular cigarettes, king-size cigarettes had more tobacco and cost a few pennies more per pack. Smokers could consume the same number of cigarettes each day but use more tobacco and pay more. The growing affluence of the U.S. population allowed smokers to pay the higher costs and contributed to the profits of the tobacco company. New brands of king-size cigarettes, such as Pall Mall, Winston, and Marlboro, became more popular than the older standard brands. Chesterfield cigarettes, in response, began to appear in both regular and king size.

Other efforts to distinguish one brand from another emerged. Cigarettes with filters grew in popularity, particularly among women, as did mentholated cigarettes. Filter cigarettes had been introduced in 1936 but did not become well liked until the publicity in the 1950s about health concerns. Although the attraction to these innovations involved more than health concerns, cigarettes with filters and menthol could, in their advertising, appeal to the health conscious. New filtered products such as Winston, L&M, Kent, and Viceroy grew in sales, in part based on advertisements that emphasized the ability of filters to purify cigarette smoke and make the habit safer and cleaner. The filters would in fact only modestly reduce the risks of cigarettes, but smokers felt reassured. Health claims were also made about mentholated cigarettes: They were cleaner, fresher, and tastier than other cigarettes. Kool cigarettes, the first popular brand to add peppermint extract to tobacco to form a menthol cigarette, used a name that implied that the cigarette smoke would be less irritating and hot.

The tobacco companies also conducted research to find a safer cigarette and successfully marketed some low-tar and low-nicotine cigarettes. During the 1950s, cigarette makers often made claims about the tar content—the particles contained in the residue or by-product of the burning of tobacco that are inhaled with tobacco smoke—of their cigarettes. Because tar was a major source of the harmful effects of tobacco use on health (but also a major source of tobacco flavor), cigarette makers hoped that low-tar cigarettes would attract smokers worried about their health. The competition among cigarette manufacturers over sales of low-tar cigarettes that occurred in the 1950s became known as the tar derby. The low-tar and health claims made on behalf of the cigarettes became so confusing that the FTC took over testing for cigarette tar. However, smokers either rejected low-tar cigarettes with filters that cleansed the smoke so much as to significantly lose flavor or puffed harder and longer to obtain the same chemicals from the low-tar cigarettes as from regular cigarettes. Efforts in the 1980s and 1990s to market smokeless cigarettes and nicotine-free cigarettes flopped altogether.

The new types and brands of cigarettes and the competition they generated led to more choices for smokers. In 1941 the top three brands captured 72 percent of the market, while in 1961 the top three sellers had 48 percent of the market.[28] Consumers less often adopted a brand for life than in the past but would switch quickly to another brand based on advertisements or new cigarette styles. Brands proliferated at an even faster pace in the 1960s and 1970s in the hope of finding a new winner; for example, Virginia Slims (which used the slogan "You've Come a Long Way Baby") targeted younger, more independent women. By 1978 smokers had their choice among 190 different brands and brand types.

The major tobacco companies remained dominant. Reynolds, American, and Liggett and Myers, products of the trust breakup in 1911, remained the top three companies in 1961. Three other companies, Lorillard, Brown & Williamson, and Philip Morris, rounded out the top six. Although still profitable, the companies recognized the need to diversify in the face of growing antitobacco sentiments. Philip Morris, for example, purchased the Miller Brewing Company and Seven-Up; R. J. Reynolds purchased several food businesses and eventually merged with Nabisco; Liggett and Myers purchased liquor distilling and other companies to form the Liggett Group and later the Brooke Group. Lorillard was acquired by a business conglomerate, Loews Corporation, which also owns movie theater and hotel companies. Diversification over the years represented an implicit recognition by tobacco companies that they needed to protect themselves from the likely decline of the cigarette business in the United States. They would in the future also employ another strategy for survival by turning their attention to new markets outside the United States—developing nations where there were few smokers and little organized opposition to the smoking industry.

RECENT TRENDS AND PATTERNS, 1990–PRESENT

A SLOWER RATE OF DECLINE

Negative publicity about the harm of cigarette smoking, the addictiveness of nicotine, and the efforts of tobacco companies to promote self-destructive behavior produced a decline in cigarette smoking. Reviewing the trends since 1964, the 1989 Surgeon General's report could point to substantial progress.[29] The number of cigarettes consumed per adult fell from 4,269 in 1964 to 2,827 in 1990. From 1965 to 1990, the percentage of male smokers fell from 51.9 to 28.4, and the percentage of female smokers fell from 33.9 to 22.8. The decline among males exceeded that among females in large part because males were at higher levels in 1965. Despite a greater decline in smoking among light and moderate smokers, who were less addicted to nicotine than heavy smokers, the trends encouraged public health officials.

Smoking among youth declined much as it did for older groups during the years from 1964 to 1990. Because youth smoking would foretell future trends at older ages, progress against smoking before age 18 had special importance. For young adults 18–24, male smokers fell from 54.1 percent of the age group in 1965 to 25.1 percent in 1990, and female smokers fell from 37.3 to 22.4 percent over the same period. Yearly surveys of high school seniors, which began in 1976, revealed a similar decline in daily smoking until 1990. For boys, such smoking fell from 28 percent to 18 percent and for girls from 29 percent to 19 percent.

The downward trends in current smoking stemmed in part from fewer people ever starting the habit but also from more people quitting. An increase in the percentage of former smokers represented progress against smoking. In 1965, 19.8 percent of males said they used to smoke but currently did not, and 8 percent of females said they used to smoke but currently did not. In 1990, 30.3 percent of males and 19.5 percent of females fit the category of former smokers. In terms of those who never smoked, the percentages rose for males from 28.3 in 1965 to 41.3 in 1990. For females, however, the trend for "never smokers" was less positive: It fell little, from 58.1 percent in 1965 to 57.7 in 1990. The drop in current smoking among females largely comes from the rise in former rather than never smokers.

Although some signs of decline continued, the rate of decline in cigarette smoking slowed. Among adults from 1990 to 2006, the percentages of current male smokers fell by only 4.5 percent—from 28.4 to 23.9. For females, the decline was similarly modest (from 22.8 to 18.0). Among smokers in the 1990s, light and moderate consumption of cigarettes increased relative to heavy smoking, but as with not smoking, the percentages appear slow to change. Overall, after some 40 years of antismoking efforts, about one-fifth of the U.S. population continues with the habit. Given the population of the United States, these percentages translate into roughly 45 million current smokers and about an equal number of former smokers.

Concerning trends among young people during the 1990s, rather than falling continuously, rates of smoking in fact showed some increases. Among high school seniors, daily smoking among boys and girls fell from about 29 percent in 1990 to 20 percent in 2006. However, the trend shows a disconcerting rise from a low point in 1992 of around 16 percent to about 25 percent in 1997. Since 1997, however, smoking among high school seniors has fallen each year, and most public officials hope that the trend will continue downward. In any case, the rise and then fall leave current levels of smoking at higher levels than many had expected.

Through its Healthy People Goals for 2010, the U.S. government strives to reduce current smoking rates among high school students to below 16 percent.[30] That goal seems unlikely to be reached. For all adults, the goal is to reduce smoking to 12 percent—a goal that is unlikely, given the experiences over the last decade. Reaching the goal would require major efforts at getting adult smokers to quit.

Why the slowdown? Continued declines may become more difficult as the remaining smokers are those most attracted and addicted to cigarettes. Those best able to resist starting to smoke and to quit once they start will likely have already done so, and those who currently smoke may have the most trouble stopping. The slowdown in cessation also likely relates to the efforts of the tobacco industry. Lower cigarette prices in the early 1990s and the increased availability of bargain brands contributed in particular to a rise in smoking rates among young people. Conversely, rising prices in the late 1990s and early 2000s help explain the decline. Advertising and promotional expenditures by tobacco companies, which grew throughout the 1990s and increased dramatically in the early 2000s, also may moderate the potential for smoking to decline. For example, an issue of *People* magazine with a cover story on "Teens and Sex"—a story likely to attract young readers—contained 14 pages of cigarette ads. Antismoking advocates argue that some of the ads would appeal especially to young people: a picture of a slim young model in tight-fighting clothes with the label "Totally Kool" and a Marlboro ad promoting adventure gear and depicting youthful mountain climbers.

Cigars have for most of the last half century declined in popularity, although they enjoyed resurgent popularity since the 1990s. In 1970, 16.2 percent of men smoked cigars. The figure fell to 3.5 percent by 1991 but rose to 8.4 percent in 1998 and continued to grow in the 2000s by another third (female cigar smoking remained negligible over the period). As shown by the popularity of *Cigar Aficionado* magazine and cigar bars, the resurgence of cigar smoking involves desires to enjoy their flavor and aroma, much as one enjoys gourmet food and quality liquor. Furthermore, the newfound status associated with cigar smoking may reflect a trend of "chic" among young men. The largest increase has thus come in the consumption of premium cigars, particularly among white males ages 25–34. Although for most, cigar smoking represents an occasional pleasure rather than a daylong habit, the health risks faced by occasional cigar smokers are greater than for those who abstain altogether from tobacco products.

Smokeless tobacco has also failed to decline in the 1990s, staying at 5 to 6 percent use among men (female use is negligible). Pipe smoking has declined among men after a brief period of popularity in the 1960s. Use of bidis, a tobacco product common in India but new to the United States, has increased among youth. Bidis are small brown cigarettes that are hand rolled in a leaf and tied at one end by a string. About 12 percent of high school girls and 17 percent of high school boys have tried the product, but few use it on a regular basis. About 5 percent of high school students have tried kreteks, a kind of cigarette that mixes tobacco and clove spice.

Use of the hookah, a water pipe common in the Middle East that filters tobacco and other smoke through water, has become fashionable among young people. The flavoring of the tobacco and the use of filtering to make the smoke milder encourages the belief that hookah smoking is safer and less addictive than use of cigarettes, cigars, smokeless tobacco, and bidis. However, public health experts say that hookah use remains dangerous.

Smoking figures have only recently began to be gathered for pregnant women but appear more favorable than the figures for smoking in general. The percent of live births in which mothers reported smoking during pregnancy fell from 18.4 in 1990 to 11.4 in 2002. The percentage of heavy smokers (more than one pack a day) among pregnant women fell from 6.6 percent to 3.8 percent. However, since many women may hide their smoking habit from physicians and researchers, the levels may be artificially low. Smoking by pregnant women harms not just the smokers themselves but also retards the growth of the fetus, increases the risk of stillbirth, and often results in low birth weight babies. The decline over time may result in part from the growing embarrassment among pregnant smokers and greater willingness to misreport their habits.

WHO SMOKES?

The decline in cigarette smoking from the 1960s involved some groups more than others, and as a result, has in recent years come to concentrate smoking among persons with certain social characteristics. The groups that now have the highest smoking rates also appear to consist of individuals whose attraction to the habit is most difficult to change. Assuming that the decline in smoking occurs among those who most strongly desire or are best able to avoid or give up the habit, those who do smoke will be the most resistant to change. Who are these people? In simplest terms they are those people whose physiology and psychology make them most prone to addiction, who find the most enjoyment from cigarettes, and who are most attracted to the image of cigarette smokers. However, these people are concentrated in some groups more than in others.

Gender and Age

Perhaps surprisingly, gender and age no longer distinguish strongly between smokers and nonsmokers. Men continue to smoke more than women, but the traditionally large differences have declined, particularly among the young. For high school seniors, smoking differences between the sexes are negligible and for all ages reach about 5 percent. The equality between the sexes reflects the faster decline among males in recent decades. This trend may come from the strong efforts of tobacco companies to appeal to women with their products and the desire of women to act in ways that assert their independence and freedom. More simply, the slow rate of decline among females may merely reflect the fact that they adopted the habit later than males and have not yet had as much time as males to reject the habit.

With regard to age, the percentages of current smokers differ little among those under age 65. At ages 18–24, 23.9 percent of persons smoke; at ages 25–44, 23.5 percent of persons smoke; and at ages 45–64, 21.8 percent of persons smoke. The percentage falls to 10.2 percent at ages 65 and over, largely because older persons have had longer to quit and face more serious health conditions that require quitting. In addition, fewer smokers than nonsmokers survive to old age. Otherwise, smoking today appears similar across ages and generations.

Socioeconomic Status

Educational attainment, occupational prestige, and income levels reflect the major components of socioeconomic status (SES). In general, the higher the SES of a person, the less likely he or she is to smoke. This trend has strengthened over the years, which increasingly concentrates smoking among low SES groups. The most recent figures available show that 35.4 percent of high school dropouts smoke, while 9.6 percent of those with an undergraduate degree and 6.6 percent with a graduate degree smoke.[31] Data on income and occupational differences in smoking are harder to come by but reveal much the same pattern. Those living at poverty level are more likely to smoke than those with income above the poverty level, and among those above poverty level, smoking declines as income increases. Similarly those in high prestige occupations with high education and high earnings—professionals (lawyers, doctors, professors), corporate managers, and technical specialists (computer programmers, engineers)—smoke the least. Persons in lower-level white-collar occupations, such as salespeople, administrators, store clerks, and secretaries, smoke more than persons in higher status occupations. And persons in lower status occupations such as factory workers, truck drivers, construction workers, and cleaning service people smoke the most.

Race and Ethnicity

Race and ethnic differences in smoking relate to SES differences, as minority groups tend to have lower education and income than whites. African Americans once smoked more than whites, but the difference has largely disappeared. In 1974, for example, 44.0 percent of blacks and 36.4 percent of whites smoked. In 2006, the percentages equaled 23.0 for blacks and 21.9 for whites. Among young people, smoking among blacks has declined dramatically and has contributed to the similar rates across races. Figures for high school seniors show that less than 10 percent of black youth smoke—a percentage substantially lower than for whites.

Among other race and ethnic groups, Native Americans have the highest rates of smoking (32.4 percent), and Hispanics (15.2 percent) and Asian Americans (10.4 percent) have the lowest rates. The low rates for Hispanics and Asian Americans may stem from the relatively large portion of recent immigrants in these groups who were not exposed to the habit as much in their country of origin as those born in the United States.

Residence

Smoking across states in the United States demonstrates no strong regional pattern. In 2006, the highest rates were in Kentucky, Indiana, Tennessee, and West Virginia, while Utah, California, and Connecticut had the lowest rates. Within states, smoking tends to be more common in rural areas, a pattern that reverses the earlier tendency for city dwellers to be smokers. Concerns over healthy lifestyles and the higher SES in cities contribute to this new pattern.

Religion

Few differences in smoking exist across religious denominations, and to the extent that they do, they likely reflect differences in education and income among members of various religions. However, attending services regularly, regardless of faith, relates closely to nonsmoking. Highly religious persons had for centuries rejected smoking as a worldly pleasure that, if not sinful, did little to bring one closer to God. Such beliefs do much today to distinguish smokers from nonsmokers.

Youth

The same factors affecting adult patterns of smoking also influence smoking of girls and boys, but the social characteristics of parents prove as important as the social characteristics of the youth themselves. Based again on data for high school seniors, youthful smokers have the following characteristics.[32]

- Those with less educated parents are more likely to smoke than those with highly educated parents.

- Those growing up in a rural area are more likely to smoke than those growing up in a large city or suburb.

- Those living alone or with only one parent are more likely to smoke than those living with both parents.

- Those performing poorly in school and not planning to go to college are more likely to smoke than those doing well in school and planning to go to college.

- Those saying religion is not important in their lives are more likely to smoke than those saying religion is important or very important in their lives.

- Those holding jobs and earning more income are more likely to smoke than those without jobs (and presumably devoting more time to academics).

- Those participating in delinquent and criminal activities are more likely to smoke than those not participating in such activities.

These relationships reflect only tendencies. Smoking cuts across all teen social groups, and many persons with characteristics that should make them prone to smoke nonetheless reject the habit, just as others not prone to smoke take up the habit. The same point holds in describing group differences in smoking adults. Still, group tendencies exist and offer insights into the social forces behind individual decisions to smoke or not to smoke.

REASONS FOR SMOKING

Information obtained from smokers on the reasons they started and continue seldom proves insightful. They state that they smoke because they enjoy it and because it is too hard to stop. That answer merely raises other questions. Why do some people enjoy it more and find it harder to stop than others? What factors underlie the attraction to smoking among the fifth of the U.S. population that continues the habit? If smoking brings addiction, physical pleasure, and psychological rewards, why do some give into these rewards but not others? The answers to the questions must consider physiological, psychological, economic, cultural, and social factors.[33]

Biological differences across individuals help explain why some smoke. Studies of twins have found that a genetic predisposition to smoke passes across generations. For example, those who start smoking at an early age have different chemical receptors in the brain than others and metabolize nicotine differently than others. Those physically prone to stronger addiction will find the withdrawal symptoms more painful and smoking more difficult to stop.

Psychological traits affect the tendency to adopt and continue smoking. Impulsive individuals may lack the ability to control their behavior in general and may lack the ability to resist the temptation to smoke in particular. Those with fewer coping skills to deal with their problems and those fatalistic about what happens to them may give into temptation to smoke more than others. Those prone psychologically to risk taking and sensation seeking may take up and continue smoking. Lastly, extroverted personality types, whose outgoing and engaging behavior is highly valued, are more likely to smoke than introverted personality types.

Prosmoking beliefs and attitudes increase the likelihood of smoking. Smokers often believe that their habit helps to control weight, improve mood, and realize a desirable image. Use of cigarettes can, among teens in particular, help smokers feel cool, confident, and part of a group. Similarly, the desire of young women to control their weight with smoking and emulate the glamorous images of thinness found in magazines, advertising, movies, and television contributes to their smoking. However, researchers understand less about why some come to accept these beliefs and others reject them; perhaps those addicted to smoking use their beliefs to justify their addiction.

Obtaining a release from social stress through the mild narcotic effect of nicotine motivates smokers to continue the habit. The propensity to smoke, despite its long-term harm and immediate financial cost, may serve as a short-term coping mechanism to deal with difficult circumstances. Smokers say that cigarettes give them a boost, help them concentrate, and make them feel better. Indulging in the addictive pleasures of nicotine may help in dealing with daily problems and tasks. Youth in particular, given the difficulties they face entering into the adult world, may find smoking helps alleviate their stress. Yet smoking may reduce stress largely because it relieves the withdrawal symptoms produced by the lack of nicotine. If smoking relieves stress, it also produces more stress.

The smoking of parents and friends can lead adolescents to take up the habit themselves. Teens may directly imitate the behavior of those they feel close to or may adopt the beliefs and attitudes of parents and friends that lead indirectly to smoking. Those whose parents smoke are much more likely to smoke themselves than those whose parents do not smoke. Similarly, those whose friends smoke are much more likely to smoke themselves than those whose friends do not smoke. In short, social influences affect the decision to smoke. If, for example, peers offer support for smoking and parents offer opposition to smoking, those with stronger ties to peers than parents will be more likely to smoke. In much the same way, lack of involvement in school, sports teams, and religious organizations—all groups that oppose tobacco use—will increase smoking.

Advertising serves as a major source of the attraction to smoking, particularly among young people. According to many experts, the attractive and glamorous images of smokers in magazine ads lead young people to imitate those images by smoking (cartoonlike characters such as Joe Camel influence even grade-school children). Advertising images may also appeal to rebellious youth by implying a connection between smoking and independence and to girls by implying a connection between smoking and sophistication.

Public health advocates have noted another source of attraction to smoking among youth. Films tend to depict smoking in positive ways and to do so often. Although smoking dropped dramatically in the population, smoking in films increased between 1980 and 2000. In earlier decades, films might use smoking to reflect actual social behavior, but today films distort reality by their portrayal of smokers. Public health groups have blamed film studios for making smoking seem normal and even attractive, and several studios responded by adopting voluntary rules to limit use of tobacco in their films. Even so, the viewing of older movies on DVD and television means images of smoking can influence teens for many years to come.

Perhaps a more useful way to understand the question of why people smoke requires considering not what attracts people to cigarettes, but what prevents them from acting on this attraction. History has shown that billions throughout the world have found the stimulating and addictive effects of cigarettes hard to resist. What gives some special motivation to resist? Reasons for not smoking might include worry about the long-term health effects, impairment of athletic performance, unpleasant smell and taste, reactions of nonsmoking friends, and monetary costs.

Lastly, a small and sometimes vocal group maintains they smoke simply because they enjoy the habit and resent the accusations of antismoking groups that their decisions are illegitimate. In the words of one writer who smokes, "I believe life should be savored rather than lengthened, and I am ready to fight [those] trying to make me switch." Another writer states, "Cigarettes improve my short-term concentration, aid my digestion, make me a finer writer and a better dinner companion, and, in several other ways, prolong my life."[34] Some smokers claim they have not been manipulated by advertising images, are not addicted and irrational, were not misled by tobacco companies, and did not act out of insecurity or impulsiveness. Such explanations give smokers the responsibility for their decisions.

NEGATIVE PUBLIC OPINIONS ABOUT SMOKING

As smoking has become concentrated in a smaller part of the U.S. population, the negative attitudes toward the habit have grown—even among smokers. In terms of their views on the harm of smoking, there is virtually unanimous agreement among smokers and nonsmokers alike. A Gallup poll found that 92 percent of respondents answered "Yes" when asked, "Does smoking cause lung cancer?" Eighty-eight percent of smokers and 93 percent of nonsmokers agreed with the statement. A clear consensus on the relationship between smoking and health has emerged, and this consensus represents a substantial change from the past. In 1954, only 41 percent agreed with the statement. The largest increase came in the 1960s, when the agreement jumped from 45 percent to 71 percent, but the steady negative publicity about smoking since then has raised agreement another 21 percent since 1969.

Other evidence suggests that smokers recognize the harm they are doing to themselves with the habit. When asked in a poll, 81 percent of smokers said they would like to quit, and 79 percent said they were addicted to cigarettes. In one study that asked smokers and nonsmokers to estimate the harm of smoking in terms of the added risk of death, the likelihood of dying from a smoking-related cause, and the years of life lost, both groups overstated the risks identified by the scientific literature.[35] Their answers demonstrate in stark terms that smokers recognize the serious health risks they face.

The public generally recognizes the right of individuals to smoke and does not favor making cigarettes illegal. That does not, however, mean that the public in general and nonsmokers in particular fully respect smokers. If people believe that smoking involves a personal choice, then they also will blame individuals for that choice and sometimes even view smoking as "deviant conduct."[36] Smokers must tolerate urgings from their family, friends, doctors, neighbors, workmates, teachers, religious leaders, media, and government to stop. Nonsmokers feel free to criticize and shame smokers for their inability to stop a destructive habit. Segregation of smokers in airports, restaurants, and office buildings makes smokers feel separate from the rest of society, even sometimes as victims of discrimination. Smokers have the right to choose to use tobacco, but that choice comes with a social as well as a personal health cost.

The negative view of smoking and smokers perhaps shows most clearly in surveys of high school seniors, whose beliefs reflect the future public opinion of adults.[37] About 66 percent prefer to date people who do not smoke, 55 percent think that being a smoker reflects poor judgment, and 70 percent see smoking as a dirty habit. Less than 10 percent of high school students think that smokers look mature and sophisticated, or cool and calm—most see smokers as insecure and foolish. These negative beliefs are more typically held among nonsmokers more than smokers but still reveal a general distaste for the habit among the general public.

A psychologist at the University of Pennsylvania has coined the term *moralization* to describe the process that translates antismoking preferences into views of cigarette use as an immoral act.[38] Moralization shows not just in the dislike of cigarette smoking but in the outrage of nonsmokers when confronted by undesired cigarette smoke, in the crusading views of antismoking advocates, and in the association of smoking with weakness. As a result of this process, smoking can produce disgust more than disagreement, criticism more than indifference, and condemnation more than understanding.

On one hand, the negative views of smoking should discourage the habit, as most people aim to follow the conventional norms of society. On the other hand, the common antismoking views may in some ways make the habit all the more attractive to some, and the sometimes zealous efforts to control individual smoking behavior can produce a backlash among those valuing independence and individualism against the forces of conformity. Smoking has always involved a sense of daring, but with the negative views of the habit these days, it may offer this appeal even more than in the past.

The negative perceptions about cigarette use have led some concerned about the potential abuse of government power to oppose public health efforts against smoking.[39] These critics see antismoking efforts as the attempt of one group to impose its own tastes and preferences on another group and to do so through the use of government force, censorship, economic penalty, and vilification. The end result of the more zealous forms of cigarette control is a form of puritanical repression much like the one that led to alcohol prohibition.[40] In answer to these accusations the 2000 report of the Surgeon General's office states, "It would be hard to deny that moral zealotry has entered into the contemporary movement to reduce smoking," but also that "it would be equally hard to argue that zealotry is the dominant element in the movement."[41] Most policymakers and voters accept tobacco control efforts because the efforts stem largely from medical and scientific evidence and aim to promote the health of the population.

LIGHT CIGARETTES

In the 1960s, public health officials concluded that if smokers could not quit using cigarettes, it would be better for their health if they smoked low-tar cigarettes.[42] A shift to these products would not eliminate tobacco-caused cancer but would reduce its prevalence. Tobacco companies created and marketed low-tar and low-nicotine cigarettes that came to be called "light" or "ultra light" cigarettes. The determination of tar and nicotine in a cigarette came from a machine that smoked the cigarette and measured the tar and nicotine yield (known as the machine measured yield).

During the last 50 years, changes in cigarette design and manufacturing have produced a 60 percent decline in machine-measured tar and nicotine yields. While cigarettes in 1955 averaged 35 milligrams of tar, they now average around 10 milligrams.[43] Nicotine in cigarettes has dropped just as much. Presently, lower-yield cigarettes dominate the market. About 98 percent of cigarettes sold are filtered, and about 65 percent of cigarettes sold are classified as low-tar products (the machine-measured tar is less than 15 milligrams per cigarette). A partial list of these products includes the following brands: Marlboro Lights, Camel Lights, Kool Lights, Merit Lights, Winston Lights, Salem Lights, Newport Lights, Now, Vantage, Carlton, Virginia Slims Lights, and Parliament Lights.

Along with light cigarettes, other types of cigarette products have increased in popularity. Several smaller companies market cigarettes that use tobacco without any additives or inorganic substances. As natural products, these cigarettes might be viewed by smokers as healthier. The Liggett Group sold their traditional brands such as Chesterfield and Lark to concentrate on developing and marketing a new low-nicotine cigarette to aid smokers wanting to quit. Still other companies sell clove cigarettes that contain some tobacco but not as much as regular cigarettes. None of these products has become a big seller, but as a group they meet demand from a growing segment of smokers who prefer nontraditional types of cigarettes.

The National Cancer Institute argues, however, that despite earlier claims, light cigarettes offer little health benefit.[44] They may in fact increase the risk to health by leading smokers to try the lighter brands rather than quit altogether. The new brands also fail to reduce the harm of tar, the absorption of nicotine, and the rates of lung cancer for two reasons. First, smokers either inhale light cigarettes more intensely to get more flavor and nicotine or they increase the number of cigarettes they smoke per day. Second, tobacco companies placed ventilation holes in the filters that could be easily blocked by a smoker's lips or fingers and therefore often fail to dilute the delivery of tar and nicotine. Cigarettes that yield low tar in machines do not always deliver the same benefit when smoked by people. As a result, recent epidemiological studies reveal little health value from the growth of light cigarettes. Smokers of light cigarettes are no more likely to quit or live longer than smokers of regular cigarettes.

Tobacco companies have recently come to deny the safety of light or low-tar yield cigarettes. Philip Morris, for example, has circulated notices with some of their brands. The notices state that the tar and nicotine levels are not necessarily good indicators of how much of these substances smokers inhale and that smokers should not assume that low-tar cigarettes are less harmful than other cigarettes. Critics of the tobacco industry claim that this effort is merely a way to absolve them of liability for the harm caused by so-called safe cigarettes. Indeed many suits have been filed on behalf of smokers of light cigarettes. Based on the claim that cigarette companies misled smokers about the safety of light cigarettes, law firms are soliciting smokers of light or safe cigarettes who have been diagnosed with smoking-related illnesses.

TOBACCO USE IN MINORITY COMMUNITIES

Compared to white non-Hispanics, Native Americans have higher levels of smoking, African Americans have similar levels of smoking, and Hispanics and Asian Americans have lower levels of smoking. Yet as smoking has declined in the general population, tobacco companies have done more to target smokers and potential smokers in the minority communities. Besides directing appeals to these communities with advertising, the tobacco industry has done much to provide economic support.

A report of the Surgeon General's office on tobacco use among minority groups notes that several actions of the tobacco industry have strengthened its standing in the African-American community.[45] Tobacco companies were among the first in the South to hire African Americans in their factories, to provide management opportunities for African Americans, and to employ African Americans as models and spokespersons for their products. By placing advertisements in African-American publications, tobacco companies have helped to support minority businesses. Companies have also contributed funding to community agencies and civil rights organizations, sponsored cultural events, and supported African-American political candidates.

Along with providing economic support, the tobacco companies have targeted certain types of advertising to appeal to African Americans. In general, cigarette ads are more common in magazines for African Americans, such as *Ebony*, *Essence*, and *Jet*, than in magazines for the general population, such as *Time*, *People*, and *Mademoiselle*. More specifically, mentholated cigarettes, which are particularly popular among African Americans, are heavily advertised in publications with a minority readership. One new cigarette product, Uptown, was by all appearances introduced by R. J. Reynolds to appeal specifically to African Americans, but protests led the company to withdraw the product after early tests. In any case, advertising targeted at minority groups may contribute to use of cigarettes in their communities.

Involvement of tobacco companies in other minority communities has not been as extensive as in the African-American community, but they do make an effort to reach all minority groups. They have sponsored activities to enhance racial or ethnic pride, such as Mexican rodeos, American Indian powwows, Chinese New Year festivities, and Cinco de Mayo festivities. They also directed advertising to Hispanic, Asian-American, and Native

American communities. Outdoor advertising of cigarettes was (until banned) more commonly located in urban minority communities than in white parts of cities and suburbs. In-store displays appear more commonly in small city convenience stores in ethnic communities. And specific brands were targeted for minority groups: Rio and Dorado for Hispanics, Mild Seven (a popular cigarette in Japan) for Asian Americans, and American Spirit for Native Americans.

On the one hand, these efforts of cigarette makers reflect economic power of minority groups. When other product makers often ignore minorities in their promotions and advertising, the attention of cigarette makers provides an economic boost to often disadvantaged communities. On the other hand, with life expectancy in most minority communities already lower than average, the promotion of cigarettes threatens to maintain that disadvantage. Critics in minority communities and government agencies have worked hard to oppose special efforts by tobacco companies to appeal to vulnerable minorities.

CHANGES IN THE TOBACCO INDUSTRY

It might seem that the negative publicity about smoking and the decline in smoking in the United States would have weakened the tobacco industry. The public increasingly views the tobacco industry and its executives as evil in their efforts to addict young people. The negative views not only have reduced sales but have led to legal judgments that have imposed billions of dollars in damages on the tobacco companies. It would seem that the industry must be facing major financial problems.

In fact, the tobacco industry is thriving. It has changed form, has suffered defeats, and lost the respect and profits it once had, but it still does well. Across the world it enjoys $300 billion in sales annually. If government and private suits raise the legal costs of tobacco firms, they can pass those costs on to consumers. If markets in the United States and other high-income countries shrink as citizens increasingly reject smoking, they can focus on new markets outside these nations. If they are portrayed as morally evil, they can justify their industry in terms of providing a legal product that adults enjoy.

In the United States, recent mergers and acquisitions of tobacco companies have made the major players more difficult to keep straight. However, four companies dominate tobacco sales:

1. The Altria Group, headquartered in Virginia, owns Philip Morris USA, Philip Morris International, and John Middleton (a cigar maker). Originally a British firm that entered the American market with a small office in New York City in 1902, Philip Morris grew to the nation's

largest tobacco company before becoming part of Altria. It enjoys its success through sales of the world's most popular cigarette, Marlboro, and also makes Parliament and Virginia Slims brands. Across the world, Altria has captured 17.6 percent of the market and has $57 billion in sales, making it the world's largest private cigarette company. Along with dominating sales in the United States and Mexico, the company is the top seller of cigarettes in France, Germany, Poland, and Russia. In America, Philip Morris was known as a vigorous opponent of tobacco controls in previous decades. However, Altria now officially recognizes the hazards of smoking and runs ads to prevent youth smoking.

2. Reynolds American, headquartered in Winston-Salem, North Carolina, was founded with the merger of the R. J. Reynolds Tobacco Company and Brown & Williamson. It also owns R. J. Reynolds International Products (worldwide distributor of cigarettes), Conwood Company (smokeless tobacco), and Santa Fe Natural Tobacco Company (additive-free products). R. J. Reynolds, maker of Camel, Winston, and Salem cigarettes, at one time led in cigarette sales in the United States. However, some unwise decisions, including an expensive leveraged buyout in 1988, saddled the company with so much debt that it had to sell much of its business and lost market share to other companies. The merger with Brown & Williamson made it the second-largest seller of cigarettes in the United States. The R. J. Reynolds Company was criticized strongly for the Joe Camel advertising campaign in the 1980s and 1990s, which critics said directly appealed to children. Brown & Williamson had the second-largest American sales until the merger. It made Kool, Lucky Strike, Pall Mall, Tareyton, and Viceroy cigarettes, all of which continue to be produced under Reynolds American. However, the company received much negative publicity after the release of its internal documents on nicotine, addiction, and youth advertising.

3. Lorillard Tobacco Company, headquartered in Greensborough, North Carolina, is the third-largest and oldest continuously operating cigarette company in the United States. It was owned by Loews Corporation through its stake in the Carolina Group. In 2008, however, Loews made Lorillard Tobacco a separate company. Loews says that the spin-off makes financial sense, but observers suggest that the company also wants to remove the stigma of association with cigarette making and selling. Lorillard makes Newport cigarettes, the number-one selling menthol brand in the United States, as well as Kent, True, and Old Gold.

4. Liggett Vector Brands, headquartered in Durham, North Carolina, is the fourth-largest tobacco company in the United States. After selling off its traditional products of L&M, Chesterfield, and Lark in 1999 to

concentrate on discount-priced and generic brands and on low-tar and -nicotine cigarettes, the Liggett Group merged in 2005 with Vector Tobacco to create this company. The company's products include Liggett Select, Eve, Grand Prix, and nicotine-free Quest. The company highlights its research on safe cigarettes and other innovative products.

Four other international companies have major sales outside the United States:

1. British American Tobacco, based in London, England, owns the brands developed by the American Tobacco Company and formerly owned Brown & Williamson. It now has a share of the new company formed from the merger of Brown & Williamson and the R. J. Reynolds Tobacco Company. It also owns the South African tobacco company Rothmans International. Across the world, it has 15.1 percent of the cigarette sales, worth about $49 billion—second in size to Altria. With 300 brands such as Dunhill and, outside the United States, Kent, Lucky Strike, and Pall Mall, its cigarettes are top sellers in Canada, India, Brazil, South Africa, and many other nations of South America and Africa.
2. Japan Tobacco, the world's third-largest tobacco company, is partly owned by the Japanese government. It expanded from the Japanese market to buy the rights to sell Camel, Salem, and Winston brands outside the United States and has 6.4 percent of world cigarette sales. In 2007, it purchased Gallaher Group Plc, a British based international tobacco company whose brands include Benson & Hedges, Silk Cut, and Mayfair. This purchase added 3.1 percent of the world market to the company.
3. Imperial Tobacco Group Limited, headquartered in Bristol, England, has 3.6 percent of world market in cigarette sales. In February 2007, it acquired Commonwealth Brands, an American cigarette maker. In February 2008, it acquired a large European company, Altadis, which had another 2 percent of world cigarette sales.
4. One other company deserves mention because of its size, although it sells few cigarettes internationally. With a monopoly on sales in China, the China National Tobacco Corporation has 33.7 percent of the world market by virtue of selling to the 350 million smokers in the country. The company also markets some of its 900 brands outside China, but foreign sales are only about 3 percent of the national market.

The continued success of these firms stems from the nature of their product. Cigarettes differ from almost all other consumer items: Their addictive nature keeps customers returning, and the unique properties of inhaling cigarette smoke and ingesting nicotine mean that no other product can take its place. Combined with the low cost of producing cigarettes, these properties make for a high profit margin. In one analysis, most of the cost of a pack of cigarettes (more than $8.00 in New York City) goes to taxes and retailer markup. The production, advertising, marketing, and legal costs of the companies equal only $1.45 per pack, and profit equals 28¢.[46]

GLOBAL SPREAD OF CIGARETTES

The expanding markets for cigarettes in low- and middle-income nations across the world offers a profitable source of sales for tobacco companies and a new worry for public health officials. A few figures from the World Health Organization (WHO) illustrate the global patterns of change in tobacco use.[47] About 1.3 billion people across the world smoke and consume about 15 billion cigarettes each day. Smokers make up about 35 percent of adult men in industrialized societies and 50 percent of adult men in developing countries. For women, the pattern is reversed. About 22 percent smoke in industrializing nations and about 9 percent in developing countries. Yet tobacco advertising increasingly targets women in developing nations to increase the low usage rate.

The trends reveal further divergence between developed and developing nations. From 1970 to 2000, cigarettes consumed per adult age 15 and over fell by 24 percent in more developed countries and rose by 46 percent in developing countries. For example, consumption per person has risen by 143 percent in China, 78 percent in Egypt, and 187 percent in Indonesia. Projections suggest that, largely because of growth in the developing world, the 1.3 billion smokers throughout the world in 1995 will rise to 1.6 billion by 2025.[48] Although women have lower smoking levels than men, they have more room to grow. Worldwide surveys of youth ages 13 to 15 show that girls smoke nearly as much as boys. Since youth smoking affects adult smoking decades later, females levels will likely rise substantially in the future. A prediction from the WHO suggests that the percentage of females who smoke will rise from 12 percent in 2005 to 20 percent in 2025.[49]

The trends in smoking in developing nations obviously concern public health officials, who now refer to a *worldwide* smoking epidemic. They decry the adoption of a behavior that will reduce longevity across the globe at the same time other forces of development, medicine, and public health serve to increase longevity. With tobacco deaths currently numbering about 5 million per year worldwide, they may plausibly reach 10 million by 2030, with 70 percent occurring in developing regions.

For tobacco companies, worldwide tobacco use presents opportunities for sales that counter the increasingly successful efforts in the United States to combat cigarette use and restrict the power of the tobacco industry. Despite facing higher taxes, judicial setbacks, negative publicity, legislative restrictions, and a declining market in many high-income nations like the United States, the tobacco industry has maintained its profitability—and its ability to promote the use of tobacco—with global sales and marketing efforts. Tobacco companies have used mergers, price cuts, advertising, and the promotion of positive images of smokers to sell more cigarettes across the world. However, they now face strengthening global public health efforts against tobacco, including an international treaty that would create consistent antismoking policies across the world.

CURRENT KNOWLEDGE ABOUT SMOKING AND HEALTH

DETAILING THE RISKS

Tobacco smoke contains more than 4,000 known compounds that enter the lungs along with various gases. These compounds include nicotine, which passes into the bloodstream through the lungs, affects cells throughout the body, and produces an addictive physical and mental reaction. They also include 43 different substances identified as carcinogens (or cancer-causing substances) and carbon monoxide, a colorless, odorless, and highly toxic gas. The exact processes of how these compounds adversely affect the body are not always well understood, but studies have clearly documented the association between absorption of these tobacco smoke compounds and health problems.

Among the known adverse consequences of cigarette smoking are increases in death from heart disease (the most common cause of death in the United States), diseases of the arteries, lung and throat cancer, cancers of numerous other organs (bladder, pancreas, kidney, stomach, and cervix), and chronic obstructive pulmonary disease (chronic bronchitis and emphysema). Numerous studies have demonstrated these relationships, but the Cancer Prevention Study II from 1982 to 1986 provides data on a large number of Americans.[50] The study examined the smoking habits of more than 1.2 million volunteers and then followed them over the next four years to record information on the cause of death for those who died during the period. The key statistics came from the rate of death for current smokers, former smokers, and never smokers. With the huge sample, the study was able to examine the effect of smoking on relatively rare causes of death.

According to the results the risks of lung cancer for current male and female smokers are 22.4 and 11.9 times higher, respectively, than they are for nonsmokers. Called relative risk ratios, these numbers indicate that for every nonsmoker who dies of lung cancer, 22 current male smokers and 12 current female smokers die. The risks of lung cancer for former smokers are lower than current smokers but still high. For every nonsmoker who dies of lung cancer, nine former male smokers and five former female smokers die. Quitting smoking reduces the risks of lung cancer but does not eliminate them altogether. Other cancers, although not as common as lung cancer, also appear more among smokers and former smokers. Compared to never smokers, current male smokers have relative risks of 27.5 for lip and mouth cancer, 7.6 for esophagus cancer, 2.9 for kidney cancer, and 2.9 for bladder cancer.

Cigarette smoking also increases the risks of heart disease. At ages 35–64, 2.8 current male smokers and 3.0 current female smokers die of heart disease for every nonsmoker who dies of heart disease. For former male and female smokers, the relative risks are 1.7 and 1.4. While these risks are lower than for lung cancer, they translate into more smoking-related deaths. Since more people in the United States die of heart disease each year than from any other cause—about 725,000 in 1998—the added risk of premature death for smokers contributes substantially to loss of life. Smoking thus accounts for roughly 20 percent of heart disease deaths.

Two other diseases deserve special attention because of their prevalence and close association with smoking. For every nonsmoker who dies of a stroke at ages 35–64, 3.7 current male smokers, 4.8 current female smokers, 1.4 former male smokers, and 1.4 former female smokers die of a stroke. Chronic obstructive pulmonary disease (COPD), which includes emphysema, chronic bronchitis, and other diseases that block the flow of air into the lungs, also occurs more commonly among smokers. For every nonsmoker who dies of COPD, 9.6 current male smokers, 10.5 current female smokers, 8.8 former male smokers, and 7.0 former female smokers die of the disease.

A 2004 Surgeon General's report summarizes these facts on the health consequences of smoking by concluding that smoking harms nearly every organ of the body. It adds the following diseases to the list of those caused by smoking: abdominal aortic aneurysm, acute myeloid leukemia, cataracts, cervical cancer, kidney cancer, pancreatic cancer, pneumonia, periodontitis, and stomach cancer.

Averaged across all causes of death, current male smokers are 2.3 times as likely to die prematurely as male never smokers, and current female smokers are 1.9 times as likely to die prematurely as female never smokers (the risks for former male and female smokers are, respectively, 1.6 and 1.3). Similarly, risks for heavy smokers to die prematurely of these diseases are higher than for light smokers, and risks for former smokers who used cigarettes for a long period are higher than those who used cigarettes for a short period. From the point of view of the individual, smokers can expect to live 13–14 fewer years on average than nonsmokers. Of course, some smokers will live as long as or longer than nonsmokers and some smokers will die at a very young age, so the 13–14 years represent an average; nonetheless, the average figure provides a useful summary.

Based on the higher risk of death among former and current smokers and on the prevalence of former and current smokers in the U.S. population, the 2004 Surgeon General's report estimated the number of deaths due to cigarettes. These numbers make the harm of smoking easy to summarize and understand. If former and current smokers had the same risks of death as those who never smoked, then there would be 263,600 fewer male deaths, 176,500 fewer female deaths, and 440,100 fewer total deaths in 1999 (the last year for which these statistics were available). From 1965 to 1999, 11.9 million deaths resulted from smoking. Smoking-related impairment from sickness and disability adds further to the health costs. Counting medical care and lost work, the estimated economic costs of smoking in the United States reached $157.7 billion.

Although traditionally less likely to use tobacco than men, women are seriously affected by smoking-related mortality, a fact that led the World Health Organization to publish a short book, *Women and Tobacco*, in 1992,[51] and the Surgeon General to publish a report of over 500 pages in 2001 entitled *Women and Smoking*.[52] Relative risks of death for female smokers are lower than for males, perhaps because they inhale less and smoke fewer cigarettes. Still, female deaths from smoking are moving closer to the higher male figure. Lung cancer has even replaced breast cancer as the most common form of cancer death among women.

The risks of death from other forms of tobacco use are also elevated, although not to the same degree as from cigarette smoking. The estimated mortality rate of cigar smokers was 39 percent higher than for those who smoked neither cigarettes nor cigars, and the estimated mortality rate of pipe smokers was 29 percent higher than for those who smoked neither cigarettes nor pipes. Smokeless tobacco, taken in the form of chew placed in the cheek or snuff placed between the lower gum and lip, experienced renewed popularity with the warnings against cigarettes. Because smokeless tobacco does not involve the inhalation of smoke and associated by-products into the lungs but still gives a nicotine kick, it seemed a good alternative to cigarettes. According to one study, however, the risks of mouth cancer were four times higher for moderate users of smokeless tobacco and seven times higher for heavy users than for nonusers. Translating the statistics into something more meaningful to potential users, a story of a 19-year-old Oklahoman received much publicity.[53] He began using smokeless tobacco as a teen, became addicted, and developed tongue cancer, which spread and killed him. Although use of smokeless tobacco never reached the levels of cigarettes, and mouth cancer is rarer than lung cancer and heart disease, users of smokeless tobacco face heightened risks of death.

The cost to life from smoking also includes nonsmokers through environmental tobacco smoke, sometimes called passive, or involuntary, smoking. Although the risks are not to the same extent as they are for smokers who directly inhale cigarette smoke, they do exist. A 2006 report from the Surgeon General entitled *The Health Consequences of Involuntary Exposure to Tobacco Smoke* relies on decades of evidence to make the case for the harm of secondhand smoke, or environmental tobacco smoke (ETS).[54] The harm of ETS appears greatest for those exposed to high levels inside homes and buildings, such as spouses and children of family members who smoke heavily at home or workers in bars and restaurants with much smoking. With such exposure, the risks of heart disease can increase by 25 to 30 percent and the risks of lung cancer can increase by 20 to 30. For those exposed only occasionally to small amounts of ETS, the health threats are smaller. Yet the Surgeon General's report concludes that that there is no risk-free level of exposure to secondhand smoke. These findings help justify segregation of smokers and nonsmokers in public places, and the banning of indoor smoking altogether in many facilities.

Children, infants, and fetuses can all suffer from the smoking of their parents. Women who smoke during pregnancy are more likely to have a miscarriage or give birth to a stillborn baby than women who do not smoke while pregnant. Smoking during pregnancy also leads to higher risks of low birth-weight babies and may slow the brain development of children as they grow older. These effects come in part from the sharing of the chemically altered blood of smoking mothers with their fetuses. Later, smoking by either one or both parents in the house can increase the risks of sudden infant death syndrome (SIDS) among infants and asthma and infections among older children who breathe the secondhand smoke.

PREVENTING SMOKING

Because youth typically try cigarettes for the first time between ages 11 and 15 (grades six through 10), and most who continue to smoke as adults have started by age 20, prevention programs must begin at young ages. Nonsmoking adults rarely take up the habit, so most resources for prevention go to school-based programs. It might seem logical that presenting information on the damage of cigarette use would prevent youths from smoking, but the evidence shows the contrary. According to the Surgeon General's 1994 report on youth and smoking, "Knowledge of the long-term health consequences of smoking has not been a strong predictor of adolescent onset . . . perhaps because virtually all U.S. adolescents—smokers and nonsmokers alike—are aware of the long-term health effects of smoking."[55] Similarly a study of trends in smoking initiation from 1944 to 1988 concludes, "The public health campaign . . . has had limited or no impact on younger persons."[56] Thus, as the World Bank has observed, "In general, young people appear to be less responsive to information about the health effects of tobacco than older adults."[57]

Besides presenting information on the risks of smoking, the programs need to recognize that youth are highly influenced by their peers, their reactions to advertising, and perceptions of the prevalence of smoking in the larger society. Understanding the risks of smoking brings little benefit if youth remain attracted by the images of advertisements and lack skills to resist pressures from others to smoke. Teaching youngsters about the social skills needed to resist manipulation by advertisements and the pressures of others to smoke needs to accompany teaching them about the physical costs of smoking.

To be successful, programs also must make an intensive effort at change. Early antismoking programs had little success in changing behavior because they tended to be short in duration, small in size, and isolated from the larger context of the school and community. More recent programs have, in contrast, been more effective because they have expanded the limited form of early programs. Programs with the best results last years rather than weeks (one program, for example, consists of 30 classes over three grades), and they incorporate antismoking efforts into general health education for students. In addition, these programs view antismoking efforts as part of school and community goals rather than as a single class. They teach social skills and give students practice in resisting pressures to smoke.

Multifaceted programs that include all these components can reduce smoking initiation by about 10 percent. Other programs that are combined with mass media and community programs can do even better. The SHOUT (Students Helping Others Understand Tobacco) program, for example, consists of 18 class sessions in seventh and eighth grade and then continued telephone and mail contact in ninth grade. The intensive effort has reduced current smoking by 33 percent by the end of grade nine. However, even these multifaceted programs can have short-lived benefits. Without continued effort, the benefits of antismoking programs disappear during high school and after. Once programs end, the influence of peers and the media can overwhelm earlier antismoking messages.

A recent report from the Institute of Medicine of the National Academies, *Ending the Tobacco Problem: A Blueprint for the Nation*, gives much attention to preventing youth from staring to smoke.[58] It makes several recommendations for new policies:

- All states should license retail outlets that sell tobacco products. The licensing process should ensure that the outlets place products behind counters, follow rules on product displays, and do not sell tobacco to underage youth.

- All states should ban sales of cigarettes through mail order or the Internet. When sales are occurring only through licensed outlets, it is easier to prevent sales to underage youth.
- School boards should require all middle schools and high schools to adopt evidence-based smoking prevention programs. Students should go through these programs annually.
- A national, youth-oriented media campaign should be funded on an ongoing basis. State and local prevention and media campaigns should supplement the national one.
- National and state legislation should prevent tobacco companies from targeting any messages, regardless of their purpose, toward youth under age 18.

The report justifies vigorous action against youth smoking by noting that youth attraction to smoking changes when they get older. By that time, however, they have become too addicted to stop easily. In a sense, youth who start to smoke act against their self-interest and later desires. This justifies some intrusion or coercion in youth prevention efforts.

SMOKING CESSATION

Although preventing youth from starting to smoke is ideal, helping those who have already begun smoking will also reduce cigarette and tobacco consumption. Specialists refer to smoking cessation as nicotine addiction management because management of the addiction that makes quitting hard can help in the process. With smoking treated as a chronic disease of addiction, those trying to stop can expect remission, relapse, and difficulty in changing. Smokers need to continue their efforts without blaming themselves or attributing their problems in stopping to character weakness.

Consistent with the addiction framework and the difficulty in stopping smoking, those smokers trying to quit have a high failure rate. In fact, only 6 percent of attempts in quitting succeed for a month, and only 3 to 5 percent succeed for a year or more. Yet the low rate of success, when accumulated over time, can do much to reduce smoking. Individuals who have failed to stop in the past may with additional attempts succeed. Thus more than 40 million Americans today are former smokers—about the same number as current smokers. Since former smokers have lower rates of death than current smokers (although the rates are still higher than never smokers), quitting can improve the health of the U.S. population.

Those groups most successful in quitting once had high rates of smoking but now have relatively low rates of smoking. More men than women, more older than younger persons, and more highly educated and affluent persons than less-educated and poor persons have successfully quit. The differences in quitting do not relate to interest, as members of all groups express the desire to give up the habit (an average of 70 percent of the total U.S. population of smokers), but some groups more than others have either stronger motivation or better ability to realize their goal.

Most former smokers ended their habit on their own, usually by simply stopping and resisting the impulse to start again (a practice known as "going cold turkey"). Those able to quit most easily may have weaker physical addictions and withdrawal symptoms or greater motivation and willpower. Over the years, however, those who can most easily quit will have already done so, leaving among the population of smokers those most addicted to the product and likely to have the hardest time quitting. As a result, long-time smokers need special help in stopping. Research has identified five approaches to aiding smokers, each of which shows some effectiveness but varies from the others in cost and efficiency.[59]

First, large-scale public health programs focus on the full population of smokers. Transmitting smoking cessation messages through the media, at work, and in the community can bring crucial information to this population and help some to quit; however, such programs work best when they extend beyond the local community to become state or nationwide. Moreover smokers may need something more tangible or personal than public health messages to motivate them. The negative reactions of family, friends, coworkers, and community members to smoking can spur quitting.

Second, the simple process of distributing self-help manuals may help some smokers stop. Antismoking organizations and the government can cheaply produce self-help manuals and distribute them easily to large numbers of smokers. They can further tailor the style and format of the manuals to specific gender, race, ethnic, and education groups. Such efforts appear to produce a small but consistent benefit, one that favors those less addicted to cigarettes and most motivated to change. Manuals listing telephone numbers that readers can call for help sometimes do better to promote cessation, but such calls again mostly help those already strongly motivated to stop and less addicted to nicotine.

Third, minimal clinical interventions that involve the efforts of health care personnel to urge smokers to stop can have modest effects. Clinicians who not only ask patients if they smoke but also advise them to quit can help provide the motivation their patients need. With 70 percent of smokers already saying they want to quit, the urging of physicians, nurses, and other health care personnel can do much to get smokers to take the first steps to stop their habit. If clinicians also appraise the willingness of smokers to stop, assist those who want to stop, and check on the progress of the patients who attempt to stop, they can then do more to aid smoking cessation. When treated as part of regular health care checkups, these minimal clinical interventions involve little cost and can do more than self-help manuals alone.

Fourth, counseling alone and in combination with other treatments is effective for treating tobacco dependence. Intensive counseling requires the most cost and effort but works better than less intensive procedures, particularly for highly addicted smokers. It also works for adolescent smokers. Such interventions should include multisession counseling over a period of at least five months to develop problem-solving or coping skills. Less intensive and expensive, telephone quit-line counseling also has some benefits and more easily reaches broad segments of smokers trying to quit.

Fifth, pharmacological approaches that treat the physical reactions to smoking cessation and nicotine withdrawal with medications can help smokers quit. Companies widely promote nicotine replacement therapy in the form of gum or patches (and less commonly nicotine nasal spray and inhalers). Abundant evidence demonstrates the value of these products, and clinicians highly recommended them. Combined with more socially based methods of support, use of nicotine replacement therapy is helpful. Antidepressant medications, notably bupropion and perhaps serotonin reuptake inhibitors such as Prozac and Zoloft, may also help. Many who quit smoking experience depression, and clinical studies of bupropion and nicotine replacement theory find that the combination increases the quit rate over those using nicotine replacement therapy alone. Combining multiple medications can help further. Use of medications is expensive, but the effectiveness and positive consequences for health suggests that health insurance should cover the cost.

Based on these results, authorities recommend that public health agencies make counseling and treatment programs available to those who need them. This might include covering the costs of the programs with insurance or providing free or low-cost programs to low-income persons. In addition they recommend large-scale public health interventions that extend local community efforts to include whole states. Statewide tobacco control programs have had some success in changing the smoking behavior of adults (less so for youth) and result in a decline in tobacco consumption. The programs not only increase public health messages and treatment opportunities but also raise taxes as a means to regulate tobacco. Combined with intensive counseling and nicotine replacement therapy for some smokers, comprehensive efforts to change the social environment that supports smoking appear promising.

REGULATING TOBACCO

ECONOMIC STRATEGIES

Outside of making the product illegal or restricting its use in public places, the government can do little directly to prevent adults from smoking. For minors the known harm of cigarette smoking and antitobacco educational campaigns will ideally prevent them from wanting to purchase cigarettes, but otherwise restrictions are necessary. States have laws to prohibit the sale of cigarettes to minors (under 18), but teens can get around the restrictions.

A potentially more effective approach to reducing smoking involves raising taxes. Economic studies have demonstrated that a 10 percent increase in price will reduce overall consumption of cigarettes by 3 to 5 percent. High prices not only reduce the average number of cigarettes consumed by smokers but lead some to give up the habit altogether. They further may prevent some young people from starting, thus helping to prevent lifelong addiction.

Although pricing relates to the decisions of the tobacco industry, governments regulate the cost of cigarettes to consumers with taxes. Federal, state, and local excise (per unit) taxes on cigarette purchases represent a substantial cost. State legislatures and local communities have been quite willing to increase taxes on cigarettes. Since 2000, nearly every state added to the per-pack tax. For example, in addition to the 39 cent federal tax, New York State adds a $2.75 tax and New York City adds $1.50 tax on a pack of cigarettes. Still, antitobacco experts call for increases in the federal tax rate and for harmonizing tax rates across states so that smuggling cigarettes from low-tax states to high-tax states is not such a problem.

The taxes on cigarettes in the United States remain well below those in most other high-income nations. In the United Kingdom, taxes make up 78.0 percent of the average price of cigarettes, in Germany they are 74.5 percent, and in France they represent 80.4 percent. European nations tend in general to tax more highly than the United States, but even Canada imposes cigarette taxes equal to 76.3 percent of the average price. These figures suggest that much room remains to raise cigarette taxes.

REGULATION OF INFORMATION

The government has some, but far-from-complete, power to regulate the information tobacco companies provide to consumers through advertising and packaging. Below is a list of major regulatory actions.

- In 1955 the FTC objected to claims made by cigarette ads that certain brands improved health.
- In 1957 Congress held hearings on deceptive ads about filter-tip cigarettes.
- In 1965 Congress required a mild warning statement on cigarette packages.
- In 1967 the FCC in enforcing its fairness doctrine required television and radio stations to air antismoking ads in order to counter the views presented in cigarette ads.

- In 1971 Congress banned tobacco ads from the public airways used by television and radio stations and required warnings in magazine advertisements.
- In 1984 the Smoking Education Act required that four strongly worded warnings be rotated on cigarette packages and advertisements.
- In 1986 the Comprehensive Smokeless Tobacco Health Education Act required three rotated warning labels on smokeless tobacco packages.

More recently the FTC leveled a complaint against R. J. Reynolds for using the Joe Camel or Old Joe cartoon character in its ads. The 1997 complaint argued that the ads appealed to minors who by law could not purchase cigarettes and were not old enough to fully evaluate or understand the information available on the harm of smoking. A 1994 suit in California had also accused the ads of violating California laws on unfair competition. After failing in the California supreme court to have the suit dismissed, Reynolds ended Joe Camel ads and promotions in California. As part of the 1998 nationwide settlement of lawsuits, the company stopped the Joe Camel campaign nationwide. However, advertising to minors continues as a major source of dispute between the tobacco companies and their opponents in the government, judiciary, and private-sector groups.

Despite their ability to regulate information, government agencies have not, in the absence of congressional legislation, been able to regulate the product itself. In the 1990s the head of the Food and Drug Administration (FDA), Dr. David Kessler, attempted such regulation but ultimately the effort failed. Claiming that cigarettes are in essence a delivery system for an addictive substance, nicotine, the FDA suggested that ads with the words *satisfaction, strength,* and *impact* were describing the pharmacological effects of cigarettes. The FDA also cited evidence from tobacco industry documents that manufacturers manipulated the levels of nicotine in their cigarettes to strengthen their addictiveness. As it did for other drugs, then, the FDA proposed to regulate cigarettes. Since the FDA already regulated nicotine in the form of patches and gum, why shouldn't it regulate the nicotine in cigarettes? The agency thus proposed to use this regulatory power to restrict the sales of cigarettes without obtaining new congressional legislation. The regulations would, among other things, require that the tobacco industry spend $150 million a year to support prevention education among children and ban promotional items, free samples, color ads in magazines with more than 15 percent of the readership under age 18, and sponsorship of sporting or entertainment events using brand names.

Joined by retailers and advertisers, the tobacco industry responded to the proposed regulations by filing lawsuits that claimed the FDA did not have jurisdiction. Proposed legislation in Congress also threatened to bar the FDA from regulating tobacco. President Bill Clinton nonetheless approved the new FDA rules on August 23, 1996. The final rules changed somewhat by emphasizing more strongly the need to protect minors and by eliminating the required $150 million payment from the tobacco companies for antismoking education but maintained the goal of regulating the industry under existing law.

However, lower courts largely invalidated the regulations by concluding that existing statutes did not give the FDA the authority it claimed. After appeals, the U.S. Supreme Court on March 21, 2000, affirmed by 5-4 the lower court decision against the FDA. Although recognizing the harm of cigarette use by minors that motivated the FDA, the Supreme Court majority agreed that Congress in previous laws did not intend to give the FDA regulatory control over tobacco. The Court noted that Congress had throughout history treated tobacco differently from other drugs under the purview of the FDA.

More than eight years after the Supreme Court decision, Congress may give the FDA regulatory power through legislation. Although it still has a way to go, the legislation to make this change appears to have enough support to become law. Even Philip Morris USA supports the legislation (after getting agreement to exclude menthol from the list of substances to be banned from cigarettes). The legislation still needs to be voted on by the House and to get approval from the Senate committee and the full Senate. And some former Secretaries of Health have criticized the legislation for not banning menthol. Still, the chances for changes in regulation look good.

CLEAN INDOOR AIR REGULATIONS

The most widely supported regulations of tobacco relate to protecting non-smokers (and, to a lesser degree, smokers) from the tobacco smoke of others. Environmental tobacco smoke, or ETS, is sometimes called secondhand smoke. Breathing such smoke is sometimes called passive or involuntary smoking and can have serious health consequences for nonsmokers. These consequences justify bans on smoking in public places.

Regulating environmental tobacco smoke has strong support. Public opinion surveys indicate that people respect the rights of smokers to enjoy their tobacco, if they are aware of the harm it does themselves, but also the rights of nonsmokers to stay free from the unwanted smoke of others and from the risks of involuntary smoking. Likewise a majority of smokers accept the need to place restrictions on where they can light up. In the private realm, stores, hotels, and restaurants have therefore done much to segregate smokers or prohibit smoking altogether. Employers also support restrictions on smoking because limiting access to cigarettes in the workplace increases the productivity of workers, reduces the risks of accidents, and limits insurance costs. They also have an obligation to protect workers from risk of injury while on the job, and protecting them from cigarette smoking fits this obligation.

Government regulations have extended and encouraged private efforts to create clean indoor air. In 1988 Congress banned smoking on domestic air flights of less than two hours and later extended the restriction to all public U.S. flights. Similar federal restrictions involving interstate commerce and travel apply to trains and buses. Federal government buildings are now also smoke-free. Numerous state and local restrictions exist as well. Most states limit smoking in public buildings such as hospitals and airports, government buildings, and many private workplaces.

Battles to implement additional smoking restrictions generally occur at the local or state level and involve banning smoking altogether in bars and restaurants. Berkeley, California, was the first such city to do so in 1977, but Los Angeles followed in 1993 and San Francisco in 1994. However, many in the food and drink industry fear a loss of business from such restrictions and have worked to prevent wider implementation of the restrictions. That resistance has weakened, with past evidence suggesting that the ban does not hurt business. Along with many cities passing bans (New York City adopted the ban in 2003), states have done so as well. Nineteen now prohibit smoking in private workplaces (not including bars and restaurants), 24 prohibit smoking in restaurants, and 18 prohibit smoking in stand-alone bars.

California has over the years been a leader in tobacco control and has comprehensive clean air laws. Smoking is prohibited in all enclosed spaces of employment (except for break rooms with direct ventilation to the outside). It is prohibited inside government buildings and vehicles, and school facilities. It is prohibited in licensed child-care centers, including private homes during hours of operation, and on playgrounds. In addition, the California Health and Safety Code has this provision related to clean air: "It is unlawful for a person to smoke a pipe, cigar, or cigarette in a motor vehicle, whether in motion or at rest, in which there is a person under 18 years of age in the vehicle. Violation is an infraction punishable by a fine not exceeding $100 for each violation. A law enforcement officer shall not stop a vehicle for the sole purpose of determining whether the driver is in violation."[60]

Today, cities and counties sometimes go beyond state laws to add stricter bans. These bans extend from inside to outside of buildings. For example, some communities ban smoking in bus shelters, on school property, downtown sidewalks, city parks, hospital grounds, and sidewalks outside public buildings. Other bans include private residences such as apartment buildings or college dorms. One plan to reduce tobacco use calls for all accredited correctional facilities such as prisons and jails and all health-care facilities including nursing homes and psychiatric hospitals to ban smoking. It further calls on states to limit smoking in cars and homes with children.

Several European countries have nationwide smoking bans. In 2004, Ireland became the first country in the world to implement a comprehensive smoking ban in indoor workplaces, including restaurants and bars. New Zealand in 2004 and the United Kingdom in 2007 followed with bans. That these countries have a long tradition of smoking in pubs makes the change one of cultural as well as public health importance. Sweden, Norway, France, and Italy also have bans but allow designated smoking rooms. Few nations in the developing world have comprehensive bans but many have partial ones. Public health officials expect that they will soon move toward the models of high-income nations.

Advocates of clean indoor air regulations suggest that protection from secondhand smoke will not only benefit the health of smokers and non-smokers but also discourage smokers from continuing the habit or consuming as many cigarettes as they would otherwise. The need to go to a separate room or outside to smoke limits, they argue, the number of cigarettes that can be consumed each day and may create enough trouble to encourage smokers to give up the habit altogether. Perhaps the inability to light up after a meal in restaurants further changes the motivation of smokers to continue the habit. A study of New York City before and after the ban on smoking in workplaces (including bars and restaurants) showed overall smoking dropped by 4.1 percentage points between 2002 and 2006 (a price increase also contributed to the decline). Regardless of their effects on the consumption of cigarettes by smokers, increasing restrictions on smoking in public indoor places will no doubt continue.

LITIGATION

Litigation involves the use of private law by victims of cigarette use or their surrogates to receive compensation for the injuries they suffered. Using the tort (a word derived from Middle English meaning "injury") system, plaintiffs bring action against tobacco companies to obtain damages for wrongful behavior. The suits are extraordinarily expensive, particularly since tobacco companies use whatever resources they think necessary to win the cases. The plaintiffs and their lawyers receive the monetary damages and gain the benefits of winning a suit, but they also bear the cost. From the point of view of policymakers, litigation is an inefficient form of regulation since court cases take a long time, are extremely costly, and usually give the awards from a victory to only a few beneficiaries. Rather than a direct form of action of the government on behalf of its citizens, litigation on behalf of individuals can only indirectly regulate tobacco.

Still, antitobacco advocates favor litigation in the absence of stronger legislation. Legal victories against tobacco companies can raise prices, which discourages smoking. A few years back, Philip Morris had to raise the prices of its cigarettes by about 10 percent to cover the costs of a legal settlement, and today about 50¢ of every pack of cigarettes go to paying legal settlements and legal fees. Legal victories can also discourage tobacco companies from making misleading claims about the safety of their products, selling products to uninformed consumers, and making unsafe products. After decades of denying the harm and addictiveness of tobacco, industry executives have admitted to these problems as part of legal settlements.

Legal victories can help educate the public about the ways tobacco companies aim to manipulate them with ads and promotions. The anger felt by victims about this treatment can motivate further action against tobacco companies. Legal victories can reduce the political and economic power of the tobacco companies. Although they enjoyed much political clout in the past, tobacco companies have lost much of their ability to influence legislators and government executives, in part because of the negative publicity that has emerged in litigation. And legal victories bring in new advocates on behalf of public health—trial lawyers. Although motivated in part by contingency fees, lawyers have brought new energy and strategies to the battle against the tobacco companies.

These public health benefits have come slowly. A review of the history of litigation distinguishes three waves of suits, with only the most recent having been successful. The first wave began in 1954 with early suits against the tobacco companies based on the emerging evidence of the harm of smoking. The suits claimed that tobacco companies were negligent in not warning smokers of the possible harm of the product, or that tobacco companies offered an implied warranty for the safety of the product. Few suits reached trial, as tobacco companies outspent their adversaries and delayed proceedings until the financial losses led the plaintiffs to withdraw. For those plaintiffs who did endure, courts did not favorably receive claims of either negligence or implied warranty. None of the suits resulted in victory against tobacco companies.

The second wave began in 1983 with two changes in strategy. Groups representing plaintiffs began to pool resources so that they could outlast the expensive delaying tactics of tobacco lawyers. Also, a new legal argument claimed that tobacco companies were strictly liable for a product that causes addiction and kills users. As with victims of a faulty automobile or electrical appliance, smokers claimed cigarette manufacturers were responsible for the harm of their product. The tobacco industry in turn responded that smokers were not harmed by cigarettes, and even if they were, they knew of the harm, at least since the warnings placed on cigarette packages in the mid-1960s, but freely chose to continue smoking. To counter claims of addiction, the lawyers could point to millions of smokers who had quit the habit. Lawyers for Rose Cipollone, a dying smoker, used the strategy of placing liability on the cigarette maker and won an award of $400,000 in 1988, but the arguments of the tobacco lawyers ultimately won in appeal and her survivors eventually dropped the suit. After the first two waves of litigation, no plaintiff or plaintiff's attorney had yet recovered any money from the tobacco companies.

The third and only successful wave began in 1992 soon after the final decision in the Cipollone case. The new approach relied more on class-action rather than individual suits in order to further pool resources. A class-action suit enables a group of persons suffering from a common injury to bring suit. The action on behalf of a large number of people increases the total amount that can be awarded. Although the injured parties must share the benefits of the class and individually receive much less than in a regular suit, a successful class-action suit would impose daunting costs on the tobacco companies. Moreover, the contingency fees for trial lawyers would reach levels high enough to motivate legal firms to invest in suits. Plaintiffs in many suits of this third wave of litigation enjoyed greater financial resources than in the past.

The legal strategy of this third wave also took a new form. Rather than merely claiming harm from cigarettes, plaintiffs accused the tobacco companies of intentional misrepresentation, concealment, and failure to disclose information about the addictiveness and harm of smoking. Supporting these accusations required evidence that tobacco companies indeed knew of the harm of their products, and this evidence came from the unlikely and unexpected public release of internal industry documents. Merrill Williams, an employee of a Louisville law firm with access to the files of Brown & Williamson Tobacco, gave copies of incriminating documents to lawyers suing tobacco companies. In addition, a professor at the University of California and zealous antitobacco advocate, Stanton Glantz, received copies of documents, as did sympathetic congressional representatives. After they appeared on the Internet, a judge ruled that the documents were in the public domain and could be used by plaintiffs in cases against Brown & Williamson and other tobacco companies. Another key to success in the third wave of suits came from Jeffrey S. Wigand, a former top research executive at Brown & Williamson. He asserted in testimony and in public that the company knew of the harm and addictiveness of cigarettes. Many other examples of likely tobacco industry misrepresentation, concealment, and failure to disclose followed. With this evidence the new legal strategy of accusing the companies of fraud had much potential for success.

Most important in terms of government regulation, the attorneys general of all states brought claims against tobacco companies to recover their Medicaid costs for tobacco-related illnesses. These efforts began with a suit brought by the state of Mississippi under Attorney General Mike Moore and represented by successful trial lawyers Richard Scruggs and Ron Motley. Mississippi and three other states negotiated their own settlements with the tobacco industry, while 46 other states and the District of Columbia negotiated a 1998 Master Settlement Agreement. The settlement involved payment of $246 billion by tobacco companies over 25 years. It also included several public health provisions, such as restricting youth access to tobacco products, ending brand name sponsorships and promotion activities, limiting outdoor advertising, and contributing to cessation and prevention programs. The agreement created an important precedent in another way: It was the first time the tobacco industry had agreed to settle a suit.

The settlement has brought dispute over how states should spend the funds, with antismoking advocates accusing government officials of using the money for purposes other than tobacco prevention. According to a report from the Government Accountability Office,[61] about 30 percent of the $52.6 billion of the awards to states went to health care, about 23 percent to cover budget shortfalls, and about 7 percent to general fund expenses. Only about 3.5 percent went to tobacco control. In turn, the tobacco companies have contested the amounts they owe. They claim that their loss of market share to smaller companies not participating in the Master Settlement Agreement reduces the amount they owe to the states. Philip Morris USA has been paying the full amount but putting a portion into a special account and calling for arbitration.

Signing the Master Settlement Agreement has not protected tobacco companies from continued lawsuits. The R. J. Reynolds web page lists dozens of suits against the company between 1999 and 2008. The company claims a strong track record in trial outcomes and promises to continue defending itself in court. According to one study, plaintiffs won about 41 percent of the 75 cases that were tried to verdict during the years from 1995 to 2005. Although tobacco companies won many cases, they paid out millions in others.

In 1999, the Clinton administration sued major tobacco companies under the Racketeer Influenced and Corrupt Organizations Act (RICO). The government argued that tobacco companies engaged in a 50-year scheme to defraud the public. After the 2004 trial held in the U.S. Court for the District of Columbia, the judge found that the tobacco companies were liable under RICO and ordered bans on the use of terms such as *light* and on any actions that minimized the addictiveness and harm of smoking.

The litigation strategy has critics, however. Believing that such efforts unfairly penalize legal businesses, remove responsibility from individuals for their actions, limit the freedom of individuals to make their own choices, and enrich trial lawyers, some oppose the tendency toward making huge and numerous awards against tobacco companies. Economists in particular view the awards as a form of tax on cigarettes and argue that such taxes should come from the legislature rather than the judiciary.[62] Yet the litigation strategy seems to be spreading. The European Commission joined in suing U.S. tobacco companies for smuggling cigarettes into Europe without paying import duties and taxes. The World Health Organization similarly recommends that other nations use the U.S.-style litigation strategy to control tobacco.

GLOBAL TOBACCO CONTROL

In response to the worldwide growth of tobacco, regulation efforts have taken a global turn. Many antitobacco organizations have become international in their goals and membership. Businessman and current New York City mayor Michael Bloomberg reinforced this trend by contributing $125 million in 2006 for fighting tobacco use in developing countries. Recipients of the funds include the Campaign for Tobacco-Free Kids, Centers for Disease Control and Prevention Foundation, the Johns Hopkins Bloomberg School of Public Health, the World Health Organization (WHO), and the World Lung Foundation. Other organizations such as the Global Partnership for Tobacco Control and the International Union against Cancer have primary goals of stopping smoking in the developing world.

The WHO has taken the lead in global tobacco control. Its Tobacco Free Initiative has advisers in regions across the world working with national antitobacco officials to reduce tobacco use. Most importantly, it led the effort to create a world antitobacco treaty called the Framework Convention on Tobacco Control. By October 2008, 168 nations had signed the treaty. It calls for nations to increase taxes and prices for cigarettes, ban smoking in public buildings and workplaces, restrict the additives manufacturers can include, support cessation programs, limit advertising and packaging, and support public education. The treaty also calls for nations to decrease the supply of tobacco by stopping illicit trade, smuggling, and sales to minors. Four years in the making, the treaty needed negotiation and persuasion to get widespread support but now faces challenges in persuading national legislatures to ratify a treaty that may be perceived as ceding control to international organizations.

Besides the treaty, other worldwide efforts for tobacco control have moved forward. To help countries fulfill the promise of the Framework Convention on Tobacco Control, the WHO recommends a set of six effective tobacco-control policies. The acronym MPOWER summarizes the six policies:

1. Monitor tobacco use and prevention policies. Good data on the use of tobacco helps nations see the extent of the problem and the benefits of prevention policies. All too little information is available now from many developing nations.

2. Protect people from tobacco smoke. Smoke-free laws are easy and inexpensive to implement and, even if smoking rates are high, can protect nonsmokers from the harm of secondhand smoke. Only 5 percent of the world's population now enjoys the protection of comprehensive smoke-free legislation.

3. Offer help to quit tobacco use. Since smokers are addicted to nicotine, they need help in stopping. Treatments involving medical advice, medications, nicotine replacement products, and support groups for quitting can help. Governments need to subsidize the costs of these treatments.

4. Warn about the dangers of tobacco. Comprehensive warnings about the dangers of tobacco can help motivate smokers to quit and prevent young people from starting. Since residents of poorer nations often have limited knowledge of the risks of smoking, packages need to carry bold and highly visible warnings.

5. Enforce bans on tobacco advertising, promotion, and sponsorship. Countering the billions spent by tobacco companies on marketing and advertising requires total rather than partial bans. For example, the bans should stop the free distribution of tobacco products, a strategy companies use to get youth to start smoking.

6. Raise taxes on tobacco. According to the WHO, a 70 percent increase in the price of cigarettes through tax increases—for example, from $2.00 a pack to $3.40 a pack—would reduce worldwide smoking-related deaths by a quarter. The taxes most discourage smoking among groups most prone to start—low-education and low-income groups, who can least afford the tax increases. The taxes raised can then help fund tobacco-control policies, cessation treatments, and health care.

The WHO also suggests that these policy changes give special attention to women, a group likely to increase smoking at a faster rate than men. For example, women are more likely than men to smoke cigarettes labeled as "light," "mild," or "low tar." Prohibiting use of such terms may help prevent women from starting to smoke. Policy changes to make cessation programs part of family health care may also help women smokers.

SMOKERS' RIGHTS

The vigorous efforts of federal, state, and local governments, the medical profession, nonprofit agencies, and trial lawyers to eliminate or control tobacco have spawned a countermovement devoted to smokers' rights. Critics of antitobacco polices argue that the goal of community health has come to conflict with and override individual liberty and freedom of choice. They argue that adults have the right to choose smoking pleasure over longevity of life, and efforts to prevent this choice can result in government tyranny.[63] Numerous smokers' rights organizations have developed over the years (often with support of the tobacco industry).

These groups have responded to policies that implement high cigarette taxes, restrict advertising, ban smoking in public places, and encourage litigation. First and foremost, smokers' rights advocates oppose special cigarette taxes. Excessively high taxes on cigarettes, they say, unfairly punish smokers and businesses that sell cigarettes. According to some, smokers do not impose special costs on society that would warrant having to pay special taxes. Because smokers tend to die younger than nonsmokers, the short-term cost of treating tobacco-related illness is more than outweighed by other savings. In the long run, nonsmokers cost the government more than smokers in expenses for social security, nursing home care, and health care in old age.

Rather than use the cigarette tobacco revenues for tobacco-related costs, governments typically use them for general expenditures. Yet critics note that these revenues often end up lower than expected, which in turn requires more increases in taxes. The low revenues stem in part from the efforts of smokers to search out cheaper prices in places where taxes are lower. For example, Native Americans can sell tax-free cigarettes at lower prices on their lands, and they advertise their prices on the Internet. Internet purchases and large-scale commercial smuggling across state borders also become common. Critics believe that these problems could be avoided with fairer tax policies.

Second, smokers' rights advocates oppose government programs to restrict the flow of information about tobacco and the choice of individuals to smoke. Limitations in certain forms of advertising represent, according to antitobacco critics, a form of censorship and a threat to freedom. They view smoking as a legal behavior and adults as free to make their choice without government restrictions on the information they can obtain. Government control of information thus represents a step toward prohibition. If government controls access to information about smoking, it may lead to a ban on smoking altogether. They believe that a ban on smoking can then lead to other threats to liberty—bans on the type of food people can eat, the movies they can watch, the alcohol they can drink, the games they can play, and the ideas they can have—and that government should have no such role in controlling the personal choices of individuals.

Smokers' rights advocates reject the claim that they are manipulated by and need protection from tobacco advertising. They believe that people rather than the tobacco companies are responsible for their choices. Indeed, it is difficult to prove scientifically that advertising causes people to smoke. The free market of ideas includes the opportunity to hear about products, even if most people oppose the use of the product.

Third, smokers' rights advocates oppose banning smoking in bars and restaurants. Although smokers recognize their responsibility to consider the wishes of nonsmokers to be free of smoky air, many view efforts to ban smoking totally in private buildings, restaurants, and bars as mistaken. Critics attack the public health literature by suggesting that the evidence of the harm of secondhand smoke is suspect. They say that the amounts of secondhand smoke faced by nonsmokers in daily life are so small as to be difficult to measure and unlikely to harm health. They believe that second-hand smoke does not present sufficient risk to warrant banning smoking in public places.

Even if the evidence were stronger, such bans create problems. They harm small businesses by keeping smokers away and creating problems of enforcement. In New York City, for example, a confrontation about smoking in a club soon after a ban had been imposed in 2003 resulted in the death of an employee. The bans also reveal a lack of understanding about economic choice and property rights. Free-market supporters suggest that business owners have the right to ban or not to ban smoking in their establishments, and patrons have the right to choose to go to smoking or nonsmoking establishments. Offering choices to both owners and patrons would create a more satisfying solution than a government-imposed ban. It would provide for those wanting smoke-free places to eat and drink and for those wanting to enjoy cigarettes with their food and beverages. (However, another issue is an employees' right to a smoke-free workplace.)

Finally, smokers' rights advocates oppose litigation against tobacco companies. They believe that such efforts distort economic incentives and hurt rather than help smokers. Perhaps more important, they reflect an unwillingness to hold individual smokers responsible for their own actions. Many people believe that smoking is a choice, just as not smoking and quitting are choices (indeed, more than 40 million Americans have quit smoking). Given the widespread knowledge of the harm of smoking, smokers should assume the risks associated with the habit. The increased litigiousness of society has, according to critics, worked to deny this individual responsibility. Even if smokers deserved some compensation for smoking, litigation has failed to provide it. Most of the funds go to the states or trial lawyers rather than to the victims of smoking (who do not survive long enough to see an award). In the end, huge awards against tobacco companies do more to punish smokers by raising cigarette prices than help smokers.

Beyond their opposition to specific policies, smokers' rights advocates worry about the increasingly negative view of smoking. Such attitudes can lead to discrimination against smokers in finding jobs, getting insurance, obtaining service in businesses, and participating in everyday activities. Rightly or wrongly smokers often feel as if they are part of a persecuted minority, and many have taken steps to organize themselves in opposition to what they view as a puritanical antismoking crusade.

---

[1] Iain Gately. *Tobacco: The Story of How Tobacco Seduced the World.* New York: Grove Press, 2001, p. 3.

[2] *Ibid.*, p. 23.

[3] Arlene B. Hirschfelder. *Encyclopedia of Smoking and Tobacco.* Phoenix, Ariz.: Oryx Press, 1999, pp. 109, 151, 225–226.

[4] Quoted in Robert Sobel. *They Satisfy: The Cigarette in American Life.* Garden City, N.Y.: Anchor Press, 1978, p. 51.

[5] Jack Gottsegen. *Tobacco: A Study of Its Consumption in the United States.* New York: Pittman, 1940, pp. 57, 65.

[6] Sobel. *They Satisfy*, p. 20.

[7] Quoted in Gately. *Tobacco*, p. 234.

[8] Joseph R. Gusfield. *Symbolic Crusade: Status Politics and the American Temperance Movement.* 2d ed. Urbana: University of Illinois Press, 1986, pp. 7–8.

[9] Gottsegen. *Tobacco*, p. 144.

[10] Quoted in Gately. *Tobacco*, p. 234.

[11] John C. Burnham. *Bad Habits: Drinking, Smoking, Taking Drugs, Gambling, Sexual Misbehavior, and Swearing in American History.* New York: New York University Press, 1993, illustration I.22.

[12] Jordan Goodman. *Tobacco in History: The Cultures of Dependence.* London: Routledge, 1993, p. 106.

[13] Gottsegen. *Tobacco*, pp. 149–150.

[14] Richard Tennant. *The American Cigarette Industry.* New Haven, Conn.: Yale University, 1950, pp. 136–142.

[15] Luther L. Terry. "The Surgeon General's First Report on Smoking and Health." In Alan Blum, ed., *The Cigarette Underworld: A Front Line Report on the War Against Your Lungs.* Secaucus, N.J.: Lyle Stuart, 1985, p. 15.

[16] U.S. Department of Health and Human Services. *The Health Consequences of Smoking: Cancer. A Report of the Surgeon General.* Washington, D.C.: U.S. Department of Health and Human Services, 1982, p. xi.

[17] Alan Kluger. *Ashes to Ashes: America's Hundred-Year Cigarette War, the Public Health, and the Unabashed Triumph of Philip Morris.* New York: Alfred A. Knopf, 1996, p. 239.

[18] Gately. *Tobacco*, p. 317.

[19] David Krogh. *Smoking: The Artificial Passion.* New York: W. H. Freeman, 1991, p. 59.

[20] U.S. Department of Health and Human Services. *The Health Consequences of Smoking: Nicotine Addiction. A Report of the Surgeon General.* Washington, D.C.: U.S. Department of Health and Human Services, 1988, p. v.

[21] Paul Slovic. "Cigarette Smokers: Rational Actors or Rational Fools?" In Paul Slovic, ed., *Smoking: Risk, Perception, and Policy.* Thousand Oaks, Calif.: Sage Publications, 2001, pp. 97–124.

[22] Kluger. *Ashes to Ashes*, p. 702.

23 U.S. Department of Health and Human Services. *Preventing Tobacco Use among Young People. A Report of the Surgeon General.* Washington, D.C.: U.S. Department of Health and Human Services, 1994.

24 Morton Hunt. *The Story of Psychology.* New York: Anchor Press, 1993, p. 347.

25 Elizabeth Whelan. *A Smoking Gun: How the Tobacco Industry Gets Away with Murder.* Philadelphia: George F. Stickley, 1984, pp. 105–106.

26 Whelan. *A Smoking Gun*, p. 110.

27 Allan M. Brandt. *The Cigarette Century: The Rise, Fall, and Deadly Persistence of the Product That Defined America.* New York: Basic Books, 2007.

28 Sobel. *They Satisfy*, p. 184.

29 U.S. Department of Health and Human Services. *Reducing the Health Consequences of Smoking: 25 Years of Progress. A Report of the Surgeon General.* Washington, D.C.: U.S. Department of Health and Human Services, 1989, p. 11.

30 U.S. Department of Health and Human Services. *Healthy People 2010.* Washington, D.C.: U.S. Department of Health and Human Services, 2000, p. 27-12.

31 "Cigarette Smoking among Adults—United States, 2006." *MMWR Weekly*, vol. 56 (November 9, 2006): 1,157–1,161.

32 "Monitoring the Future." In U.S. Department of Health and Human Services, *Women and Smoking. A Report of the Surgeon General.* Washington, D.C.: U.S. Department of Health and Human Services, 2001, pp. 59–63.

33 U.S. Department of Health and Human Services. *Women and Smoking*, pp. 453–527.

34 Quoted in Jacob Sullum. *For Your Own Good: The Anti-Smoking Crusade and the Tyranny of Public Health.* New York: Free Press, 1998, p. 6.

35 W. Kip Viscusi. *Smoking: Making the Risky Decision.* New York: Oxford University Press, 1992, pp. 7–8.

36 Kluger. *Ashes to Ashes*, p. 678.

37 U.S. Department of Health and Human Services. *Women and Smoking*, pp. 68–69.

38 Paul Rozin. "The Process of Moralization." *Psychological Science* 10 (May 1999): 218–221.

39 Sullum. *For Your Own Good*, p. 13.

40 Richard Klein. *Cigarettes Are Sublime.* Durham, N.C.: Duke University Press, 1993, p. 3.

41 U.S. Department of Health and Human Services. *Regulating Tobacco Use: A Report of the Surgeon General.* Washington, D.C.: U.S. Department of Health and Human Services, 2000, p. 49.

42 National Cancer Institute. *Risks Associated with Smoking Cigarettes with Low Machine-Measured Yields of Tar and Nicotine. Smoking and Tobacco Control Monograph 13.* Washington, D.C.: U.S. Department of Health and Human Services, 2001, pp. 1–10, 193–198.

43 National Cancer Institute. *Risks Associated with Smoking Cigarettes with Low Machine Measured Yields of Tar and Nicotine*, p. 2.

44 National Cancer Institute. *Risks Associated with Smoking Cigarettes with Low Machine-Measured Yields of Tar and Nicotine*, pp. 1–10.

45 U.S. Department of Health and Human Services. *Tobacco Use among U.S. Racial/Ethnic Minority Groups: African Americans, American Indians and Alaskan Natives,*

Asian Americans and Pacific Islanders, and Hispanics. A Report of the Surgeon General. Washington, D.C.: U.S. Department of Health and Human Services, 1998, pp. 213–224.

[46] Tara Parker-Pope. *Cigarettes: Anatomy of an Industry from Seed to Smoke.* New York: New Press, 2001, p. 27.

[47] "Tobacco Facts." Framework Convention Alliance for Tobacco Control. Available online. URL: http://www.fctc.org/docs/factsheets/fca_factsheet_001_en.pdf. Downloaded in June 2008.

[48] The World Health Organization. *Tobacco or Health: A Global Status Report.* Geneva: World Health Organization, 1992.

[49] "Gender and Tobacco Control: A Policy Brief." World Health Organization. Available Online. URL: http://www.who.int/tobacco/resources/publications/general/policy_brief.pdf. Downloaded in June 2008.

[50] U.S. Department of Health and Human Services. *Reducing the Health Consequences of Smoking: 25 Years of Progress,* pp. 140–141.

[51] Claire Chollat-Traquet. *Women and Tobacco.* Geneva: World Health Organization, 1992.

[52] U.S. Department of Health and Human Services. *Women and Smoking,* 2001.

[53] Hirschfelder. *Encyclopedia of Smoking and Tobacco,* p. 199.

[54] U.S. Department of Health and Human Services. *The Health Consequences of Involuntary Exposure to Tobacco Smoke: A Report of the Surgeon General.* Atlanta: Centers for Disease Control and Prevention, 2006.

[55] U.S. Department of Health and Human Services. *Preventing Tobacco Use among Young People,* p. 135.

[56] E. A. Gilpin, L. Lee, N. Evans, and J. P. Pierce. "Smoking Initiation Rates in Adults and Minors: United States, 1944–1988." *American Journal of Epidemiology* 140 (September 15, 1994): 535–543.

[57] World Bank. *Curbing the Epidemic,* p. 45.

[58] Richard J. Bonnie, Kathleen Stratton, and Robert B. Wallace, eds. *Ending the Tobacco Problem: A Blueprint for the Nation.* Washington D.C.: National Academies Press, 2007.

[59] U.S. Department of Health and Human Services. *Regulating Tobacco Use,* pp. 100–128.

[60] "State Legislated Action on Tobacco Issues: 2007." American Lung Association. Available online. URL: http://www.rwjf.org/files/research/20080422slati.pdf. Downloaded in June 2008.

[61] "States' Allocations of Payments from Tobacco Companies for Fiscal Years 2000 through 2005." Government Accountability Office. Available online. URL: http://www.gao.gov/new.items/d07534t.pdf. Posted on February 27, 2007.

[62] W. Kip Viscusi. *Smoke-Filled Rooms: A Postmortem on the Tobacco Deal.* Chicago: University of Chicago Press, 2002, p. 8.

[63] Sullum, *For Your Own Good,* p. 13.

CHAPTER 2

THE LAW AND THE TOBACCO INDUSTRY AND SMOKING

FEDERAL LAWS AND REGULATIONS

Given the importance throughout history of tobacco to the American economy, of cigarettes to individual consumers, and of smoking to the health and well-being of the U.S. population, it is surprising that only a few federal laws and regulations govern the product and activity. The limited legal intervention of the government stems in part from the view of Americans that the purchase of cigarettes and smoking is a personal choice and individual right. It also stems from the power of the tobacco industry to block the actions that the legislative and executive branches might take against the industry. The most important recent actions against the tobacco industry have come from the judiciary; however, this appears to be changing. The public has become more supportive of controls on tobacco advertising to youth and on indoor smoking in public places, and the government has become increasingly active in implementing these controls. This section of the chapter describes the federal laws and regulations that have most affected the tobacco industry and smoking.

FEDERAL CIGARETTE LABELING AND ADVERTISING ACT (1965)

As the first modern federal legislation to address the perils of smoking, the 1965 Federal Cigarette Labeling and Advertising Act signaled an important beginning to the government's battle against the tobacco industry and smoking. Although the law placed only modest requirements on cigarette makers and actually prevented more stringent regulations from going into effect, the entrance of Congress into the realm of tobacco control set a precedent that in years to come would lead to stronger legislation.

The Law and the Tobacco Industry and Smoking

After the release of the 1964 Surgeon General's report on health and smoking, the Federal Trade Commission (FTC), which had for some time struggled with the tobacco companies over misleading advertisements about the health benefits of cigarettes, proposed tough new rules. These rules would require warnings about the health risks of smoking on cigarette packages, print advertisements, and broadcast commercials as well as the listing of the tar and nicotine content of cigarettes. With a mandate to restrain unfair and misleading business practices, this agency of the executive branch of the government had the potential to seriously threaten the interests of the tobacco industry.

To forestall such action the tobacco industry proposed to regulate its own advertising. It developed a code to curb ads that appealed directly or indirectly to young people, made unverified claims of health benefits, and implied smoking was essential to sexual attractiveness, social success, virility, and sophistication. Bowman Gray, chairman of the board of R. J. Reynolds Tobacco Company, testified in Congress, "This advertising code represents a sincere effort by the industry to respond to criticisms of the industry's advertising."[1] However, the FTC had little confidence that self-regulation would work.

Believing that it had more clout with Congress than with President Lyndon Johnson and members of the FTC, representatives of the tobacco industry urged various legislators to pass legislation that would override the FTC regulations. The pieces of legislation debated by the House and Senate aimed to provide some sort of warning to consumers but varied in the form the warnings would take. Some legislators favored turning the FTC regulatory proposals into law, while others acting more in concert with the tobacco industry wanted something weaker. At the time antismoking groups had not yet emerged as a strong political force, and groups such as the American Cancer Society and the American Medical Association (AMA), which doubted if warnings would have much effect on smoking, did not lobby for the law. In the end the weaker version of the legislation passed.

The legislation required that cigarette packages include the following (somewhat mild) statement: "Caution: Cigarette Smoking May Be Hazardous to Your Health." The statement did not use more frightening words such as *death* and *lung cancer* and qualified its impact with the words *may be hazardous*. The packages would list the warnings on the side in small type rather than on the front in larger type. Unlike the original FTC proposals, the legislation did not include any provisions for warnings on advertisements or commercials and did not require statements of the tar and nicotine content of cigarettes. Two other provisions that seemed less important at the time were included instead. One provision denied all federal and state agencies the power over the next four years to require any additions or revisions to the warning. This provision aimed to produce uniform statements on cigarette packages but also to keep the FTC and other government agencies out of the issue and to assert Congress's power. Another provision required the FTC and the Department of Health, Education, and Welfare through the Office of the Surgeon General to report annually to Congress on cigarette advertising and on smoking and health.

Despite its opposition to the warning, the tobacco industry enjoyed, according to most observers, a victory with the legislation. It preempted more stringent regulations with modest requirements for a warning statement and allowed advertisements to continue as they had in the past. The legislation also allowed the industry to drop its efforts at self-regulation that, if followed, would have done much more to change the nature of cigarette advertising. Although less clearly realized at the time, the warnings on cigarette packages had the advantage of serving in the future to protect the industry from lawsuits. Smokers would not easily be able to claim in a suit that they had lacked knowledge of the health risks of smoking or that the tobacco companies had hidden the danger of their product. Warnings would play an important role in suits to follow.

However, the provision requiring annual reports to Congress by the FTC and the Surgeon General allowed antismoking forces in the government to continue their steady criticism of smoking and cigarette advertisements. Year after year, the Surgeon General published reports listing the harm of cigarette use. These reports would become increasingly critical over the years, eventually concluding that nicotine was an addictive drug and claiming that 400,000 persons a year died prematurely from smoking. The FTC also continued its condemnation of tobacco advertising as misleading and manipulative and recommended in the years to come that the government mandate more strongly worded warnings and exert greater control on advertisements.

FAIRNESS DOCTRINE APPLIED TO TOBACCO (1967)

Extending the fairness doctrine to issues of tobacco by the Federal Communications Commission (FCC) represented an important victory for antismoking forces. The decision gave them free television and radio air time to counter claims made on behalf of cigarettes in paid advertising. By most accounts the antismoking ads effectively persuaded many consumers not to smoke. The benefit of the antismoking ads did not last long, as banning all cigarette television and radio ads in 1971 ended free air time for anticigarette ads. Still the use of the fairness doctrine to battle tobacco companies offered a new and valuable form of smoking regulation.

The fairness doctrine had since 1949 required television and radio stations that presented material on important and controversial issues to give air time to both sides of the issues. Since television and radio stations used the public airwaves (unlike magazines and newspapers), and broadcast frequencies in the years before cable were relatively scarce, the government had a responsibility to ensure that stations used their airwaves for the good of the public. One way to do so involved the fair treatment of opposing viewpoints. The doctrine initially applied largely to politicians and interest groups representing competing sides of political issues and prevented stations from bias in favor of one political party or set of interests.

Angered by a cigarette commercial he saw on television in 1966, John Banzhaf III, a young New York City lawyer, requested air time from WCBS-TV in New York City to rebut the cigarette ads the station carried. After being turned down by the station, he filed a complaint with the FCC, which enforced the doctrine. In 1967 the FCC ruled in Banzhaf's favor by requiring that stations provide a significant amount of air time for the other side of the controversial issue of the health hazards of smoking. The commission did not force stations to air an equal number of anti- and prosmoking commercials but threatened to revoke their licenses if they did not give significant time to the antitobacco side. After a court ruled in support of the commission's decision, Banzhaf and others proceeded to set up organizations that monitored the compliance of stations with the ruling.

The rule had a considerable impact. In practice about one antismoking commercial appeared for every three smoking commercials, which translated into donations by broadcasters of $75 million in air time.[2] In one effective commercial, William Talman, a well-known actor from the *Perry Mason* television show, appeared. He was sick and dying from lung cancer after decades of smoking three packs of cigarettes a day. Introducing his wife and children, he stated he was battling for his life and to enjoy more time with his family. He then urged others not to smoke. His death by the time many of the commercials aired lent power to the ads. Reviewing these antismoking ads, a leading tobacco control scholar claimed that they were more effective than any other technique of persuading people to stop smoking.[3]

PUBLIC HEALTH CIGARETTE SMOKING ACT (1969)

Moving beyond warnings on packages, this act banned cigarette advertising from television and radio (all media subject to the authority of the FTC) beginning on January 2, 1971. It also strengthened the wording of the warnings on cigarette packages and led to the inclusion of warning statements on print advertisements. Although not part of the legislation, a later consent decree from the FTC required warnings on advertisements in newspapers, magazines, and outdoor displays.

The 1965 Federal Cigarette Labeling and Advertising Act included no provisions on tobacco advertising, but the FTC continued its criticism of the tobacco industry for misleading practices in promoting its product. In 1967 the FTC noted that despite warnings on packages, cigarette sales had continued to rise, in large part because advertisements depicted images of healthy smokers. Particularly disconcerting, these images appealed to young people and thereby led teens to start smoking before they fully understood the risks. The FTC first called for stronger warnings on packages and new warnings on ads to counter the influence of the ads. In 1969, however, the FTC took another approach: Six of seven commissioners voted to prohibit cigarette advertising from television and radio. Such a ban had been implemented in England in 1965 and seemed an effective way to moderate the influence of the tobacco companies in promoting smoking.

Addressing the issue in 1969, the House of Representatives responded to concerns of both the tobacco industry and the National Association of Broadcasters (which received 10 percent of its advertising revenue from tobacco companies) with a bill. In exchange for acceptance of stronger warnings by the tobacco industry, the bill would prohibit state and federal agencies from taking any action on cigarette advertising. However, stronger opposition to the tobacco industry had emerged in the Senate, and it appeared that a bill to ban advertising would pass in that chamber. Recognizing defeat, the tobacco industry accepted the proposed ban, and the act passed in 1969.

The act specified that cigarette advertising on television and radio would cease on January 2, 1971. The date chosen allowed cigarette companies to flood the airwaves with commercials during the New Year's Day football games. The act also strengthened the warning on cigarette packages to state:

WARNING: The Surgeon General has Determined that Cigarette Smoking is Dangerous to Your Health.

The warning replaced *may be* with *is* and cited the Surgeon General's office as the source of the claim. As in earlier legislation the 1969 act also preempted other government agencies from requiring changes in the warning. A group of broadcasters rather than the cigarette companies challenged the restrictions on their right to free speech with the television and radio ban on tobacco ads, but in *Capital Broadcasting v. Mitchell*, the D.C. district court affirmed the constitutionality of the prohibition.

The law effectively and quickly eliminated ads from television and radio but did little to slow the advertising efforts of tobacco companies. The companies saved more than $200 million on electronic advertising and could use these savings for promotions and space in magazines, in newspapers, and on outdoor billboards. Before the ban tobacco companies spent $205 million on television advertising, $12.5 million on radio advertising, $14 million on newspaper advertising, and $50 million on magazine advertising. By 1979 newspaper advertising had soared to $241 million and magazine advertising to $257 million.[4] Tobacco companies spent other funds on promotional items such as coupons, lighters, key chains, and clothing with brand names, and on sponsorship of sporting and entertainment events. The continued growth in advertising led the American Cancer Society, the American Medical Association, the American Public Health Association, and the American Heart Association to advocate (unsuccessfully) a ban on all advertising.

Not only did the ban not appear to harm tobacco companies with the shift of advertising to different media, but it may have actually helped them in another way. The ban also eliminated free airtime given to antismoking groups. The cigarette counteradvertising appeared effective, and tobacco industry executives admitted that they accepted the ban in part to end free antismoking commercials. The fairness doctrine did not apply to magazines and newspapers, and antismoking groups did not have the resources to pay for ads to balance those of the tobacco industry. The act ended the application of the fairness doctrine to tobacco and ultimately appeared to benefit more than it harmed the tobacco industry.

COMPREHENSIVE SMOKING EDUCATION ACT (1984)

The 1984 Comprehensive Smoking Education Act strengthened the wording of the warnings placed on cigarette packages and required that the warnings also be displayed prominently on advertisements. Its importance comes not only from further efforts to limit the ability of tobacco companies to attract new smokers but also from the emerging signs that the tobacco industry had lost much of its traditional influence on the political process in Washington, D.C. The 1980s saw the emergence of new leaders in Congress who had the skill and political power to guide antitobacco legislation through both the Senate and House of Representatives.

As in earlier legislation, the impetus for this act came from the FTC. In monitoring advertisements in magazines, newspapers, posters, and billboards, the FTC once again accused the tobacco industry of misleading business practices. Ads tended to appeal to young people by depicting smokers as youthful, healthy, active, and confident (even though the known harm of cigarettes contradicted these images). A 1981 report concluded that the existing warnings did little to counter these positive images, and regulations needed to limit more forcefully the appeal of cigarettes.[5]

Taking up the recommendations of the FTC, Representative Henry Waxman of California, a Democrat, held hearings on the business practices of the tobacco industry and developed a bill in the House of Representatives that would more stringently control tobacco advertising. In the Senate, Al Gore, a new Democratic senator from Tennessee, managed to negotiate a milder form of the bill by finding a way to compromise between antismoking and tobacco interests. In the end a bill emerged that was weaker than the one envisioned by Henry Waxman but still represented a victory for antismoking forces.

The public most noticed the provision of the bill that required the rotating of four new warning statements on both packages and on advertisements. The four warning statements used more direct, specific, and unqualified wording than the early ones:

SURGEON GENERAL'S WARNING: Smoking Causes Lung Cancer, Heart Disease, Emphysema, and May Complicate Pregnancy.

SURGEON GENERAL'S WARNING: Quitting Smoking Now Greatly Reduces Serious Risks to Your Health.

SURGEON GENERAL'S WARNING: Smoking by Pregnant Women May Result in Fetal Injury, Premature Birth, and Low Birth Weight.

SURGEON GENERAL'S WARNING: Cigarette Smoke Contains Carbon Monoxide.

The warnings stated that smoking causes specific diseases (rather than stating smoking is hazardous or dangerous). These warnings would appear not just on cigarette packages but also on ads. Countering pictures of smokers having fun, the noticeable insert in the ad would remind readers of the result of smoking.

Other provisions would prove significant in years to come. The act required tobacco companies to provide the government with lists of the additives put in cigarettes during the manufacturing process; government officials would analyze the information on additives but keep it confidential. In 1994, however, the government reversed course and released the lists. The publicity about the additives, many of which are harmful, embarrassed the tobacco industry. In addition the warnings chosen for the packages and advertisements preempted efforts of state and most federal agencies to develop other warnings but did not prevent the FTC from continuing its own efforts to control tobacco advertising.

In some ways the act did not go as far as antismoking advocates would have liked. The warnings did not mention death and addiction and did not include information on the amounts of tar, nicotine, and carbon monoxide inhaled with a cigarette. Still the act represented a substantial change in the willingness of the government to control the tobacco industry.

COMPREHENSIVE SMOKELESS TOBACCO HEALTH EDUCATION ACT (1986)

Although it was slow in coming, strong evidence had accumulated by the mid-1980s that smokeless tobacco caused oral cancer and nicotine addiction. The evidence worried public health officials because smokeless tobacco use had been rising among adolescents, in part because they thought it would not cause cancer and was not addictive. The law banned advertising of smokeless tobacco on electronic media and required three rotated warnings on smokeless tobacco packaging and all advertising except billboards:

WARNING: This product may cause serious mouth cancer.

WARNING: This product may cause gum disease and tooth loss.

WARNING: This product is not a safe alternative to cigarettes.

The FTC implemented the act, later coming to decide that T-shirts, jackets, hats, and lighters represented a form of advertising and should not include brand names or logos.

MASTER SETTLEMENT AGREEMENT (1998)

This agreement between 46 state attorneys general, as well as the District of Columbia, and major U.S. tobacco companies settled pending lawsuits by the states for recovery of Medicaid costs they incurred in treating smoking-related illnesses. Its importance shows in the huge size of the award—$246 billion over 25 years—and in the willingness of the tobacco industry to settle rather than fight the suits. In addition four other states settled suits separately.

The initial events leading to the Master Settlement Agreement (MSA) began with a suit filed by the state of Mississippi against tobacco manufacturers, wholesalers, and trade groups. The Mississippi attorney general, Mike Moore, working with successful trial lawyers Richard Scruggs and Ron Motley, led the effort. In a major shift in strategy the suit did not request damages on behalf of injured smokers. After all, courts and juries had not in the past been willing to absolve smokers of their responsibility for choosing to smoke despite knowing the harm of the product. Rather the state, which itself had never assumed the risks of smoking that individuals did, wanted to recover the costs taxpayers had to pay for tobacco-related illnesses. Officials noticed that of the Mississippians whose medical costs the state covered with Medicaid, half were smokers. In this way the state rather than the smokers themselves had been injured by the tobacco companies. In addition to these costs, the state requested costs for reimbursement of legal expenses. In the meantime a group of private plaintiff law firms rather than the state itself fronted the expenses of bringing the suit. The states of Minnesota, Florida, and West Virginia filed their own suits soon after. The new legal approach appeared promising enough that attorneys general from nearly all the other states and the District of Columbia would seek recovery of their own costs for tobacco-related illnesses.

The states made the case that the companies had violated antitrust and consumer fraud laws by withholding information about the harm of smoking, had manipulated nicotine levels to maximize addiction, and conspired to withhold lower risk products from the market. Given these fraudulent actions, the companies were, according to the suits, responsible for the costs to taxpayers of public Medicaid costs for smoking-related illnesses.

Bennett LeBow, the CEO of the Brooke Group, which owned the smallest of the big tobacco companies, Liggett Tobacco, broke ranks first by negotiating with the states. Although the other manufacturers vowed not to give in to the state demands for payment, LeBow believed that fighting would harm the nontobacco parts of his company and saw little chance of winning. Tobacco industry documents on the Internet provided examples of deception and manipulation and also made settlement seem sensible. In 1996 the company agreed to pay up to $50 million, publicize the ingredients of its cigarettes, and strengthen its warning labels. The settlement, although small, shifted the balance of power against the tobacco companies.

The other tobacco companies, Philip Morris, R. J. Reynolds, Brown & Williamson (part of the British-American Tobacco Company), and Lorillard, soon followed in reaching agreements. On July 2, 1998, they settled with Mississippi by agreeing to pay $3.4 billion over 25 years. Separate agreements were also reached with Minnesota, Florida, and West Virginia. More important, the companies proposed a settlement with other states that would end all pending lawsuits brought by government agencies and all other pending class-action lawsuits. Given the goal of ending certain types of lawsuits, the agreement needed the force of national law to make it work; however, Congress could not agree on the terms for such legislation, and the proposed agreement failed.

From this failure both sides accepted the Master Settlement Agreement on November 23, 1998. Dealing directly with the state attorneys general (except for the four states that negotiated agreements separately), 11 tobacco companies made concessions to the states in return for dropping the suits for Medicaid reimbursement. The major concession of the tobacco companies was to pay $246 billion to the states over 25 years; however, the agreement included many other provisions.

- **Youth access:** Tobacco companies would provide no free samples where underage persons are present, would provide no gifts to youth in return for purchases, would provide no gifts through the mail without proof of age, and would offer no cigarettes in packages of fewer than 20.

- **Marketing:** Tobacco company brand names would not sponsor sporting events, concerts, and events with a significant youth audience, paid underage spectators, or underage participants; in addition tobacco companies would ban the display of tobacco names in stadiums and arenas, the use of cartoon characters in ads, payments to promote tobacco products in movies, and distribution of merchandise with tobacco logos.

- **Lobbying:** Tobacco companies would not advocate for diversion of settlement funds for nonhealth uses, lobby against restrictions of advertising on school grounds, or challenge state and local tobacco control laws enacted before June 1, 1998.

- **Outdoor advertising:** Tobacco companies would ban outdoor advertising such as billboards and transit ads and would pay for ads discouraging youth smoking.

- **Cessation and prevention:** Tobacco companies would contribute $25 million annually for 10 years to charitable programs devoted to preventing teen smoking and the diseases associated with teen smoking, and would contribute $1.45 billion over five years to support a national sustained advertising and education program to counter youth tobacco use.

The payment of the funds to the states has created debate about their use. In some cases the funds have gone for government programs unrelated to tobacco control. Ideally states would use them to prevent youth smoking. Given the potential for statewide prevention and education programs to work better in halting cigarette use than local or school-based programs, the settlement funds used for statewide programs would do much to discourage cigarette use. Settlement funds could also pay for the kind of antismoking ads that had so much success in the past. Debate over the use of the funds continues to the present.

Critics of the settlement point to the fact that it represents a financial windfall for the states but otherwise does little to improve the health of citizens. The funds gained from the tobacco companies go not to the victims of smoking-related diseases but to lawyer's fees and the state budgets controlled by politicians. In one sense, the ultimate costs of the settlement fall on smokers. Because the settlement raises the costs of cigarettes, it in essence imposes additional taxes on those who smoke. Some recommend that states replace these hidden taxes imposed by judicial agreements with unconcealed taxes passed by democratic legislation.[6]

From the point of view of the tobacco industry the settlement has done little to ease its litigation problems. Without national legislation from Congress to prevent future suits, the agreement with the states does not prevent others from filing similar suits. Health care organizations such as Blue Cross/Blue Shield, the federal government, state agencies, and individuals continue to file suits based on the same legal principles as those that led to the Master Settlement Agreement.

FAMILY SMOKING PREVENTION AND TOBACCO CONTROL ACT (2008)

Since the 2000 Supreme Court decision in *Brown & Williamson Tobacco Corporation v. U.S. Food and Drug Administration* to overturn efforts of the FDA to regulate tobacco, Congress has considered and rejected several pieces of legislation to explicitly give the FDA regulatory power over tobacco. Legislation introduced in 2007 by Henry Waxman (D–California) in the House and Edward Kennedy (D–Massachusetts) in the Senate may be more successful, however. Although not yet passed by either chamber, the legislation appears to have wide support.

In the House, the Energy and Commerce Committee approved the bill by a bipartisan vote of 38-12 and now has more than 200 cosponsors for consideration by the full chamber. In the Senate, the companion bill is under consideration by the Committee on Health, Education, Labor, and Pensions but has 56 cosponsors, including several Republicans. Experts believe that the legislation has its best chance yet of passing both the House and Senate. Perhaps surprisingly, the bill even has support from some tobacco companies. On its web page, Philip Morris said that the legislation would provide clear standards for cigarette makers and protection for consumers. Other tobacco companies objected to the broad authority the legislation would give to the FDA in regulating them, but objections seem less intense than in the past.

What changes would occur with the legislation? According to a summary from Senator Kennedy,[7] it would give the FDA authority to:

- Restrict advertising that targets children and makes misleading claims about cigarette safety;
- Enforce laws that prevent sale of cigarettes to minors;
- Require stronger warning labels on tobacco products;
- Take steps to prevent companies from adding hazardous ingredients to their tobacco products;
- Analyze and approve any new reduced-risk cigarettes developed by tobacco companies; and
- Help smokers overcome their addiction.

Should the legislation pass and be signed by the president, it will change tobacco regulation considerably.

However, one part of the legislation has created controversy and some opposition from prominent antitobacco advocates. The proposed legislation bans most fruit, candy, and spice flavorings because they are seen as attracting youth. However, it exempts menthol, an ingredient of many popular cigarette brands, in return for the support of the legislation by

Philip Morris. Yet, seven former health secretaries joined to oppose the exemption. Menthol cigarettes are popular in the African-American community and the exemption may most harm minorities.

STATE AND LOCAL LAWS AND REGULATIONS

In the absence of major federal legislation concerning tobacco since 1986, much of the initiative has moved to states and localities. States have always had laws restricting access to minors but in more recent years have strengthened these laws. In addition states have expanded their taxes on cigarettes to reduce the demand for the product and to bring in government revenues. Both states and localities have also addressed issues of clean indoor air with laws and regulations banning or limiting smoking inside buildings. Since the 50 states and the District of Columbia differ greatly in their smoking laws and regulations, this section reviews only the broad outlines of the differing approaches in three areas: access of minors, clear indoor air, and taxes.

Access of Minors

All states restrict the sale of tobacco to youth under age 18 (Alabama, Alaska, New Jersey, and Utah restrict sales to youth under 19) but vary in the procedures they use to enforce the rules. Regulations in most states require retailers to have a license to sell cigarettes over the counter and post a sign indicating the minimum age of purchase. A smaller number of states also regulate the minimum age for salespersons, and a few attempt to educate employees of the seriousness of the problem of youth cigarette sales. Without strong enforcement efforts and severe punishments, however, these regulations lack power. Historically little effort has gone into policing sales to youth, and significant numbers of minors could purchase cigarettes with little trouble. More recent attempts to strengthen enforcement make youth cigarette purchases more difficult, but studies found 22 to 33 percent of sales went to minors.[8]

With the commercial availability of cigarettes from retailers declining, youth can attempt to obtain the product from older friends or by other means. This shifts laws and regulations away from sellers to the youth who purchase, possess, or use cigarettes. Although all states prohibit sales by retailers, fewer states have laws and regulations concerning the buyers. Public health advocates tend to blame retailers for sales to minors more than the minors themselves, who by reacting to advertising seem more like victims than criminals.

The federal government has become involved in these efforts. The U. S. Congress in 1992 passed an amendment sponsored by Representative Mike Synar, a Democrat from Oklahoma as part of the Alcohol, Drug Abuse, and Mental Health Administration Reorganization Act. The amendment required states to adopt and enforce a minimum age for tobacco sales, as well as demonstrate reductions in the retail availability of tobacco products to youth. The federal government does not have authority over state laws, but failure of states to follow these strictures would result in the loss of federal block grant funds for substance abuse. States followed the requirements by increasing random unannounced inspections, measuring retailer violations of the rules, and restricting access of youth to vending machines.

Some state laws take a more active approach to fighting youth smoking. Effective January 1, 2002, a set of laws in California prohibiting sales of cigarettes to minors added some new requirements: The laws prohibit smoking of tobacco products within a playground or sandbox area, the sale or display of cigarettes without the supervision or assistance of a clerk, and the sale or importation of bidis. To enforce rules about the sales of cigarettes to minors, the laws make business owners as well as clerks liable for infractions. The state can use sting operations to determine if retailers sell tobacco products illegally and to investigate sales of cigarettes to minors through the Internet, phone, or mail. Some cities in California have gone even further. In San Diego, for example, ordinances prevent advertising displays in places where children may see them, and cigarette displays near candy and nonalcoholic beverages are not allowed.

Clean Indoor Air

As of January 1, 2008, most states had adopted some form of clean-air law: 29 states prohibited smoking in public places, 30 prohibited smoking in state or local government buildings, 19 prohibited smoking in private workplaces (not including bars and restaurants), 24 prohibited smoking in restaurants, and 18 prohibited smoking in stand-alone bars.[9] Arizona, Delaware, the District of Columbia, Hawaii, Illinois, Massachusetts, New Jersey, New Mexico, New York, Ohio, Rhode Island, and Washington have prohibitions in all five types of locations. In 2007 alone, five states approved new clean-air legislation. Even Tennessee, a tobacco growing state with strong prosmoking sentiments, passed such a law. Although not comprehensive, it prohibits smoking in many public places and workplaces.

The spread of these prohibitions across the country represents a major change. Minnesota became the first state, in 1975, to ban smoking in most public places. Adoption of bans by other states followed slowly and usually applied to public buildings but not bars and restaurants. Although restaurants often had to have separate smoking sections, the habit of smoking with food and drink, disputes over the harm of secondhand smoke, and concerns over the freedom of choice of bars and restaurants slowed adoption of comprehensive bans. However, when California banned smoking in all workplaces, including restaurants, in 1994 and added bars to ban in 1998, it provided a model for other states to follow.

In the absence of state laws, local ordinances remain a source of tobacco control. By 1988, nearly 400 local ordinances had been enacted to protect indoor air from cigarette smoke, and 820 ordinances in 1998 restricted or banned smoking in public places. For workplaces not covered by state or local laws, private firms have increasingly decided to restrict smoking in their facilities. By 1992, 87 percent of worksites with 50 or more employees had a smoking policy of some kind. A large employer itself, the federal government stringently regulates smoking in its buildings. With state laws, local ordinances become less important, but past success at the local level helps smooth passage of state laws. Today, cities and counties sometimes go beyond state laws to add stricter bans. For example, some communities ban smoking within apartment buildings, bus shelters, school property, college dorms, downtown sidewalks, city parks, cars with children present, hospital grounds, and sidewalks outside public buildings.

Taxes

Although used historically to raise revenues, taxes also help to reduce smoking through raising the price of a pack of cigarettes. Two sorts of taxes can apply to cigarettes. Excise taxes specific to tobacco products are added by states, counties, or cities before purchase, and sales taxes on products in general are added at the time of the purchase. The excise taxes are generally larger. As of January 1, 2008, New Jersey had the highest excise tax, at $2.575 per pack.[10] However, New York State jumped to the top with a $2.75 tax on June 3, 2008. Rhode Island, Washington, Alaska, Arizona, Connecticut, Maine, Maryland, and Michigan all have excise taxes of at least $2.00 per pack. South Carolina has the lowest excise tax, only 17 cents per pack.

Other taxes can, in addition, add significantly to the cost of cigarettes. The federal cigarette tax is 39 cents per pack. City excise taxes can add further to the costs of cigarettes. Combined with the $2.75 state tax, the New York City tax of $1.50 means smokers in the city pay $4.25 in taxes—the highest combined state/local tax in the country. Chicago follows with a combined city/state tax of $3.66.[11] On top of the other taxes, general sales taxes apply to cigarettes in all but a few states. For example, the 7.25 percent sales tax in California and the 7.0 percent sales tax in New Jersey further raise the prices of cigarettes.

COURT CASES

Suits against the tobacco industry began in the 1950s, but few reached a jury, and none until the 1990s resulted in monetary damages awarded to the plaintiffs. In the 1990s the number and variety of suits increased greatly, and enjoyed more success. This section reviews court cases involving the tobacco industry and smoking that have set legal precedents for the treatment of both victims of smoking and the tobacco industry.

GREEN V. AMERICAN TOBACCO COMPANY (1957)

Background

This suit against a major tobacco company over the effect of smoking on lung cancer was the first of its type to go to jury. Dr. Larry Hastings, a physician and lawyer specializing in product liability, filed suit in December 1957 against the American Tobacco Company on behalf of Edwin M. Green. A navy veteran of World War II, Green had begun smoking in the 1920s at age 16 and continued the habit for 32 years until he was diagnosed with lung cancer. The American Tobacco Company manufactured Lucky Strike, the brand Green had smoked all those years. Although he died at age 49, only two months after the filing, the case continued on behalf of his survivors.

A flurry of lawsuits had followed the early publicity about the harm of smoking for lung cancer. The Surgeon General had not yet published his 1964 report on health and smoking, and warning labels were not yet required on cigarette packages. Yet enough information had emerged about the likely harm of cigarettes for smokers to seek redress for their injuries. Green's and other suits comprised a first wave of litigation over the harm of cigarettes.

Legal Issues

The court case revolved around the issues of implied warranty and negligence of the tobacco companies. The plaintiffs argued that by selling Lucky Strike to the public, the American Tobacco Company implied that the product was safe, and this warranty was breached when it turned out that cigarettes caused cancer. Cigarette manufacturers were thus liable for their negligence in selling a harmful product just like makers of a defective car were liable for the injury caused by the car. The defendants argued that no proof existed that cigarettes caused cancer. The defense acknowledged a statistical association, as smokers tended to die younger than nonsmokers, but argued that association does not prove causality. Many physicians and researchers, although well aware of the association, admitted that they did not understand the causes of cancer and testified for the defense. Also in favor of the defense, the nature of the harm of cigarettes differed from that of other products used in liability cases. The harm of a defective car brake on the driver who as a result crashes and dies is immediate and obvious, but the harm of cigarettes takes decades to emerge, and for many smokers does not emerge at all. To understand the connection between smoking and lung cancer, a jury would have to rely on the testimony of medical experts rather than their own perceptions.

The plaintiffs called as witnesses many of the pioneering researchers on the link between smoking and lung cancer, but the defense countered the testimony with its own experts. At this early date the plaintiffs had no incriminating documents from the tobacco industry to prove the manufacturers knew of the potential harm of smoking. To the contrary, tobacco industry representatives denied the validity of claims about the dangers of smoking.

Decision

Deliberating for 10 hours, the Florida jury concluded on August 2, 1960, that Edwin M. Green did indeed die of lung cancer caused by smoking Lucky Strikes but declined to award damages because they believed the American Tobacco Company did not and could not know of the harm of the cigarette in 1956 when Green learned he had lung cancer. They therefore concluded the company was not liable under laws of implied warranty. Neither the plaintiffs nor the defendants were happy with the decision. Counsel for the tobacco company worried that the jury had, in concluding cigarettes caused the lung cancer of Green, come close to making a financial award. Hastings felt that it made no sense to hold the company accountable for the lung cancer but not to award damages on the basis of that accountability. The plaintiffs appealed the decision and gained a new trial, but the second jury in 1964 clearly sided with the defendants.

Impact

Along with similar verdicts in similar cases, the tobacco industry victory ended suits based on implied warranty and negligence. Reflecting the nature of the first wave of lawsuits against the tobacco industry, *Green* was about as close to a victory as any others at the time. In other similar trials such as *Lartigue v. Liggett and Myers* in Louisiana and *Ross v. Philip Morris* in Missouri, juries showed even stronger resistance to the claims of smokers. They tended to view smoking as a personal choice that did not implicate the manufacturers in ultimate health problems and death. Suits against the tobacco industry would have to employ other strategies.

CIPOLLONE V. LIGGETT GROUP, PHILIP MORRIS, AND LOEWS (1992)

Background

Marc Z. Edell, a lawyer involved in asbestos litigation, thought that the case law used by victims of asbestos products to sue the manufacturers might also apply to victims of tobacco products. With the support of his law firm, he sought a client who suffered from the ill effects of smoking and lived in New Jersey, the state where the case law seemed best for bringing the suit. He found a resident of Little Ferry, New Jersey, named Rose Cipollone who agreed to file suit.[12]

Cipollone was a 57-year-old smoker with lung cancer. She had started smoking at age 16 because it looked cool and glamorous to her, and by 18 was smoking a pack a day, later moving up to one and a half packs each day. She began with Chesterfield cigarettes, manufactured by Liggett and Myers (later the Liggett Group), but switched to the company's filtered L&M cigarettes in the hope that they would be milder and safer. She later switched to Philip Morris's Virginia Slims because she thought the style looked glamorous. Later still she changed to Lorillard's low-tar brand, True. In 1981 an X ray showed a lesion in her lung that upon biopsy proved to be a malignant growth. Despite two lung operations the cancer returned to her lungs by 1984 and soon spread to her brain and the rest of her body. At the time she met Marc Edell she was undergoing chemotherapy but was clearly dying. Alive to file the suit in 1983, she died on October 21, 1984. The suit specified three defendants, the Liggett Group, Philip Morris, and Loews Corporation (owner of Lorillard), each a maker of cigarettes that Cipollone had smoked.

Legal Issues

The case for the plaintiff relied on changes in product liability laws that had occurred during the 1960s and 1970s. In the past, companies were responsible for damages incurred by users of a defective product, and courts required evidence of negligence on the part of the manufacturers to award damages. Later, however, courts had come to accept claims that inherently dangerous products, even when not defective, could make the manufactur ers liable for harm done to users. Under the new reasoning manufacturers who profited from risky products such as tall ladders and sharp tools should share the costs of the use of the risky product. In other words manufacturers should be strictly liable for their products. If extended to cigarettes, the logic of strict liability could result in damages to smokers dying of smoking-related illnesses. The plaintiff avoided the accusations of negligence or making a defective product but thought the tobacco companies might be liable for the inherent risks of cigarettes.

The fact that warnings had been placed on cigarette packages in 1965 might, however, remove the liability. If smokers knew of the risks they then shared fault in starting or continuing to smoke, and this absolved the manufacturers of liability. The plaintiffs would address this issue in their case against tobacco companies. They claimed that when Cipollone began smoking, she and most everyone else did not know of the full extent of the possible harm of cigarettes. By the time the risks became widely known and makers included warnings on the packages, she was too addicted to stop. Worse, if the tobacco companies themselves had known of the harm and addictiveness of their product, yet reassured the public that despite scientific studies their product was safe, they prevented Cipollone and others from making an informed choice about the product. The plaintiff argued that in trusting what the companies said, she had been deceived. Although she had a choice in smoking, she did not have an informed choice.

A key component of the case of the plaintiff involved showing that the tobacco makers knew of the harm of cigarettes and deceived the public by denying such harm. Edell and his staff thus devoted much effort to requesting and reviewing private documents of the tobacco companies. If the tobacco companies admitted in private that cigarettes were harmful, it would imply that their public claims were dishonest. For example, memoranda from the Philip Morris chief Helmut Wakeham urged the company to develop a "medically acceptable" cigarette and to stop denying the existence of persuasive evidence of the harm of cigarettes.

The tobacco lawyers presented several arguments in response. Only a statistical association existed between smoking and lung cancer, and scientists did not really know the causes of cancer. After all, many smokers never get lung cancer, and some nonsmokers get lung cancer. Moreover the type of lung cancer of Cipollone rarely occurs among smokers and did not fit the statistical association. No proof therefore existed that the manufacturer's products had caused the health problem.

Even if she had proof, the plaintiff knew of the risks, according to defense attorneys. Well before packages started to include warnings Cipollone had repeatedly received advice from family and friends to stop smoking; she had also adopted filtered cigarettes in the hope that they would not present the same health risks as unfiltered cigarettes. Had the warnings on cigarette packages begun earlier, she would have continued her habit, just as she did in the 1960s and 1970s, after the warnings were added. Cigarettes remained a legal product that contributed to the enjoyment of individuals, the finances of the government, and the growth of the economy. Whatever the risks associated with this beneficial product, individuals had the choice to smoke or not smoke, and Cipollone chose to smoke, argued the defense.

Attorneys for the tobacco companies presented one other legal issue that would cause dispute through the course of the trial and later appeals. The defense claimed that the 1965 and 1969 acts of Congress that required warning labels also blocked liability claims against cigarette manufacturers. The legislation prevented federal and state agencies from changing or adding to the warnings specified by Congress. While some claimed that this provision merely ensured the use of standardized warnings across all states, the tobacco industry had another interpretation. It argued that liability awards involved a form of state regulation that negated the warnings placed on packages by Congress and therefore violated congressional intent.

Decision

Before giving the case to the jury for a decision the presiding judge of the New Jersey federal court, H. Lee Sarokin, ruled on the claim of the tobacco lawyers that congressional legislation prohibited liability suits. He rejected the claim, noting that if Congress wanted to do this it would have stated explicitly that the law would prevent later tort claims. However, an appeals court reversed Sarokin's decision and required the judge to allow the defendants to include this argument in their case. This prevented the plaintiffs from introducing evidence of the dishonesty of tobacco companies after the 1965 warnings and during the last 18 years of Cipollone's life.

The 1988 decision of the six-person jury, handed down four years after the death of Cipollone, appeared on first look as a loss for the tobacco industry. The jury awarded $400,000 to Cipollone's husband, Tony, making this the first case ever in which the tobacco companies had to pay damages. Immediate news reports highlighted this aspect of the decision, but in all other ways the tobacco companies came out victors.

The jury had in fact made no award to Cipollone through her survivors. It had concluded that Philip Morris and Lorillard had no responsibility for her death because Cipollone did not start smoking their cigarettes until after the 1965 warnings. They held the Liggett Group partly responsible (20 percent) for Cipollone's death because she smoked their cigarettes before 1966, but most of the responsibility fell on the plaintiff herself. Since the law allowed damages only when a manufacturer was more than 50 percent responsible for the harm, no award could be given to the plaintiff. The jury awarded the husband $400,000, but this made little sense when the victim of the lung cancer received nothing.

Both the Liggett Group and Edell on behalf of Cipollone's survivors appealed the decision. The Liggett Group claimed it could not be liable for $400,000 to the husband if it was not liable for the death of his wife. Edell appealed Judge Sarokin's decision to prohibit evidence concerning tobacco industry behavior after 1965. After a complex appeals process the case ultimately ended up with the U.S. Supreme Court. In a 1992 decision of 7-2, the Court held for the tobacco companies in determining that a damage award based on actions after 1965 would frustrate Congress's efforts to establish a single nationwide standard of warning. They did allow for Edell to bring suit on other grounds, but both Edell's law firm and Cipollone's survivors had neither the resources nor the will to try again—the odds of success seemed too low to continue.

Impact

Cipollone v. Liggett Group, Philip Morris, and Loews ultimately gave a victory to the tobacco companies. The strict liability arguments offered by the plaintiff failed, as had earlier implied warranty and negligence arguments, to supply a satisfactory basis for receiving damages. With the Supreme Court's decision, the tobacco companies had maintained their perfect record of never paying out damages. However, the case's relatively close brush with triumph, particularly given the imbalance of the resources in favor of the tobacco companies, would embolden others to continue the efforts to sue the companies. Plaintiffs would need to find some argument to overcome the tendency of juries to hold smokers largely responsible for their behavior, but solutions would come soon. The case represented the end of a second wave of lawsuits based on strict liability and the beginning of a third wave that, with new legal arguments, would prove more successful for plaintiffs.

CARTER V. BROWN & WILLIAMSON (1996)
Background

After *Cipollone*, a case leading to an award against tobacco companies helped define a third wave of tobacco litigation incorporating new strategies. Grady Carter, a 66-year-old retired air traffic controller living in Florida, had started smoking Lucky Strike cigarettes in 1947, had switched brands in 1972, and continued the habit until his diagnosis of lung cancer in 1991. He had tried hard to quit but felt hooked by the habit. Upon hearing claims made in 1994 by tobacco company executives that cigarettes were not addictive, he decided to sue. In the suit he and his wife named Brown & Williamson, the maker of Lucky Strike cigarettes, as defendants and requested $1.5 million in damages. Represented by Jacksonville, Florida, lawyer Norwood S. Wilner, who would file hundreds of lawsuits against tobacco companies over the years, they claimed the company was liable because it knew of the harm of cigarettes but did not warn consumers until required to do so by the government.

A key difference between this case and previous ones related to the public release of internal documents from Brown & Williamson that the plaintiff's lawyers could use in the trial. In the past the discovery process compelled plaintiff attorneys to go through the time-consuming process of requesting and reviewing tobacco company documents, a process hindered whenever possible by the companies. However, copies of such documents came from Merrill Williams, a paralegal at a Louisville, Kentucky, law firm. He came across Brown & Williamson documents indicating that tobacco company executives had knowledge of the harm of tobacco products. He made copies of the documents and contacted a lawyer in Mississippi, Richard F. Scruggs, who was suing tobacco companies. A professor at the University of California and zealous antitobacco advocate, Stanton Glantz, also received copies in the mail of 4,000 pages of the documents from an unknown source. The documents eventually made their way to Congress and appeared on the Internet. A judge then ruled that the documents had become part of the public domain and could be used by plaintiffs in cases such as the Carters' against Brown & Williamson.

Legal Issues

Florida law had some advantages for the plaintiff and made the state a useful place to bring suit. It allowed a damage award even when the plaintiff had major responsibility for the injury. Unlike in New Jersey where an award could be made only if the defendant was at least 50 percent responsible, a Florida plaintiff could receive an award if the defendant was less than 50 percent responsible. This moved legal issues away from whether the smoker, Grady Carter, held primary responsibility for his habit—he would admit that he did. Rather it focused on whether the tobacco industry was also partly responsible.

The legal issues concerned the knowledge Brown & Williamson had of the harm of cigarettes, and the fraud and misrepresentation that occurred when the company refused to admit the harm. Unlike previous cases the plaintiffs did not claim that the company was liable because of the nature of its product but because it misled users about that nature. The plaintiffs presented newly released documents that demonstrated knowledge of the addictiveness of nicotine and the risks of smoking for health that dated back to years before cigarette packs added warnings. For example, one document dated July 17, 1963, from the chief legal counsel for Brown & Williamson stated that "we are, then, in the business of selling nicotine, an additive drug effective in the release of stress mechanisms."[13] Yet the companies did not inform the public of this fact or distribute a safer, less addictive cigarette when it would have benefited the public.

Brown & Williamson responded that the responsibility for the decision to smoke fell on the individual, particularly when cigarette packages had included warning labels for some 30 years. The labels absolved the company of liability for the hazards of smoking. Moreover the defendant claimed that the cigarettes manufactured and sold by the company provided just what smokers wanted.

Decision

Siding with the plaintiff, the Jacksonville, Florida, jury awarded $750,000 to the Carters in 1996. Jurors commented that the tobacco company's dishonesty bothered them, and they wanted to send a message that such dishonesty would no longer be tolerated. The decision represented a defeat for the tobacco company. However, a Florida appeals court overturned the verdict on an issue unrelated to the culpability of the tobacco industry. The higher court ruled that Carter in waiting for some time after the diagnosis of lung cancer to file the lawsuit, exceeded the four-year statute of limitations for such cases.

Impact

The victory against the tobacco industry in *Carter*, even though a statute of limitations violation overturned the verdict, presented a strategy for success that would guide hundreds of lawsuits in the years to come. Taking an approach that differed from previous cases, the *Carter* case suggested that juries would respond more favorably to arguments about the deception of tobacco companies than they would to arguments about the harm of smoking by itself. The strategy would not invariably bring victory, as it failed in some other cases. For example, in another case brought by Norwood S. Wilner, the jury rejected the claims for damages of Jean Connor against R. J. Reynolds. She had died at age 49 of lung cancer in 1995 after having smoked Winston and Salem cigarettes for most of her adult life. Despite arguments of Connor's attorneys that tobacco companies had deceived and addicted her, the jury sided with the defendants because the plaintiff had given up smoking several years before getting lung cancer. Juries would consider the facts at hand carefully before siding with the plaintiffs against the tobacco companies. Still *Carter v. Brown & Williamson* set a precedent that would have much importance for future cases against the tobacco companies.

BROWN & WILLIAMSON TOBACCO CORP. V.
U.S. FOOD AND DRUG ADMINISTRATION (2000)

Background

In 1994 Dr. David A. Kessler, the head of the Food and Drug Administration (FDA) as appointed by President Bill Clinton, suggested in a letter to the Coalition on Smoking OR Health that the FDA might have jurisdiction over tobacco. The coalition then formally petitioned the FDA to declare all cigarettes a drug under the Federal Food, Drug, and Cosmetic Act. The wording in the act defined a drug as a product that manufacturers intended to affect the structure or function of the body. Congress had not explicitly intended to include tobacco under this definition, and the FDA had previously claimed it had no authority over tobacco. However, Kessler thought he had new reasons to change the agency's approach to regulating cigarette products.

Several key points of evidence demonstrated the druglike pharmacological and physiological effects of smoking. First, the addictiveness of nicotine made smokers use cigarettes primarily as a nicotine delivery system. The need for smokers to replace dwindling levels of nicotine in their body by lighting another cigarette demonstrates that the product affects the functioning of the body. Indeed, the FDA regulated nicotine gum and patches as drug delivery systems, and cigarettes differed from these products (besides presenting greater health dangers) largely in the way the nicotine gets into the body. Second, the manufacturers knew that cigarettes were addictive. They had supported research on the nicotine levels in their cigarettes and manipulated the level of nicotine in their products by developing strains of tobacco with high levels of the chemical and by including additives such as ammonia that boosted the efficiency of the delivery of nicotine. Tobacco company executives had testified in Congress that they did not believe cigarettes were addictive, but new documents from the internal files of tobacco companies contradicted their contention. Third, advertising highlighted the nicotine benefits of cigarettes by using code words such as *satisfaction*, *strength*, and *impact*. Appealing to youth with misleading images of health and activity, cigarette ads would contribute to a lifelong addiction to the product.

On August 10, 1995, the FDA announced the results of its investigation of whether nicotine in cigarettes fit the definition of a drug and needed regulation. Concluding that it did, the FDA proposed to oversee the sale and distribution of cigarettes and smokeless tobacco, particularly in regard to underage buyers. After undergoing some revisions in response to public comment the proposed regulations required tobacco companies to support tobacco prevention education for children, take actions to ensure underage youth would not have access to cigarettes through vending machines or other unsupervised sales, ban gift or promotional items bearing cigarette brand names, eliminate outdoor advertising near schools, and limit advertising in publications with more than 15 percent of the readership under age 18. President Clinton announced the publication of the final FDA rules on August 23, 1996.

Tobacco companies filed numerous suits against the FDA. In one major suit heard in federal court in Greensboro, North Carolina, the plaintiffs included the major tobacco companies (Brown & Williamson, Liggett Tobacco, Lorillard, Philip Morris, and R. J. Reynolds), a smokeless tobacco company (United States Tobacco), parts of the advertising industry concerned about restrictions on advertising and free speech, and trade groups representing convenience stores that would have to follow new rules in selling cigarettes.

Legal Issues

The legal issues involved whether the Federal Drug and Cosmetic Act passed by Congress applied to cigarettes. The plaintiffs claimed that cigarettes were not drugs or devices, that congressional legislation did not give the FDA authority to regulate tobacco, and that the agency had exceeded its authority in the regulations. They also claimed that the restrictions on advertising violated First Amendment rights to free speech. In defense of the regulations, the government asserted that the evidence used by the FDA to declare cigarettes a drug-delivery system met the definition of a drug in the congressional legislation.

Decision

The initial decision in April 1997 from the federal court in Greensboro agreed that the FDA had regulative authority but limited the actions the agency could take. In favor of the FDA, the decision supported the claim that tobacco fit the legal definition of a drug or drug-delivery device but did not find the justification for all the regulatory proposals to be convincing. The court put a stay on all regulations except those prohibiting sales to minors and requiring proof of age with a photo ID for purchasing cigarettes. It concluded that in doing more than restricting sales to minors, the agency had exceeded its jurisdiction. The FDA did not have the authority to restrict advertising or promotion of the product.

When appealed by both sides to the United States Court of Appeals for the Fourth Circuit, in Richmond, Virginia, the initial decision was overturned in 1998 in a 2-1 decision. The court ruled that the interpretation of the FDA might fit the specific congressional wording but ignored the history of the legislation, which provided no evidence of the intent of Congress to treat cigarettes as a drug. Having lost this round, the government appealed to the U.S. Supreme Court. On March 21, 2000, the Supreme Court by a 5-4 vote affirmed the decision of the appeal's court. While recognizing the case made concerning the harm of tobacco, the majority in a decision written by Judge Sandra Day O'Connor concluded that Congress never intended its act to apply to tobacco. It had instead set up its own special regulatory scheme for tobacco rather than give authority for regulation to the FDA. As a result the FDA could not enforce its regulations and had to drop even the requirements concerning sales to minors.

Impact

The importance of the court case against the FDA comes not from blocking the proposed regulations. States implemented most of those anyway with the Master Settlement Agreement. Rather, it comes from the inability of the executive branch to take action on its own to control tobacco. The decision meant regulation of tobacco must come from specific legislative action by Congress. With Congress thus far unable to agree on such legislation, and executive branch agencies barred from imposing their own regulations, actions to control tobacco would have to come from litigation and the judicial branch. The decision thereby accelerated the trend of using lawsuits to deal with a contentious issue left unresolved by legislation. Individuals, trial lawyers, judges, and jurors rather than elected legislators and government officials have largely taken over the task of regulating the tobacco industry, and the reliance on litigation rather than legislation continues.

FRENCH V. PHILIP MORRIS (2002)

Background

The tobacco companies' first defeat in a suit involving secondhand smoke came in June 2002. Lynn French had served as a flight attendant since 1976 for TWA on both domestic and international flights. Since the U.S. government did not ban smoking on domestic flights less than six hours until 1990, she was exposed to environmental tobacco smoke on her job for 14 years, which resulted in chronic sinus problems, according to her complaint. She sought damages of $980,000 from the major tobacco companies in a case heard in the Florida circuit court.

The suit was brought under an agreement stemming from a 1991 class-action suit brought on behalf of nonsmoking flight attendants by Stanley M. Rosenblatt in *Broin v. Philip Morris*. As with the other 8,000 flight attendants who had chosen to be included in the suit, Norma Broin, a nonsmoker who developed lung cancer after 13 years as a flight attendant, claimed she was the victim of secondhand tobacco smoke. The lawyers in the *Broin* suit negotiated an agreement in which the tobacco companies donated $300 million for research on smoking-related diseases in Norma Broin's name, and Rosenblatt and his wife received $49 million. The flight attendants received no damages but obtained the right to bring suit to recover individual compensatory (not punitive) damages. Under this agreement French (and eventually 2,800 other flight attendants) brought suit.

Legal Issues

As a nonsmoker, French did not have to face the problem of most smokers in suits against the tobacco companies. Since the plaintiff had never made the decision to smoke, the tobacco companies could not claim she had individual responsibility for her use of cigarettes. Moreover she could not have known of the risks she faced from secondhand smoke since neither the tobacco companies nor the Surgeon General had provided such warnings. In the defendants' favor, the evidence of the harm of secondhand smoke was not as strong as for direct smoking, and the class-action issues in the case were complex. Several previous efforts to sue tobacco companies had failed on these grounds.

The judge in the case, Robert P. Kaye, had overseen the earlier settlement agreement and used the settlement to justify a different criterion than usual to determine product liability. Over the objections of tobacco company lawyers, he relieved the flight attendant of the burden of proving that cigarettes and secondhand smoke caused her health problems. The defense presented testimony that the sinus problems experienced by French were more commonly caused by bacteria and allergies than by secondhand smoke. However, the jury could presume under the settlement, according to Judge Kaye, that secondhand smoke can cause debilitating illness. The tobacco lawyers argued that in making $300 million available for research on diseases suffered by flight attendants, they never admitted that environmental tobacco smoke could cause health problems.

Decision

The six-person Miami jury awarded French $5.5 million in compensatory damages—more than five times as much as requested in the suit. The jury gave $2 million for injuries suffered in the past and $3.5 million for injuries she would suffer in the future. However, a Miami-Dade circuit judge reduced the award to $500,000 three months later in September 2002. The judge called the original amount "shocking," noting that French appeared composed and in no physical distress and had shown little evidence that her sinus problems significantly restricted her activities as a flight attendant, wife, and mother. Tobacco company lawyers viewed the ruling as justification for further appeals to overturn the decision altogether.

Impact

As the first defeat for the tobacco companies in a secondhand smoke case, *French v. Philip Morris* could have a potentially great impact on future cases. With thousands of other suits by flight attendants pending, the precedent of the award to French, even after being reduced by Judge Fredericka G. Smith, would open up tobacco companies to liability to nonsmokers as well as smokers. In November 2005, the Florida Supreme Court refused to consider an appeal of the case. With the failed appeal, trials for about 3,000 other claims by flight attendants against tobacco companies can proceed.

SHARON A. PRICE V. PHILIP MORRIS (2005)

Background

In a class-action suit filed on February 10, 2000, in the Madison County, Illinois, Circuit Court, Sharon Price and others alleged that the Philip Morris USA tobacco company violated the Illinois Consumer Fraud Act. After responding to objections of the defendant, the plaintiffs submitted a second complaint on February 11, 2003, that made the following points:

- Philip Morris USA sold Cambridge Lights and Marlboro Lights under claims that the cigarettes had decreased tar and nicotine;
- Such claims, based on tests using cigarette smoking machines, were misleading because people smoking the cigarettes actually get higher levels of tar and nicotine than shown by the machines and are harmed more than smoking regular cigarettes;
- The company modified the tobacco blend, used reconstituted tobacco, and added dangerous chemicals such as ammonia to deliver more tar and nicotine to smokers buying the light cigarettes.

Philip Morris USA denied the claims, arguing that the U.S. Federal Trade Commission (FTC) authorized use of the term *light* and, indeed, required manufacturers to provide information on the tar and nicotine content of their cigarettes.

In 2001, for purposes of the suit, the court certified (or gave legal standing too) a class of about 1.14 million smokers who purchased Cambridge Lights or Marlboro Lights in Illinois for personal consumption. The class consisted not of persons whose health was harmed by the cigarettes but of persons who were economically defrauded when they purchased the cigarettes under the belief that they were safer. This class differed from classes of smokers suing tobacco companies on the basis of physical harm and health problems. The plaintiffs still sought large economic damages, however. With the large number of smokers who bought the products, both healthy and unhealthy, the cost of damages to Philip Morris USA for economic fraud would be substantial.

After the circuit court rejected motions by Philip Morris USA to decertify the class and have the court make a summary judgment without going to trial, the trial went forward in 2002. Having heard witnesses, the circuit court issued its judgment on March 21, 2003. It ruled that Philip Morris USA was liable under the Illinois Consumer Fraud Act for making false statements or concealing facts. Based on expert testimony and evidence from public health researchers, the court determined that the term *light* falsely conveyed the idea of lower tar and nicotine and greater safety to consumers. Further, neither the right to free speech nor actions of the FTC protected Philip Morris USA from making such false statements. The court awarded $7.1 billion in actual damages to be paid to the plaintiffs and $3 billion in punitive damages to be paid to the state (or the plaintiffs if laws barred the state from receiving the damages).

Philip Morris USA then appealed the decision directly to the Illinois Supreme Court, which considered the case.

Legal Issues

The legal issues of the case relate to interpretations of consumer fraud—the key contention of the plaintiffs and the basis for the circuit court decision—under the Illinois Consumer Fraud Act. The facts concerning sales of the light products, the inhalation of tar and nicotine, the actions of Philip Morris, and the measurement of tar and nicotine using smoking machines had less relevance to the legal issues examined by the Illinois Supreme Court.

Philip Morris USA argued in its appeal that section 10b(1) of the act makes an important qualification. It says that nothing in the act shall apply to "[a]ctions or transactions specifically authorized by laws administered by any regulatory body or officer acting under statutory authority of this State or the United States." According to Philip Morris, laws and regulations of the federal government did in fact authorize use of the term *light* for cigarettes with certain levels of tar and nicotine. They pointed to the Federal Cigarette Labeling and Advertising Act and various consent decrees (or agreements) between the FTC and the tobacco companies to support their claim. Former employees of the FTC testified that the agency certainly intended to regulate use of labels for cigarettes. Federal regulations therefore preempt the state law. By complying with the federal government, Philip Morris USA satisfies the qualification in section 10b(1) of the state law. It cannot be held liable for actions sanctioned by the federal government. To further support its case, the defendants cited previous rulings by the Illinois Supreme Court that limited state consumer action on the basis of federal laws and regulations.

The plaintiffs responded that the FTC never sanctioned fraudulent use of the term *light*. While setting general guidelines, the agency never gave specific approval to the actions of Philip Morris USA. Indeed, the agency would certainly oppose the direct misrepresentation that the suit alleged. The Illinois law therefore is not preempted by federal law, and the state court does not need to defer to the federal government. Further, the Illinois Supreme Court precedents have little relevance to the case because they apply to different industries and circumstances.

Decision

By a vote of 4-2, the Illinois Supreme Court reversed the judgment of the circuit court, ruling in favor of Philip Morris USA that section 10b(1) of the Illinois Consumer Fraud Act bars such a judgment. The ruling thus dismissed the $10 billion verdict.

The decision focused specifically on the actions of the FTC with regard to cigarette labeling and advertising: "If the FTC has specifically authorized the use of the terms 'lights' and 'lowered tar and nicotine' by PMUSA [Philip Morris USA] in its labeling and advertising, PMUSA may not be held liable under the Consumer Fraud Act, even if the terms might be deemed false, deceptive, or misleading." The Illinois Supreme Court concluded that the FTC did authorize use of these terms. Although the agency never adopted formal trade regulations, it did use terms like *light* in is publications, testimony to Congress, and consent decrees made with tobacco companies. According to the ruling, these unofficial actions are enough to trigger the state law exemption.

The ruling added that it in no way approved of the actions of Philip Morris USA. To the contrary, it expressed concerns about the devastating harm done to public health by smoking. Yet the court's duty to interpret the existing law as developed by the legislature took precedence. The plaintiffs must go the Illinois General Assembly to change consumer protection laws rather than rely on the courts to punish tobacco companies.

Two other justices concurred in the decision but for a different reason: The plaintiffs failed to demonstrate that they sustained actual damages. The claim that they lost money by buying Cambridge Lights and Marlboro Lights assumes they would have not bought any cigarettes had the tobacco company not made light products. More likely, the light products substituted for regular products that had the same price. Buying light cigarettes instead of regular cigarettes did not increase the costs of cigarettes and did not result in economic damages. The plaintiffs cannot recover damages they did not sustain.

The Law and the Tobacco Industry and Smoking

Impact

The U.S. Supreme Court denied a petition for review of the ruling on November 27, 2006. With the failed appeal, the decision in this case limits the ability of smokers of light cigarettes to sue on grounds of economic fraud and deception. It sets a broad standard in Illinois for defining whether the federal government authorized various actions of businesses. In addition, given the unwillingness of the U.S. Supreme Court to review the Illinois ruling, suits filed on the same grounds against tobacco companies in many other states will fall under the same legal reasoning as the Illinois suit. Smokers, public health officials, and attorneys will need to use other legal theories, such as those based on actual or potential health damages from smoking, to punish tobacco companies. Altria, the parent group of Philip Morris USA, viewed the decision as a victory, as did stock analysts, who predicted better future performance for tobacco stocks.

Critics of the tobacco industry decried the decision. They viewed it as excusing the abhorrent behavior of tobacco companies. By focusing on a technical issue of what the FTC authorized, the court ignored a more important issue—the immoral and deceptive actions of the tobacco companies. Worse, according to critics, the ruling has implications for consumer fraud in areas other than tobacco. Suing companies for fraud within states will be increasing difficult if agencies in the federal government previously intervened to regulate the companies. The ruling thus favors corporations more generally over the interests of consumers.

However, the Supreme Court gave new hope to tobacco opponents with a December 2008 ruling. It said that smokers in Maine could sue for fraud because tobacco companies falsely claimed light or low-tar cigarettes were safer. Much as in Illinois, a class action was brought in Maine on behalf of smokers in the state who purchased light cigarettes. Lawyers for the tobacco company in this case, Altria, argued that the Federal Trade Commission approved use of the terms *light* and *low tar* and that the federal Cigarette Labeling and Advertising Act prevented suits by the states over actions falling under the law. The court rejected those claims, however, allowing the class action to proceed in Maine. In response to the ruling, lawyers in Illinois filed a motion to reopen *Price v. Philip Morris*.

---

1 U.S. Department of Health and Human Services. *Reducing Tobacco Use. A Report of the Surgeon General.* Washington, D.C.: U.S. Department of Health and Human Services, 2000, p. 164.

2 Jacob Sullum. *For Your Own Good: The Anti-Smoking Crusade and the Tyranny of Public Health,* New York: Free Press, 1998, p. 88.

3 Kenneth E. Warner. "Clearing the Airwaves: The Cigarette Ad Ban Revisited." *Policy Analysis*, vol. 5 (Fall 1979): 435–450.

[4] Elizabeth Whelan. *A Smoking Gun: How the Tobacco Industry Gets Away with Murder.* Philadelphia: George F. Stickley, 1984, p. 130.

[5] M. L. Myers, C. Iscoe, C. Jennings, W. Lenox, and E. Sacks. *A Staff Report on the Cigarette Advertising Investigation.* Washington, D.C.: Federal Trade Commission, 1981, pp. 229–239.

[6] W. Kip Viscusi. *Smoke-Filled Rooms: A Postmortem on the Tobacco Deal.* Chicago: University of Chicago Press, 2002, pp. 1–10.

[7] "Kennedy, Waxman, Cornyn, and Davis Introduce Tobacco Legislation." Senator Edward Kennedy, United States Senator for Massachusetts. Available online. URL: http://kennedy.senate.gov/newsroom/press_release.cfm?id=30D49497-D37D-4C82-87E1-3B6C9C51E4F1. Downloaded in May 2008.

[8] U.S. Department of Health and Human Services. *Reducing Tobacco Use*, p. 208.

[9] "State Legislated Actions on Tobacco Issues: 2007." American Lung Association. Available online. URL: http://www.rwjf.org/pr/product.jsp?id=28611&typeid=136. Downloaded in June 2008.

[10] "State Legislated Actions on Tobacco Issues: 2007."

[11] "Top Combined State-Local Cigarette Tax Rates." Campaign for Tobacco-Free Kids. Available online. URL: http://tobaccofreekids.org/research/factsheets/pdf/0267.pdf. Downloaded in June 2008.

[12] Alan Kluger. *Ashes to Ashes: America's Hundred-Year Cigarette War, the Public Health, and the Unabashed Triumph of Philip Morris.* New York: Alfred A. Knopf, 1996, pp. 639–677.

[13] Court TV Case Files. *"Carter v. Williamson."* Available online. URL: http://courttv.com/casefiles/verdits/carter.html, posted December 26, 2002.

CHAPTER 3

CHRONOLOGY

This chapter presents a chronology of important events relating to the tobacco industry and smoking. Tobacco has a long history, but the chronology focuses in particular on events of the last 40 years—those beginning with the report of the Surgeon General on health and smoking, leading to the development of antismoking laws and regulations, and ending with the legal battles against the tobacco industry. Unless otherwise stated the listed events occurred in the United States.

5000–3000 B.C.

- Tobacco is first cultivated in the Andes Mountains in South America in current-day Peru and Ecuador.

A.D. 1492

- Sailors on the first expedition of Christopher Columbus are the first Europeans to smoke tobacco, sharing a pipe with local Indians on the modern-day island of Cuba. Columbus returns to Spain with only a few tobacco seeds and leaves, but stories of smoking intrigue many in Europe.

1550s

- Tobacco is grown in Portuguese and Spanish palace gardens for its beauty and ease of growth but is also studied and nurtured by physicians who suspect that it has medicinal properties.

1560

- Jean Nicot, the French ambassador to Portugal, experiments with tobacco as a medicine and claims in a letter to the queen of France that it has curative powers.

1565

- Nicolás Monardes, a physician in Seville, Spain, authors a pamphlet called *Joyful News of Our Newe Founde Worlde* that lauds the wonderful healing properties of tobacco. He claims that smoking cleanses the brain and cures among other things bad breath, kidney stones, and wounds from poison arrows.

- Naval commander John Hawkins and his crew bring tobacco from the West Indies to England, but few besides sailors use the product.

1586

- Walter Raleigh returns to England from an expedition to Virginia, where he became a habitual smoker. He brings with him American Indians who can cultivate tobacco and prepare it for smoking. Raleigh enthusiastically advocates use of the product, and tobacco use spreads quickly throughout England.

1595

- The first English-language book on tobacco, *Tabacco*, is published.

1600

- Walter Raleigh persuades Queen Elizabeth I to take a puff of tobacco smoke.

1604

- Newly crowned king of Great Britain James I publishes a pamphlet entitled *Counterblaste to Tobacco* that decries the habit as filthy, harmful, and addictive. In part motivated by his dislike of Walter Raleigh, King James nonetheless uses his views on tobacco as justification for taxing imports of the product.

1612

- John Rolfe, an English settler in Jamestown, Virginia (who later married the Wampanoag princess Pocahontas), plants tobacco, which will become the major crop of the new settlement. The following year he sends the first shipment of the product to England.

1632

- Less enthused about tobacco than colonists in Virginia, the Massachusetts Bay colony, established by Puritans, bans tobacco sales and public smoking.

1676

- Angered by the heavy taxes placed on tobacco by the Virginia governor as well as a number of other issues, planter Nathaniel Bacon leads a brief rebellion against colonial administrators.

Chronology

1700

- Tobacco exports from Virginia reach 38 million pounds. During this period tobacco can be used as currency and to pay salaries.

1713

- An Italian physician, Bernardino Ramazzini, notes that tobacco workers suffer from headaches and stomach troubles because of the tobacco dust they breathe.

1727

- Tobacco notes that attest to the quality and quantity of the product stored in warehouses become legal tender in Virginia.

1753

- Swedish botanist Carolus Linnaeus gives the name *Nicotiana tabacum* to the tobacco plant commonly smoked in Europe.

1761

- English physician Dr. John Hill cautions against the immoderate use of snuff, noting for the first time in a published document that tobacco can cause cancer.

1762

- General Israel Putnam introduces imported cigars from Cuba to the United States.

1776

- Benjamin Franklin uses tobacco as collateral when he obtains loans from France to support the American Revolution's war effort.

1789

- The French Revolution makes the tobacco habits of the aristocrats—snuff and pipes—unfashionable. Many Frenchmen attempt to identify with the working class by smoking cigarettes, a cheaper and smaller product used by those with little money.

1794

- U.S. Congress passes the first excise tax on tobacco products.

1798

- Dr. Benjamin Rush, a signer of the Declaration of Independence, writes an essay claiming that tobacco causes disastrous effects on the stomach, nerves, and mouth. He also suggests that tobacco use leads to drunkenness.

1809

- French scientist Louis-Nicolas Vanquelin isolates nicotine from tobacco smoke.

1829

- A pipe smoker, Rachel Jackson dies soon after her husband, Andrew, is elected president.

1839

- The discovery of a new way of curing the bright tobacco leaf with heat from charcoal produces a particularly mild and pleasant flavor when the tobacco is chewed or smoked.

1848

- The founder of the Seventh-Day Adventists, Ellen Gould Harmon White, comes to see abstaining from tobacco (and coffee and tea) as a crucial part of healthful living. Opposition to tobacco later becomes a central tenet of the Adventist religion.

1849

- The American Anti-Tobacco Society is founded.
- American doctor Joel Shew publishes a book, *Tobacco: Its History, Nature, and Effects on the Body and Mind*, in which he notes that cancers and tumors occur more commonly among men than women. Since men smoke more than women, he infers that smoking may be the cause.

1857

- George Trask begins publishing the *Anti-Tobacco Journal* in Fitchburg, Massachusetts.
- The prestigious British medical journal *Lancet* publishes a series of articles that debate the medical risks of tobacco but fails to offer a clear statement of the harm of smoking.

1863

- Cigarette tobacco is used by soldiers fighting for the North and the South, and returning Union soldiers popularize cigarette smoking in northern U.S. cities.

1864

- President Abraham Lincoln signs a bill that places a tax of $1 per thousand on all manufactured cigarettes. With limited production of cigarettes in the United States, the tax applies largely to foreign imports.

1866

- George Webb, an Ohio farmer, develops a new tobacco leaf product called white burley that turns out to have an unusual ability to absorb other flavors and additives. Used initially in chewing tobacco, it becomes a popular type of tobacco for cigarettes.

1868

- F. S. Kinney begins to sell prerolled cigarettes in New York City.

1874

- James Buchanan Duke, soon to dominate the tobacco industry, joins his father and brother in founding a tobacco firm, W. Duke and Sons.

1875

- Lewis Ginter, the first major figure in the business of cigarette production, begins producing cigarettes in Richmond, Virginia. Among the first to add flavors to cigarettes, he would become dominant in the production, marketing, and sale of cigarettes in the decades to come.

1878

- Manufacturers begin including trading cards in their cigarette packages, and in the years to come these cards will include pictures.

1880

- Figures show consumption of large cigars to have reached 47.1 per person, while consumption of cigarettes equals only 8.2 per person.

1881

- James Albert Bonsack invents and patents a cigarette-rolling machine that can produce 40 times as many cigarettes as a skilled production worker who rolls by hand.

1883

- To advocate its opposition to the use of tobacco, as well as alcohol, the National Women's Christian Temperance Union establishes the Department for Overthrow of the Tobacco Habit (renamed the Department of Narcotics in 1885).
- After reaching a peak of $5 per thousand, taxes on cigarettes fall to 50¢ per thousand. The change reduces the price and helps increase the popularity of cigarettes.

Tobacco Industry and Smoking

1884

- James Buchanan Duke installs two Bonsack machines in his cigarette factory, thereby increasing production without raising costs and gaining a substantial advantage over his competitors. He soon arranges a leasing agreement with James Bonsack to use more machines to manufacture his cigarettes.

1885

- An inveterate cigar smoker, former president Ulysses S. Grant dies of throat cancer. Upon discovering the cancer in 1884, doctors had encouraged Grant to limit his smoking to three cigars a day.

1890

- Following a price war stimulated by the increasing use of cigarette manufacturing machines to lower production costs, Duke merges several competitors with his business to form the American Tobacco Company and monopolizes cigarette sales and production.

1893

- Attempting to monopolize sales of chewing tobacco as well as cigarettes, Duke buys several chew producers, forms the National Tobacco Works, cuts prices, and invites other producers to joint his company. Most companies agree to join, further increasing Duke's power in the tobacco industry.

1895

- North Dakota becomes the first state to prohibit cigarette smoking by youth and adults. Many other states follow in the next five years with anticigarette legislation.

1896

- The Diamond Match Company begins freely distributing small matchbooks with paper rather than wood matches. The matchbooks allow for advertising on the outside and prove popular with cigarette smokers, who do not need to hold the flame as long as cigar and pipe smokers.

1899

- Lucy Page Gaston, who will become the nation's leading antismoking advocate, sets up the Chicago Anti-Cigarette League (changed to the National Anti-Cigarette League in 1901 and the Anti-Cigarette League of America in 1911).

1902

- A British cigarette manufacturer, Philip Morris, opens a small office in New York City. It will in the next century become the largest and most powerful U.S. tobacco company.

1904

- A woman is arrested for smoking in a car on Fifth Avenue in New York City.

1909

- Dr. Charles Pease succeeds in getting smoking banned in New York City subways.
- Responding to the failure of laws to stop its citizens from smoking, Indiana becomes the first state to repeal cigarette prohibition. Antismoking advocates aim to use education and persuasion in the absence of legislation and prohibition.

1911

- The U.S. Supreme Court affirms use of the Sherman Anti-Trust Act by the Justice Department to dissolve the American Tobacco Company and Duke's trust. The breakup results in four smaller firms—Liggett and Myers, Reynolds, Lorillard, and American—that will dominate cigarette production and sales for the following decades.

1912

- Liggett and Myers Tobacco Company introduces Chesterfield cigarettes, which use a mixture of American white burley and foreign leaf. Emphasizing its Turkish blend of tobacco and its English name, the company makes the new brand a top seller.

1913

- Richard J. Reynolds introduces Camel cigarettes. Although as cheap as other American cigarettes, Camels have a premium Turkish flavor based on a blend of American and foreign tobaccos. An extensive and intriguing advertising campaign helps make the cigarette a top-selling brand.

1916

- Duke's successors at American Tobacco introduce Lucky Strike cigarettes, whose tobacco is promoted with the slogan "It's Toasted." The cigarette is an instant success and along with Chesterfields and Camels dominates cigarette sales in the United States.

1917

- Despite the introduction of new cigarette brands, cigars still remain popular enough that production passes a new record. More than cigarettes, cigars are viewed as a stylish, leisurely form of smoking that appeals to affluent men.

1918

- Cigarettes are among the rations of U.S. soldiers fighting in Europe in World War I. Charitable organizations such as the International Red Cross and the Young Men's Christian Association (YMCA) send cigarettes to soldiers as a way to support the war effort. Many soldiers return to the states after the war with an attachment to cigarettes and support efforts to repeal anticigarette laws.
- Murad brand cigarettes build on feelings of patriotism in an advertisement that, under the drawing of a soldier with a cigarette, has the CAPTION "Murad—After the Battle, the Most Refreshing Smoke is Murad."

1919

- To promote its Helmar brand of cigarettes, Lorillard becomes the first company to picture a woman in a cigarette advertisement. In the ad the woman is seen holding but not smoking a cigarette.

1920

- Lucy Page Gaston announces she will run for the Republican presidential nomination on an antitobacco platform.

1922

- Michigan State Normal College expels an 18-year-old woman for smoking cigarettes, a decision later upheld by the Michigan supreme court.

1924

- *Reader's Digest* publishes the article "Does Tobacco Injure the Human Body?"

1927

- Aiming to appeal to a female audience, an ad from Philip Morris claims its new Marlboro cigarettes are "as Mild as May."
- In response to the growing use of cigarettes and steady repeal of state laws prohibiting cigarettes, the Department of Narcotics of the Women's Christian Temperance Union sponsors thousands of antismoking events.

- An ad from the American Tobacco Company claims that according to a survey of 20,679 physicians, Lucky Strikes are less irritating to the throat than other cigarettes.

1928

- Lucky Strike cigarettes are advertised with a picture of a women and the slogan "Reach for a Lucky Instead of a Sweet."

1930

- The *Journal of the American Medical Association (JAMA)* criticizes health claims made for cigarettes in advertisements.

1933

- To save tobacco farmers from ruin the Agricultural Adjustment Act limits tobacco production, offers government loans, and develops price supports.

1936

- Brown & Williamson introduces Viceroy filter-tip cigarettes but has little success with the new product. It will become popular in the 1950s as information on the negative effects of tobacco tar on health begins to emerge.

1938

- Raymond Pearl publishes an article in the prestigious scientific journal *Science* that is one of the first to show an association between cigarette smoking and a shorter life.

1941

- A jury finds the American Tobacco Company, Liggett and Myers, and R. J. Reynolds guilty under the Sherman Anti-Trust Act of conspiring to fix prices and create a monopoly. After the Supreme Court upholds the verdict, the companies pay a fine totaling $250,000.

1942

- Claiming that the green pigment used in its packaging is needed for the war effort, American Tobacco changes its Lucky Strike package to white. The cigarette successfully uses the slogan "Lucky Strike Green Has Gone to War."

1944

- The military's share of cigarette consumption rises to 85 billion, a quarter of all cigarettes produced in the nation. Given the high demand among soldiers for cigarettes, a shortage develops and retailers begin to ration their sales. A production decrease due to tobacco growers, who in aiming to obtain higher prices allow land to lie fallow, contributes to the shortage.

1945

- U.S. soldiers in Europe make extra money selling cigarettes to Russian soldiers and German citizens who lack access to the product. The price Europeans pay for cigarettes greatly exceeds the cost to American soldiers.

1948

- An article in the *Atlantic Monthly* describes the use of cigarettes by actors and actresses to show thoughtfulness, irritation, anxiety, and anger. Indeed, smoking in movies has become common and serves to promote cigarettes.

1950

- Studies by Ernest Wynder and Evarts A. Graham in the United States and by Richard Doll and A. Bradford Hill in England demonstrate links between smoking and lung cancer.

1952

- An antismoking article, "Cancer by the Carton," is published in the popular magazine *Reader's Digest*. The scare created by this article and several others like it temporarily results in lower purchases of cigarettes. It also leads tobacco companies to push new brands of filtered cigarettes.

1953

- Dr. Ernest Wynder and Dr. Evarts A. Graham report that they produced skin cancer in 44 percent of the mice they had painted with tobacco tar condensed from cigarette smoke. Defenders of smoking note that the results using animals, tar paint, and skin cancer do not apply to humans who inhale cigarette smoke into their lungs.

1954

- The American Cancer Society's Tobacco and Cancer Committee adopts a resolution recognizing an association between smoking and lung cancer.
- Tobacco groups establish the Tobacco Industry Research Committee to respond to negative publicity about the damage of cigarette smoking. The committee authors an ad entitled "A Frank Statement to Cigarette Smokers" that calls for more study of the possible dangers but also reassures smokers of its belief that cigarettes are safe

Chronology

1955

- The Marlboro Man ad campaign first associates the cigarette brand with cowboys, masculinity, and outdoor activity. It will make the underperforming brand one of the nation's most popular in years to come and contribute to the growth of Philip Morris.
- The Federal Trade Commission bans advertising claims about the health effects of smoking.

1957

- Congress holds hearings on deceptive filter-tip cigarette advertising.
- Surgeon General Leroy F. Burney issues a statement that evidence points to a causative effect of smoking on lung cancer.

1958

- After having earlier expressed some mild concerns about the harm to health of smoking, the Consumer's Union asserts that a definitive link exists between cigarette use and lung cancer. The organization notes that filter-tip cigarettes provide little protection from cancer and urges smokers to quit or cut down.
- The Tobacco Institute is established in Washington, D.C., to oversee lobbying and public relations efforts.

1959

- An editorial in the *Journal of the American Medical Association* holds research on cigarette smoking to the highest standards of scientific validity in claiming that no authoritative evidence exists either for or against the harm of smoking and lung cancer.

1960

- A Florida jury concludes in a suit against the American Tobacco Company that Edwin M. Green did indeed die of lung cancer caused by smoking Lucky Strikes but declines to award damages. A retrial in 1964 rejects claims against the tobacco company altogether.

1961

- President John F. Kennedy requests that the Surgeon General form a committee to assess the current knowledge on smoking and health, which Surgeon General Luther L. Terry does the next year.

1962

- The surgeon general for the U.S. Air Force orders an end to the distribution of free cigarettes in air force hospitals and flight lunches.

1964

- The Surgeon General releases his report on smoking and health, which marks the beginning of a change in attitudes toward smoking and the use of cigarettes.
- The Federal Trade Commission proposes that tobacco companies include warning labels on cigarette packages and in advertisements, but Congress proposes legislation of its own that will supersede the proposals.
- The American Medical Association's Alliance House of Delegates refuses to endorse the surgeon general's report. Used to clinical demonstrations of medical causality, such as symptoms that appear in an infection or fever, many physicians are not ready to accept statistical association as evidence of causality.
- State Mutual Life Assurance Company of America becomes the first life insurance company to offer discount policies for nonsmokers.

1965

- Congress passes the Federal Cigarette Labeling and Advertising Act, which requires a mild warning statement on cigarette packages but no warning on advertisements. The act overrides the 1964 Federal Trade Commission rules.

1966

- John F. Banzhaf III requests that the Federal Communications Commission apply the fairness doctrine to cigarette advertising on television and radio. In the following year the commission agrees with the petition and orders stations to provide airtime for antismoking ads. The policy, which lasts until 1971, leads to several influential antismoking ads.

1967

- The Federal Trade Commission begins publishing tables of the tar and nicotine content in manufactured cigarettes.
- Philip Morris launches an ad campaign for a new cigarette product, Virginia Slims, that uses the slogan "You've Come a Long Way Baby" to appeal to younger, more liberated women.

1969

- In a congressional hearing, all four physicians invited to testify on the hazards of cigarettes, including the surgeon general, are themselves smokers. Along with the rise in cigarette consumption after a few years of decline, this incident illustrates the difficulty smokers will have in quitting and public health advocates will have in eliminating the tobacco problem.

- Following recommendations from the Federal Trade Commission to ban cigarette ads from television and radio, Congress passes the Public Health Cigarette Smoking Act. It specifies the ban to begin on January 2, 1971, and new wording for the warnings on cigarette packages.

1970

- A press conference sponsored by the American Cancer Society announces the results of a research study it funded. In the study Oscar Auerbach finds that among 86 beagles taught to smoke, 12 developed tumors. Although scientific reviewers have questions about the study, its results receive much public attention.

1971

- United Airlines becomes the first to divide seating into smoking and non-smoking sections.
- The Group Against Smokers' Pollution (GASP) is founded to lobby for nonsmokers' rights.
- In *Capital Broadcasting v. Acting Attorney General and Capital Broadcasting v. Mitchell*, the U.S. Court of Appeals upholds the constitutionality of the ban on cigarette ads on television and radio.

1972

- The Surgeon General's annual report reviews the effects of environmental tobacco smoke on nonsmokers and leads to new efforts to protect nonsmokers from the smoke of others.
- The Civil Aeronautics Board requires smoking sections on commercial air flights.

1973

- Arizona becomes the first state to ban smoking in public places.
- After fluctuating since 1964, the level of cigarette consumption peaks before beginning a downward trend that continues to the present.

1975

- Minnesota passes the first statewide act to keep indoor air free of smoke by requiring no-smoking areas in all buildings open to the public.
- Cigarettes are removed from military field rations.

1976

- A New Jersey court rules that an office worker who is allergic to tobacco smoke has the right to a smoke-free office.

1977

- Berkeley, California, becomes the first city to limit smoking in restaurants and other public places.

1978

- A New Jersey administrative rule restricts smoking in restaurants and public places, the first to do so without legislative backing.
- Joseph Califano, head of the Department of Health, Education, and Welfare under President Jimmy Carter, proposes several actions to fight cigarette smoking: raising taxes on cigarettes and using the proceeds for antismoking campaigns and programs, eliminating smoking on airplanes and in restaurants, and ending government subsidies to tobacco growers. With little support for the proposals from others in the Carter administration, the opposition from tobacco growers, retail establishments, and the tobacco industry is sufficient to block the proposals.

1979

- Smoking is restricted in all federal buildings.

1981

- At a national conference of antismoking groups, delegates develop a "Blueprint for Action" that defines the start of a more aggressive antismoking movement.
- Dr. C. Everett Koop becomes surgeon general. He emerges as a powerful antismoking advocate, authoring reports on environmental tobacco smoke, addiction, and the negative health consequences of smoking for women.

1982

- The American Cancer Society, the American Lung Association, and the American Heart Association combine to form Coalition on Smoking OR Health to lobby in Washington, D.C., against smoking.

1983

- According to documents released some years later, Sylvester Stallone, actor and writer of the *Rocky* films, agrees to use Brown & Williamson cigarette products in five feature films in return for a payment of $500,000. The documents illustrate the common practices among producers of including cigarette products—otherwise prohibited from being advertised on television and radio—in their movies and films in return for payment from tobacco firms.

1984

- The Food and Drug Administration approves nicotine gum products to help smokers quit.
- The 1984 Comprehensive Smoking Education Act requires that four strongly worded warnings be rotated on cigarette packages and advertisements and requires that the warnings also be displayed prominently on advertisements.

1985

- The American Medical Association calls for a complete ban on cigarette advertising and promotion.
- Los Angeles bans smoking in most public places and in businesses employing four or more persons if nonsmokers request the ban.
- A rotating series of warnings in more specific and severe language, and in larger print, begins to appear on cigarette packages.

1986

- The Comprehensive Smokeless Tobacco Health Education Act requires three rotated warning labels on smokeless tobacco packages.
- Reports from the National Research Council and the Office of the Surgeon General review evidence that indicates nonsmokers living with smokers have an increased risk of lung cancer, and children living with smoking parents have an increased risk of respiratory problems.

1988

- The Surgeon General's report describes nicotine as a highly addictive drug and cigarettes as an efficient means of delivering the drug.
- Congress bans smoking on domestic air flights of less than two hours.
- R. J. Reynolds introduces Premier cigarettes, a virtually smokeless product that reduces cancer-causing compounds, but smokers reject the product.
- Aiming to counter the success of Marlboro cigarettes, R. J. Reynolds decides to introduce the Joe Camel (or Old Joe) cartoon character in its ads. The new ads will produce a jump in sales for Camel cigarettes and are followed with the distribution of free Joe Camel products, some of which become collector's items years later.
- California voters approve the Tobacco Tax and Health Protection Act (Proposition 99), which increases the excise tax on cigarettes by 25 percent.
- The husband of Rose Cipollone wins a $400,000 judgment against the Liggett Group for the failure of the cigarette manufacturer to warn

his wife about the dangers of its product, but the award is later over-turned.

1989

- Philip Morris introduces Next, a cigarette that has the nicotine removed from the tobacco (much like caffeine is removed from coffee beans for decaffeinated coffee). The product flops.
- The Surgeon General's report, *Reducing the Health Consequences of Smoking, 25 Years of Progress*, reports that more than 400,000 smokers a year die prematurely.

1990

- The ban on smoking in airplanes is extended to all U.S. domestic commercial air travel lasting six hours or less.
- Tobacco companies announce the sale of American cigarettes to the Soviet Union. Wall Street analysts view the move as highly profitable for the industry.

1991

- The Food and Drug Administration approves nicotine patches as an aid to smoking cessation.
- The Federal Trade Commission reaches an agreement with Pinkerton Tobacco Company, maker of Red Man chewing tobacco, which allows the company to continue sponsoring its tractor pull event on cable television but without extensive use of its brand name product and logo.
- Health and Human Services secretary Louis W. Sullivan calls for fans to shun sporting events sponsored by tobacco firms and for promoters to reject tobacco sponsorship.

1992

- The Environmental Protection Agency classifies environmental tobacco smoke as belonging to the most dangerous class of carcinogens.
- The U.S. Congress passes the Synar Amendment as part of the Alcohol, Drug Abuse, and Mental Health Administration Reorganization Act. The amendment requires states to adopt and enforce minimum age requirements for tobacco sales and to demonstrate reductions in the retail availability of tobacco products to minors. The federal government does not have authority over state laws, but failure of states to follow these strictures will result in the loss of federal block grant funds for substance abuse.

Chronology

1993

- Smoking is banned in the White House.
- Vermont extends its smoking ban in public buildings to include restaurants, bars, hotels, and motels (except those holding a cabaret license).
- Major League Baseball announces that all minor league players, coaches, and umpires will be banned from smoking or chewing tobacco in their ballparks or team buses.

1994

- Philip Morris experiments with Eclipse, a cigarette that reduces secondhand smoke by 85–90 percent. However, possible attempts by the Food and Drug Administration to regulate the product keep it off the market.
- The government releases a list of 599 ingredients added by tobacco companies to manufactured cigarettes.
- *February 28 and March 3:* An ABC television show, *Day One*, alleges that tobacco companies added nicotine to their cigarettes but later retracts the statement in response to a suit by the tobacco companies.
- *April 1:* In testimony under oath, seven leading U. S. tobacco company executives state their belief that cigarettes and nicotine are not addictive.

1995

- New evidence discloses that Philip Morris conducted research for 15 years on nicotine and that the research found the chemical to affect the body, brain, and behavior of smokers. Representative Henry Waxman of California tells company president William I. Campbell that the disclosures contradict his sworn testimony the previous year.
- Dr. Jeffrey Wigand, former vice president for research at Brown & Williamson, testifies in a deposition that the company knew cigarettes were harmful and addictive. Other sworn statements from former tobacco company employees assert that Philip Morris manipulated the nicotine levels in its cigarettes.
- *July 24:* A class-action lawsuit is filed in Wichita, Kansas, against manufacturers of smokeless tobacco on behalf of all users of the product in the state.
- *August 16:* A federal appeals court rules that congressional representatives do not have to turn over internal company documents of Brown & Williamson, which the company claims were stolen from it.

1996

- The Food and Drug Administration approves nicotine patch products for over-the-counter sales.

- Papers released in a suit brought by the state of Minnesota against tobacco companies to recover Medicaid costs of treating tobacco-related illnesses show that a Philip Morris researcher in 1977 suggested a cover-up if results about nicotine's effects prove damaging.
- Merrill Williams, a paralegal who provided antitobacco lawyers with internal documents about the health dangers of cigarettes from Brown & Williamson, admits that lawyers on the antismoking side gave him more than $100,000. Tobacco industry lawyers call the payment a bribe, while antismoking lawyers call it charity.
- *June:* Republican presidential candidate Robert Dole says he believes that tobacco may not be addictive for some people and that the government should not regulate it. Strong criticism of the statement comes from President Bill Clinton, the media, and antismoking groups.
- *August 9:* A Jacksonville, Florida, jury awards $750,000 to Grady Carter and his wife in a suit against Brown & Williamson based on claims that the tobacco company deceived the public in denying the harm and addictiveness of its products.
- *August 23:* President Clinton approves Food and Drug Administration regulations that restrict the sale, distribution, advertising, and promotion of cigarettes, but tobacco companies sue to prevent implementation of the regulations.

1997

- The Liggett Group, the smallest of the tobacco companies, after having become the first to settle with plaintiffs' attorneys, admits that nicotine is addictive and that the industry targeted minors, and turns over incriminating documents.
- A group of 41 state attorneys general and the tobacco companies propose a settlement of $360 billion to recover state Medicaid costs for treating smokers for smoking-related illnesses. However, the agreement needs the support of national legislation to enforce the provisions.
- *May 28:* The Federal Trade Commission files a complaint against R. J. Reynolds over its Joe Camel ads, accusing the company of advertising to children.
- *July 11:* In response to a suit that the company violated California consumer protection laws by targeting minors with its Joe Camel campaign (*Mangini v. R. J. Reynolds*), R. J. Reynolds agrees to restrict advertising and to fund antismoking ads for teens in California.
- *August 9:* President Bill Clinton signs an executive order establishing a smoke-free environment for federal employees and members of the public visiting federally owned facilities.

Chronology

1998

- *January 1:* California becomes the first state in the nation to ban smoking in bars.
- *June 17:* A bill introduced in the Senate to codify the provisions of the proposed tobacco settlement fails to pass. The initial agreement is thus dropped, which forces the sides to negotiate further.
- *November 11:* A U.S. appeals court overrules the lower court in finding that the Food and Drug Administration lacks authority to regulate cigarettes and smokeless tobacco.
- *November 23:* The attorneys general from 46 states and the major U.S. tobacco companies negotiate a Master Settlement Agreement that does not require legislative affirmation from Congress. Among other provisions, the tobacco companies agree to pay a total of $246 billion over 25 years to the states in order to settle suits to recover Medicaid costs of treating smoking-related illness.

1999

- *March 9:* R. J. Reynolds announces it will sell its international tobacco unit to Japan Tobacco and split its tobacco and food divisions.
- *July 7:* In the first part of the *Engle v. R. J. Reynolds* class-action suit, a Florida jury concludes the tobacco companies are liable for the harm of their product because they conspired to conceal information about the health effects of smoking. The verdict represents the first successful class-action suit against the major tobacco companies, but determination of damages will follow in later parts of the trial.
- *September 15:* Worried that it might be subject to federal prosecution, online auction site eBay decides to prohibit the sale of tobacco.
- *November:* Payments to the states from the tobacco industry under the Master Settlement Agreement are set to begin.

2000

- *March 21:* The Supreme Court ultimately determines that the Food and Drug Administration does not have legislative authority to regulate tobacco as a drug.
- *July 14:* In a second verdict in the *Engle v. R. J. Reynolds* case, a Florida jury makes a record-setting award of $144.8 billion in damages.
- *October:* Officials from 150 nations meet at a World Health Organization summit in Geneva, Switzerland, to lay the groundwork for a global tobacco treaty.
- *November 3:* The European Commission files a civil racketeering lawsuit in the United States against Philip Morris and R. J. Reynolds.

123

The suit alleges that the companies are involved in efforts to smuggle cigarettes into Europe, and as a result European nations lose billions in import duties and taxes.

- *December 11:* Philip Morris acquires Nabisco Holdings, creating the world's second-largest food maker.
- *December 19:* Cigarette prices rise by about 17¢ a pack due to increases in the prices Philip Morris and R. J. Reynolds charge to wholesalers. The price rise stems in part from the costs of the tobacco settlement.

2001

- *June 28:* Acting on a Massachusetts case, the Supreme Court places limits on the ability of state and local governments to regulate tobacco advertising. The decision to give First Amendment protection is viewed as a victory for tobacco companies.
- *June 28:* Efforts of the Bush administration to settle the lawsuit brought against tobacco companies by the Justice Department lead to accusations that it has stepped back from Clinton administration efforts to protect the public's health against cigarette makers.
- *July 31:* Maryland's program to pay farmers to stop growing tobacco proves successful enough to eliminate much of the crop.
- *August 11:* The National Conference of State Legislators reports that states are spending most of the money from the Master Settlement Agreement on programs other than for smoking prevention and cessation.

2002

- *February 19:* Lorillard Tobacco Company sues the American Legacy Foundation for ads that vilify the tobacco companies. The suit claims that direct attacks on tobacco companies violate the 1998 Master Settlement Agreement.
- *March 21:* Given the successful tactics of antismoking advocates in the United States, the World Health Organization encourages other nations to use litigation in their antismoking efforts.
- *April 11:* The Centers for Disease Control and Prevention report estimates that smoking costs the nation $150 billion a year in health costs and lost work. That amount equals $3,391 a year for each smoker.
- *June 7:* A California judge rules that the R. J. Reynolds Tobacco Company continues to pursue advertising targeted at youth, which violates the 1998 Master Settlement Agreement. The company is fined $20 million.

Chronology

2003

- *March 5:* Weeks before a tough citywide antismoking ban goes into effect, Philip Morris announces that it will move its headquarters from New York City to Richmond, Virginia.
- *April 1:* Legislation signed earlier by New York City mayor Michael Bloomberg to ban smoking in bars, restaurants, prisons, and city-owned buildings goes into effect. The law depends largely on owners and patrons of bars and restaurants to voluntarily enforce the ban, but city inspectors begin issuing fines on May 1.
- *April 9:* Norway's parliament votes to make the country among the first in the world to outlaw smoking in bars and restaurants nationwide but delays the ban until spring 2004 to make the transition for smokers less difficult.
- *May 21:* In Geneva, Switzerland, more than 190 countries approve the first international treaty against smoking. The treaty requires countries to restrict tobacco advertising, sponsorship, and promotion within five years; lays down guidelines for health warnings; recommends tax increases on tobacco products; and calls for a crackdown on cigarette smuggling.
- *June 17:* To restrict the ability of smokers to purchase cigarettes over the Internet without paying state and city taxes, the state of New York begins enforcing a new law that prohibits shipping of cigarettes to anyone but a licensed dealer. The state, which has lost billions in taxes through Internet purchases over the past years, now faces the issue of how to enforce the law.
- *June 24:* Responding to the ban on Internet cigarette sales in New York State, Native American cigarette retailers challenge the law in state court. Native American businesses have been selling cigarettes over the Internet without charging state taxes.
- *July 15:* In a controversial raid that resulted in scuffling and arrests by police, agents of the state of Rhode Island entered the reservation of the Narragansett tribe and confiscated cigarettes from a store that had been selling them without charging taxes. Governor Don Carcieri defended the raid, which had a court-approved search warrant, as necessary given the illegal sales of cigarettes.

2004

- *May 28:* In releasing a new report, the U.S. Surgeon General Richard H. Carmona issues the government's strongest warning against smoking. Adding diseases newly shown to result from smoking, such as cataracts, pneumonia, and stomach cancer, to the long list of previously identified diseases, the report concludes that smoking harms nearly every organ in the body.

- *July 29:* R. J. Reynolds approves a $3 billion acquisition of Brown & Williamson Tobacco, a unit of British American Tobacco. The acquisition combines the second- and third-largest cigarette makers in the United States. While the details are complex, the purchase reflects the trend toward mergers as tobacco companies deal with a hostile environment for their products.

2005

- *February 7:* Cuba bans smoking in public places—including smoking of its famous cigars. In instituting the ban, the government and its leader, Fidel Castro, hope to convince the Cuban public of the dangers of tobacco.
- *February 27:* A global antitobacco treaty called the Framework Convention on Tobacco Control goes into effect. Though many have not yet ratified it, the treaty has been signed by 168 nations.
- *March:* Major credit card companies and eBay's PayPal service announce they will no longer accept payment for Internet cigarette purchases. State and federal government agencies had told the companies that their services were being used to make illegal cigarette purchases or to avoid state taxes on cigarette purchases. The companies' change in policy will largely end online purchases of cigarettes.
- *December 9:* A law goes into effect in Washington State that officials call the toughest statewide smoking ban in the nation. The law not only bans smoking indoors in public buildings, including bars and restaurants, but also requires smokers outside to stand 25 feet away from the entrance to a smoke-free building when lighting up. Business owners must enforce the law or face fines.

2006

- *February 9:* The American Cancer Society reports the first drop in the number of cancer deaths in 70 years. The drop reflects lower tobacco-related cancer deaths among men.
- *March 8:* In resolving a dispute between New York City and Internet sellers of cigarettes, the city obtains a list of customers of one company, eSmokes. To enforce its law taxing Internet sales of cigarettes, customers will be pursued to pay back taxes. The company also agrees not to sell cigarettes to residents of New York State.
- *July 26:* Altria, the parent company of Philip Morris, reports strong earnings, in part from international tobacco sales. The company sees long-term potential for profit in its international tobacco and food business

- *August 17:* A U.S. district judge rules that tobacco companies engaged in federal racketeering when, over many decades, they misled the public about the risks of light and low-tar cigarettes. The ruling requires tobacco companies to buy ads describing the dangers of smoking and stop using terms that imply safety in cigarettes.
- *October 12:* R. J. Reynolds reaches an agreement with 38 state attorneys general to stop selling sweetened or flavored cigarettes that, according to experts, appeal to young people. The attorneys general contend that these cigarettes violate the 1998 Master Settlement Agreement.
- *November 15:* Michael Bloomberg, New York City mayor and wealthy businessman, announces that he will donate $125 million to five organizations—the Campaign for Tobacco-Free Kids, Centers for Disease Control and Prevention Foundation, the Johns Hopkins Bloomberg School of Public Health, the World Health Organization, and the World Lung Foundation—to promote worldwide freedom from smoking.
- *November 27:* The Supreme Court lets stand an Illinois Supreme Court ruling that overturned a verdict against Philip Morris for misleading advertising about the safety of light cigarettes. After the Illinois Supreme Court decision, plaintiffs had hoped the Supreme Court would reinstate the $10.1 billion verdict given by a lower court. That it does not do so is a victory for the tobacco industry.

2007

- *February 15:* The Family Smoking Prevention and Public Health Protection Act is introduced in the Senate. The bill would give the U.S. Food and Drug Administration regulatory authority over tobacco, including control over sales, advertising, and marketing of tobacco products. Similar bills failed to pass earlier Congresses, but advocates expect that enough support exists to pass this one.
- *July:* Walt Disney Studios announces that it will eliminate smoking from its movies targeted at families. Other companies that make films for Disney will discourage, though not eliminate, smoking. Although hopeful, public health advocates say that the announcement needs to be followed with real action to prevent children from imitating actors smoking in films.
- *October 14:* California governor Arnold Schwarzenegger vetoes a bill that advocates say will close loopholes in the state's 1994 smoke-free workplace law. The American Cancer Society criticizes the veto, saying the bill would have made it easier to enforce smoking restrictions and protect workers from secondhand smoke.
- *November 1:* Altria Group, the parent company of Philip Morris, buys the John Middleton company, the maker of Black & Mild cigars, for $2.9

127

billion. The purchase reflects efforts of the company to respond to lower American cigarette use with investment in the growing market segment of cigars.

2008

- *January 1:* A French ban on smoking in public places, first instituted in February 1, 2007, now applies to cafés, bars, nightclubs, and restaurants. In response to lobbying, places of entertainment receive an extra 11 months to prepare for the ban. Smoking in French cafés had been a part of the nation's cultural folklore, and France waited longer than many other European Union nations to begin the ban.
- *January 1:* California extends its ban on smoking in public places to include smoking in cars with minor children present. The ban responds to evidence that children inhale dangerous fumes when in a car with a smoker. The fine for violation is $100, but police officers may not pull over a vehicle for the sole purpose of enforcing the ban.
- *February 1:* The U.S. Food and Drug Administration issues warnings that Chantix, an antismoking medication prescribed by physicians, can cause anxiety, nervousness, tension, depressed mood, unusual behaviors, suicidal thoughts, or suicide attempts. The maker of the drug, Pfizer, agrees to place warnings more prominently on the packaging, but critics say the company should withdraw the drug from the market.
- *May 1:* Following its promise to make the 2008 Beijing Olympics smoke free, Chinese authorities impose a partial smoking ban. Schools, hospitals, and offices in the capital city, but not restaurants and bars, fall under the smoking ban. With 350 million smokers, a government-owned tobacco company, and a culture that encourages smoking, even the partial ban signifies a step forward in tobacco control.
- *May 2:* An Oregon court rejects claims against tobacco companies based on future harm. A class-action suit requested that the companies pay for tests to detect lung cancer, but the court rules that the plaintiffs wanting to claim compensation must first prove that harm occurred. Had the suit succeeded, it would have greatly increased the liability of the tobacco industry.
- *July 1:* A law to ban cigarette smoking in public places, including restaurants, bars, and coffee shops, goes into effect in the Netherlands. In an unusual twist, the ban does not apply to smoking marijuana and hashish, which is legal in the country, as long as the drugs are not mixed with tobacco. Coffee shops selling marijuana and hashish objected strongly to a proposed ban of all smoking.
- *December 15:* In *Altria v. Good,* the Supreme Court rules that tobacco companies are liable for fraud because they made claims in the past that their light or low-tar cigarettes were safer than regular cigarettes. The

ruling clarifies disputes over whether Congress and the Federal Trade Commission had protected tobacco companies from such suits with laws requiring warnings on cigarette packs and policies defining terms such as *light* and *low tar.* The case goes back to Maine to be heard, but the ruling significantly favors smokers in their actions against tobacco companies.

CHAPTER 4

BIOGRAPHICAL LISTING

This chapter offers brief biographical information on people who have played major roles in developments since the 13th century in the tobacco industry and smoking. Historical figures include those who popularized the product in Europe and the United States, who built the modern tobacco industry, and who changed the perceptions of tobacco with research and antismoking advocacy. Current figures include those involved in litigation over tobacco, nonsmokers' rights movements, and legislation and regulation to control tobacco.

Dr. Oscar Auerbach, principal researcher in a 1967 project funded by the American Cancer Society. After teaching 86 beagles to smoke through small holes in their throats, he found that 12 of the dogs developed tumors. This finding received much public attention, despite some scientific questions about the validity of the study.

John F. Banzhaf III, New York City lawyer who petitioned the Federal Communications Commission (FCC) in 1966 to apply the fairness doctrine to cigarette advertising. The commission accepted the position and until the end of television and radio advertising of cigarettes, required that stations provide free airtime for anticigarette advertising. Much to the concern of the tobacco industry, these early antismoking ads proved effective. Banzhaf left New York City to become a law professor at George Washington University and found an antismoking organization, Action on Smoking and Health (ASH).

Michael Bloomberg, businessman, philanthropist, and mayor of New York City since 2001. As a former smoker, Bloomberg has shown strong support for public health in general and tobacco control more specifically. As mayor, he extended the city's smoking ban to all commercial establishments. As a wealthy citizen, he donated $125 million to American and worldwide charitable organizations for promoting freedom from smoking.

James Albert Bonsack, Lynchburg, Virginia, mechanic. He won a $75,000 contest in 1881 by inventing and patenting a cigarette-making machine that could roll more than 200 cigarettes a minute. The machine would replace skilled workers who hand rolled cigarettes and make James Buchanan Duke's cigarette business the most successful in the country.

Leo F. Burnett, founder and president of a Chicago-based advertising agency. He and his firm developed the highly successful Marlboro Man and Marlboro Country ad campaigns in the 1950s and 1960s that would for decades push Marlboro to among the nation's most popular cigarettes. The masculine, independent outdoorsman depicted in the ads became a cultural icon, a symbol of both the attraction to cigarettes and the misleading images advanced by the tobacco companies.

Dr. Leroy F. Burney, surgeon general in 1957. His early and mild statement that prolonged cigarette smoking could cause lung cancer received more in the way of harsh attacks from critics than recognition of the problem by the public. Yet the statement represented the start of efforts that would culminate in the 1964 Surgeon General's report on the harm of smoking.

George W. Bush, 43rd president of the United States. Antismoking critics of President Bush, who took office in 2001, claim that he backed away from the antitobacco efforts of the Clinton administration. As evidence to support their criticisms, they point to the nomination of Tommy Thompson, who as governor of Wisconsin had ties to the tobacco industry, to head the Department of Health and Human Services, and to the willingness to settle the Justice Department suit against tobacco companies to recover Medicare costs for smoking-related illnesses.

Joseph Califano, head of the Department of Health, Education, and Welfare under President Jimmy Carter. He proposed several actions in 1978 to fight cigarette smoking: raising taxes on cigarettes, using the government proceeds for antismoking campaigns and programs, eliminating smoking on airplanes and in restaurants, and ending government subsidies to tobacco growers. With little support from others in the Carter administration, opposition from tobacco growers, retail establishments, and the tobacco industry was sufficient to block these proposals.

Richard H. Carmona, a physician and former surgeon general of the United States from 2002 to 2006. As surgeon general, Carmona sponsored several reports on the health dangers of smoking. One report concluded that secondhand smoke represents a serious health hazard and advocated smoking bans in bars and restaurants. Another report concluded that smoking harms nearly every organ in the body. He later accused the Bush administration of attempting to water down his conclusions on secondhand smoke.

Fidel Castro, leader of an armed revolution that brought him to power and president of Cuba from 1959 to 2008. A smoker of Cuban cigars since age 15, Castro often appeared in public with a cigar in hand. In 1986, he quit the habit for health reasons, and in 2005 Cuba announced a ban on smoking in some public places.

Rose Cipollone, smoker who died of lung cancer shortly after filing suit against several tobacco companies. Her husband became the first person to win damages against tobacco companies (but lost the award on appeal). Growing up in New York City, Cipollone had started smoking at age 16 and eventually smoked a pack and a half each day. In 1981 an X ray showed a lesion in her lung that upon biopsy proved to be a malignant growth. Despite two lung operations, the cancer returned to her lungs by 1984 and soon spread to her brain and the rest of her body. Alive to file the suit in 1983, she died on October 21, 1984.

William J. Clinton, 42nd president of the United States (1993–2001), the first to take an active stand against smoking and the tobacco industry. In his administration smoking was banned in the White House; regulations to control tobacco sales, advertising, and promotions were implemented (although later disallowed by the Supreme Court); and a Justice Department suit was filed against tobacco companies to recover Medicare costs for smoking-related illnesses.

Christopher Columbus, explorer who, in aiming to sail west to reach the Near East, discovered the New World. Supported in his 1492 expedition by King Ferdinand and Queen Isabella of Spain, he landed on a small island in the Bahamas and later sailed to Cuba. There some of his crew became the first Europeans to smoke tobacco. Columbus returned with some tobacco leaves and seeds, but Europeans paid little attention to the product until nearly 60 years later.

Robert Dole, former Republican senator from Kansas and presidential nominee of the Republican Party in the 1996 election. He stated during the presidential campaign that tobacco is not addictive for some people and that the government should not regulate it. Strong criticism of the statement came from President Bill Clinton, the media, and antismoking groups.

Sir Francis Drake, English explorer who circumnavigated the globe between 1577 and 1580. During his expedition he obtained tobacco from native peoples off the southwestern coast of North America and returned to England with samples.

James Buchanan Duke (Buck Duke), entrepreneur most responsible for the shape of the modern tobacco industry. In 1874 he joined his father and brother to found a tobacco firm in Durham, North Carolina. Eventually taking over, Duke showed his tremendous organizational and managerial skills in creating a successful cigarette business. He mechanized production, spent lavishly on advertising, cut prices significantly, and became the nation's largest cigarette manufacturer. Having pressured his major competitors to join him, he formed the American Tobacco Company in

1890 and became, at age 33, the first president. Although wildly successful and rich from his efforts, the trust he created was dissolved in 1911 for violating antitrust laws. The breakup created most of the companies that would dominate the industry over the 20th century.

Marc Z. Edell, lawyer who applied the case law used in suits by victims of asbestos products to suits by victims of smoking and tobacco. On behalf of his client, Rose Cipollone (and her surviving husband), in her suit against the Liggett Group, Philip Morris, and Loews Corporation (owner of Lorillard), each a maker of cigarettes that Cipollone had smoked, he became the first lawyer to win damages in a smoking case, in 1988. His arguments relied on changes in product liability law that had occurred during the 1960s and 1970s. These changes made companies more responsible for damages incurred by use of a dangerous product. Edell had more success against the tobacco companies than others before him, but he ultimately failed in his efforts when the initial award was overturned on appeal.

Dr. Hans Eysenck, well-known and respected psychologist in England. He suggested that persons with certain personality traits were prone to both smoking and early death. His research, published in 1965, showed that those unable to express anger, fear, and anxiety had a high risk of getting cancer. If those same traits led to smoking, the association between smoking and lung cancer might be spurious.

Benjamin Franklin, American patriot and pipe smoker. Using tobacco as collateral, he negotiated loans from France to support the Revolutionary War (1775–83).

Lucy Page Gaston, schoolteacher who nearly halted the fast spread of cigarette use around the turn of the 20th century. In 1899 she used the model of antialcohol groups in founding the Chicago Anti-Cigarette League. Two years later she founded the National Anti-Cigarette League and soon became one of the country's most well-known reformers. She held rallies in schools and towns in which she decried the poisons brought into the body by cigarettes and noted cases of known murderers and criminals who smoked. She further recruited converts to her organization, promoted health clinics in cities that smokers could use to quit the habit, and urged legislatures to ban the product. In 1920 she ran for the Republican Party presidential nomination. The movement led to the outlawing of cigarettes in 21 states during the first two decades of the 20th century but ultimately failed to stop the growth of cigarettes.

Lewis Ginter, leading U.S. tobacco producer until the 1880s. First using bright tobacco to produce cigarettes, he found success with his excellent marketing and sales skills. However, his major contribution came from the use of a new tobacco leaf, white burley, in cigarettes. Ginter used the new leaf, which could incorporate more flavoring than others, in several types of cigarettes. The new blends created a distinctively American style of cigarette that differed from Turkish and Russian cigarettes and could be sold at a cheaper price than the foreign imports.

Stanton Glantz, professor at the School of Medicine, University of California, San Francisco. The longtime critic of tobacco received more than 4,000 pages of secret internal industry documents in the mail from an unknown source in 1994. He publicized the damaging information contained in the documents, which increased the ability of plaintiffs to make the case that industry leaders misled them about the risks of smoking. Although he played a role in pushing the tobacco companies toward a settlement with the states over Medicaid cost reimbursement, he ultimately opposed any bargaining and urged states to do all they could to bankrupt tobacco companies.

Al Gore, senator from Tennessee, vice president of the United States (1992–2001), and presidential candidate in 2000. As a senator, he helped to negotiate the 1984 Comprehensive Smoking Education Act and prevent the blockage of the bill by tobacco interests. The act required more stringent warnings on cigarette packages.

Ulysses S. Grant, 18th president of the United States (1868–76) and victim of throat cancer. He smoked cigars throughout his life as a farmer, soldier, general in the Civil War, and president of the United States. Upon making a diagnosis that Grant had throat cancer, his doctor recommended cutting down on cigars to three a day, but Grant soon died of the disease.

John Hawkins, admiral in the English navy who with his sailors brought tobacco to England after a voyage to the Caribbean in 1562. The use of chewing tobacco became common among sailors but did not spread yet to the English population.

George Washington Hill, a successor of James Duke as president of the American Tobacco Company. Hill fully exploited the potential of advertising to increase sales of cigarettes. His efforts made Lucky Strike, a brand introduced in 1916 with the slogan "It's Toasted," tops in sales by the end of the 1920s. He also appealed to the new market of women smokers by linking cigarettes to youth and beauty—a strategy cigarette advertisers would continue. His efforts helped make cigarettes widely fashionable.

King James I, king of England (1603–25) and one of the first to speak out against tobacco. In 1604 he wrote *A Counterblaste to Tobacco*, which described smoking as filthy, stinking, vile, sinful, shameful, dangerous, and loathsome. The pamphlet contested the claims of the most famous English advocate of smoking, Walter Raleigh, and aimed to stop the growth of a habit of rising popularity. Having had little influence with the pamphlet, however, James I took steps to tax the import of the product.

Biographical Listing

John F. Kennedy, 35th president of the United States (1961–63). He made a request in 1962 to the surgeon general to convene a group that would evaluate the evidence on smoking and health. The action led two years later to the Surgeon General's report on smoking and health that warned the public of the dangers of cigarettes.

Dr. David Kessler, commissioner of the Food and Drug Administration (FDA) in the Bill Clinton administration. Proposing regulations to treat tobacco as a drug, he argued that cigarettes served as a nicotine-delivery system, that tobacco companies used their knowledge of the addictiveness of nicotine to make their cigarettes more addictive, and that the FDA could control the product based on existing legislation, much as it controlled nicotine gum and patches. The regulations would restrict the sale and distribution of cigarettes and smokeless tobacco products to children and adolescence. They would also require tobacco companies to support tobacco prevention education for children, take actions to ensure underage youth would not have access to cigarettes through vending machines or other unsupervised sales, ban gift or promotional items bearing cigarette brand names, eliminate outdoor advertising near schools, and limit advertising in publications with more than 15 percent of the readership under age 18. President Clinton announced the publication of the final FDA rules on August 23, 1996. However, suits by tobacco companies against the regulations led to a decision by the Supreme Court that existing law did not allow regulation of tobacco as a drug.

F. S. Kinney, first tobacco producer to successfully mix American bright tobacco with foreign tobaccos. After opening a small cigarette shop in Lower Manhattan in 1868, he hired foreign-born cigarette rollers to make his product, sold cigarettes in paper packages, and became the leading manufacturer in the new industry. His brand, Sweet Caporal, which contained a mix of flavors and sweeteners, became the first with a national rather than local following. As the business grew, he relocated the factories to Richmond, Virginia; the town would become a center of the tobacco industry.

Dr. C. Everett Koop, pediatric surgeon and evangelical Christian appointed as surgeon general during the Ronald Reagan administration. Although first known for his antiabortion views, he became a forceful and charismatic antismoking advocate. During the 1980s he authored reports calling cigarette smoking the nation's number one public health problem, identifying environmental tobacco smoke as a cause of cancer, and emphasizing the strongly addictive nature of nicotine. He fiercely and relentlessly attacked smoking and tobacco makers, and his leadership helped promote antismoking efforts.

Bennett LeBow, CEO of the Brooke Group, which owned the Liggett Group and Liggett Tobacco, the smallest of the major tobacco companies.

He broke ranks with the larger companies in deciding to negotiate with state attorneys general who sued to recover Medicaid costs for treating smoking-related illnesses. He worried that the suits would bankrupt the company and had little confidence that the legal strategy of the tobacco companies would prove successful. His defection in settling with the state attorneys general in 1997 led to the eventual settlement with all the major tobacco companies. He admitted on behalf of his company that cigarettes are addictive and included such a warning on the cigarettes his company manufactured.

Mike Moore, Mississippi attorney general since 1988. In 1994 he filed the first state Medicaid suit against the tobacco industry and helped convince other state attorneys general to file their own suits. Based on the suggestion of a friend, he proposed the new strategy of using litigation on behalf of taxpayers rather than smokers. Along with Richard Scruggs and Ron Motley, he brought tobacco companies to the negotiating table and to settlements with the state of Mississippi and with 46 states in the Master Settlement Agreement.

Ron Motley, plaintiff's attorney in state Medicaid suits against tobacco companies. He helped develop the legal strategy with Richard Scruggs for the 1994 case in Mississippi and represented nearly every state that brought a similar suit. Known for his brilliant courtroom tactics, he had already made millions suing asbestos companies. As he told interviewers, he jointed the antitobacco suits because he wanted to expose the dishonesty and damage of the tobacco industry and because his mother (and hundreds of thousands of others like her) had died from a smoking-related disease.

Jean Nicot, appointed French ambassador to Portugal in 1559 under Henri II and Catherine de Médicis. After learning to raise tobacco in the French embassy in Lisbon and concluding that it had strong curative powers, he sent plants and seeds to the queen of France, who was attracted to herbs and potions. Taken as snuff, tobacco soon became popular in the French court and spread quickly throughout the country. In recognition of his role in promoting the product, scientists named the tobacco plant— *Nicotiana*—after him.

Dr. Raymond K. Pearl, medical researcher at Johns Hopkins University. In 1938 he published the first study in the United States to scientifically identify a link between smoking and life expectancy. Based on his access to the medical records of a sample of 6,813 men, he found that only 45 percent of smokers lived to age 60, compared to 65 percent of nonsmokers.

Walter Raleigh, English soldier, explorer, and favorite of Queen Elizabeth I who helped popularize tobacco smoking in his country. After returning from an expedition in 1586 to Virginia, Raleigh used smoking as a symbol of adventure. Pipe smoking spread to the court of England and then to the rest of society. However, he ran afoul of King James I, who detested the habit and Raleigh's independence, and was executed in 1618 for disobeying the king's orders.

Richard J. Reynolds, founder of R. J. Reynolds Tobacco Company. He was forced by economic pressure to merge his company with James Buchanan Duke's to form the American Tobacco Company. With the breakup of the trust in 1911, Reynolds gained back his old company but started out as the smallest of the four new tobacco companies. The introduction in 1913 of Camel cigarettes, a brand with an appealing mix of American and foreign tobaccos and an intriguing advertising campaign, made his company one of the nation's most successful.

John Rolfe, early English settler of Jamestown, Virginia, who married the Wampanoag princess Pocahontas. He helped cultivate, cure, and ship to England the first successful tobacco crop. Although Jamestown would not survive, the production of tobacco would become the major crop of Virginia and a source of much profit when sold in England.

Theodore Roosevelt (Teddy Roosevelt), 26th president of the United States (1901–09) who reformed the regulation of business by attacking trusts that reduced competition. Under his administration efforts began to dissolve the cigarette and tobacco trust that James Buchanan Duke had formed with the American Tobacco Company. The efforts ended in 1911, after Roosevelt had left the presidency, with the breakup of the trust into four tobacco companies that would dominate the industry for the next 50 years.

Benjamin Rush, prominent physician and signer of the Declaration of Independence. He authored the first significant antitobacco document in the United States, "Observations upon the Influence of the Habitual Use of Tobacco upon Health, Morals, and Property," in 1798.

H. Lee Sarokin, a New Jersey federal court judge who presided over the *Cipollone* case. Seen as an opponent of the tobacco industry, he made decisions in the *Cipollone* case in 1988 that higher courts overruled. Still later, tobacco industry defendants accused him of having shown bias against the industry and had him removed from tobacco cases.

Arnold Schwarzenegger, bodybuilding champion, actor, businessman, and governor of California since 2003. An avid cigar smoker, Schwarzenegger has set up outdoor tents where he can conduct state business while complying with smoking bans in government buildings. Some antismoking groups have criticized the governor for not doing more to enforce and expand California's antismoking laws, which are among the toughest in the nation.

Richard Scruggs, Mississippi lawyer who played a crucial role in the Master Settlement Agreement. After making millions suing asbestos companies on behalf of injured workers, he worked with the state of Mississippi in its 1994 litigation to recover state costs for treating Medicaid patients with smoking-related illnesses from tobacco companies. Scruggs brought in famous trial attorney Ron Motley and fronted the costs of the suit in return for contingency fees. During the process Scruggs protected whistle-blowers Merrill Williams and Jeffrey Wigand and convinced Bennett LeBow, the head of Liggett Tobacco, to defect from other companies that wanted to fight the suit. In the end Scruggs negotiated an agreement in Mississippi, worked on the Florida suit to recover its Medicaid costs for smoking-related illnesses, and helped broker the Master Settlement Agreement in 1998.

Mike Synar, Democratic representative from Oklahoma who sponsored an antismoking amendment to the Alcohol, Drug Abuse, and Mental Health Administration Reorganization Act. His 1992 amendment required states to adopt and enforce minimum age laws for tobacco sales and to demonstrate reductions in the retail availability of tobacco products. The federal government does not have authority over state laws, but failure of states to follow these strictures would, under the amendment, result in the loss of federal block grant funds for substance abuse prevention and treatment.

Dr. Luther E. Terry, surgeon general during the administrations of John F. Kennedy and Lyndon Johnson. He convened a panel of experts to evaluate the evidence on the health risks of smoking in 1962 and sponsored in 1964 *A Report of the Surgeon General on Health and Smoking.* More than a summary of scientific findings, the report and the recommended actions bluntly told people interested in their health and a long life to give up or avoid smoking. The publicity received by the report created a stir among the public and serious problems for tobacco companies. Moreover future surgeons general would follow with additional reports that became increasingly strong in their criticism of the use of tobacco and helped to galvanize antismoking movements.

Henry Waxman, Democratic representative from California and persistent foe of the tobacco industry. He held hearings in the House of Representatives on the business practices of tobacco companies and developed a bill that would more stringently control tobacco advertising. Although he did not obtain all the provisions he wanted, Waxman with the aid of Senator Al Gore was able to get an antismoking bill passed (the 1984 Comprehensive Smoking Education Act) that required rotating of four new warning statements on both packages and advertisements. Waxman also was largely responsible for bringing chief executives of the major tobacco firms to a congressional hearing and having them state their belief that smoking was not addictive—testimony that was later contradicted by internal industry documents.

Jeffrey Wigand, biochemistry Ph.D. who worked as vice president of research at Brown & Williamson Tobacco. He became the highest-level industry executive to speak to the media about the industry's efforts to strengthen the nicotine chemical in its cigarettes. He testified in 1995 on behalf of the state of Mississippi in its suit against tobacco companies, claiming that Brown & Williamson hid damaging scientific information about addiction. After appearing on the television news show *60 Minutes* in 1996, he was accused by Brown & Williamson of misconduct, but his testimony proved crucial in the successful suits against the tobacco industry since then. His story was depicted in the movie *The Insider*, starring Russell Crowe.

Merrill Williams, a smoker and paralegal at a Louisville law firm who leaked damaging tobacco industry internal documents. Given the task in 1994 of cataloguing documents from Brown & Williamson in preparation for suits against the company, he found information in the documents that revealed company knowledge of the addictiveness of cigarettes as early as in 1963, the use of carcinogens in cigarettes, and efforts to target young people. He made copies and passed them to Richard Scruggs, the lawyer representing the state of Mississippi in its Medicaid suit against the tobacco companies. Although the documents were stolen, they eventually became public information and were used in suits against tobacco companies.

Dr. Ernest Wynder, pioneering researcher on the health consequences of smoking and outspoken critic of tobacco use. As a medical student at Washington University in St. Louis, he demonstrated with his professor, Dr. Evarts A. Graham, that a connection existed between smoking and lung cancer. His influential study, published in 1950, showed that 96.5 percent of the lung cancer patients smoked compared to 73.7 percent of the other patients. Other studies by E. Cuyler Hammond and Daniel Horn and by Richard Doll and A. Bradford Hill in the 1950s further contributed to the early evidence of the harm of smoking, but more than other researchers, Wynder became a strong and forceful critic of cigarette use. Despite much resistance from other medical researchers at the time, Wynder continued research to demonstrate the harm of smoking for health.

CHAPTER 5

GLOSSARY

Some terms, phrases, and organizations used in the previous chapters have specialized meanings relating to the tobacco industry and smoking. This chapter lists and defines these words and names in terms appropriate for general readers.

Action on Smoking and Health (ASH)   A national charitable antismoking and nonsmokers' rights organization that primarily brings legal action in support of a smoke-free society.

addiction   A compulsive need for a substance that produces withdrawal symptoms when stopped and requires increasingly larger amounts to produce the desired response. The Office of the Surgeon General similarly defines addiction as behavior controlled by a substance that causes changes in mood from its effects on the brain.

additive   A product, such as flavors and chemicals, that does not naturally occur in the tobacco plant but is added to cigarettes and other tobacco products in the manufacturing process.

American Cancer Society (ACS)   A nationwide, community-based voluntary health organization dedicated to eliminating cancer as a major health problem. It early on expressed concerns about the potential for smoking to cause cancer and has campaigned against smoking.

American Heart Association (AHA)   A national voluntary health agency committed to reducing disability and death from cardiovascular diseases and strokes. Given the connection between smoking and heart disease, the organization has played an active role in antismoking efforts.

American Medical Association (AMA)   An organization of physicians that advocates on behalf of the medical profession and has since the 1980s taken a strong position of opposition to smoking and tobacco advertising.

American Public Health Association (APHA)   An organization of professionals concerned with a broad set of public health issues, including advocacy of a smoke-free society.

Glossary

ammonia A chemical compound with a noxious aroma that is often used with water for cleaning. Small amounts have sometimes been added to cigarettes to boost the impact of nicotine on the human body.

antidepressant A drug such as bupropion, Prozac, or Zoloft that is used to relieve symptoms of psychological depression and may also moderate withdrawal symptoms from stopping smoking.

asthma A condition often caused by allergies that involves coughing, breathing problems, and feelings of constriction in the chest. Children living with smoking parents are at higher risk of asthma than others.

bidi A small brown tobacco product used commonly in India and occasionally used by youth in the United States. It consists of tobacco that is hand rolled in a leaf and tied at one end by a string.

Blue Cross/Blue Shield (BC/BS) A private health care insurance company that through its many chapters provides health insurance to more than 80 million people. It has pursued tobacco companies legally to recover its costs for treating smoking-related illnesses.

Bonsack machine A 1880 invention that pours tobacco from a feeder onto a small strip of paper, rolls a single continuous tube, and cuts the tube into equal length cigarettes. The machine did much to help increase cigarette production and sales.

bright tobacco A popular American tobacco grown in Virginia and North Carolina that, when cured with heat, develops an unusually sweet and pleasant taste and can be smoked in greater quantities than other tobaccos.

bronchitis In its chronic form, the serious inflammation of the bronchial tubes that lead to the lungs.

cancer A disorderly, uncontrolled growth of abnormal body cells that, as they multiply, invade and push aside the organs of the body. Malignant cancerous growths eventually interfere with normal body functions and result in death. Tobacco and smoking cause cancer in the lungs, esophagus, mouth, throat, and a variety of other organs.

carbon monoxide A colorless, odorless, and highly toxic gas that is contained in small amounts in tobacco smoke.

carcinogen A substance or agent producing or inciting cancer.

Centers for Disease Control and Prevention (CDC) A federal agency with the mission to promote health and quality of life by preventing and controlling disease, injury, and disability. It has been active in protecting health and safety through antismoking research.

chewing tobacco (chew) A form of smokeless tobacco that is placed as a small clump inside the mouth and next to the cheek. Usually flavored, it allows nicotine to be absorbed through the tissue of the oral cavity and requires spitting to eliminate tobacco juices from the mouth.

chronic obstructive pulmonary disease (COPD)   A category of illnesses typified by chronic bronchitis and emphysema that block the flow of air to the lungs. The disease is often caused by smoking.

cigar   A dried, prepared, and rolled tobacco leaf used for smoking. Unlike cigarettes, cigar smoke is seldom fully inhaled, but nicotine from the smoke can, though less efficiently than in the lungs, be absorbed in the mouth.

cigarette   A slender roll of cut tobacco used for smoking. The tobacco for cigarettes makes inhaling pleasurable and absorption of nicotine through the lungs efficient.

Civil Aeronautics Board (CAB)   An independent agency of the federal government that regulates airline activities, include smoking on airplanes.

class action   A legal action undertaken by one or more plaintiffs on behalf of themselves and all other persons who have an interest in the alleged wrong.

class certified   To bring a class-action suit, a class must be certified by showing that the class members share the same interests, can be fairly represented as a class, and is too large to allow lawsuits to be tried individually for each member.

compensatory damages   Damages awarded for injury or loss, including expenses, loss of time, and physical and mental suffering.

curing   The drying process used to prepare tobacco for market. The different methods of curing—flue cured (by heat from pipes or flues connected to a furnace); air cured (from air while suspended in barns for five weeks); fire cured (by heat from wood fires underneath); and sun cured (while outside in the sunshine for four weeks)—help give different flavor and texture to tobacco products.

emphysema   A type of chronic obstructive pulmonary disease that involves dilation of air spaces in the lungs and makes absorption of oxygen difficult.

Environmental Protection Agency (EPA)   A federal agency that protects human life and the natural environment. It has labeled cigarette smoke as a dangerous carcinogen.

environmental tobacco smoke (ETS)   Smoke in the air exhaled by smokers or emitted from the burning tips of cigarettes in between puffs. Most public health experts believe it poses a health risk to nonsmokers who breathe it in. It is also called secondhand smoke.

excise tax   A tax added to a product before sale. Used specifically to gain revenue from and increase the price of cigarettes, excise taxes differ from sales taxes, which are placed on products in general and are added after the sale.

fairness doctrine   A guiding principle that the Federal Communications Commission (FCC) employed to regulate electronic media before cable television. Based on the view that the airways are a public resource, the doctrine required equal time for presentation of competing views, usually by politicians and political parties. However, the FCC extended the doctrine to require the airing of antismoking ads as a means to balance smoking advertisements.

Federal Communications Commission (FCC)   An independent agency of the federal government that regulates television and radio broadcasting and in so doing ruled under the fairness doctrine that stations presenting cigarette ads must provide airtime for antismoking commercials.

Federal Trade Commission (FTC)   A federal agency that enforces laws against unfair business practices and since the 1950s has battled with tobacco companies over misrepresentation in cigarette advertising.

filters or filter tips   Fibrous material placed within one end of the cigarette tube that removes some of the harmful matter when tobacco smoke passes through it.

First Amendment   The amendment to the U.S. Constitution that specifies Congress will make no law abridging the freedom of speech or of the press. The interpretation of the amendment proved crucial in allowing congressional legislation to ban television and radio cigarette ads.

Food and Drug Administration (FDA)   A federal agency devoted to promoting and protecting the nation's public health by approving and monitoring food ingredients, drugs, and medical products.

globalization   The process of creating greater ties across nations of the globe through exchange of products through trade, information through the media, and people through travel and immigration. As part of this process, cigarettes and cigarette advertising have rapidly spread across the globe in recent years.

Group Against Smokers' Pollution (GASP)   A nonsmoker's rights organization that works to eliminate tobacco smoke from the air, educate the public about secondhand smoke, and promote smoke-free policies.

Havana cigar   A premium type of cigar made from Cuban tobacco and highly prized for its flavor. Since an embargo on Cuban products, this cigar type has been difficult to obtain in the United States.

heart disease   A life-threatening illness that typically involves blockage of the arteries that feed blood to the heart by a fatty substance called plaque. Smoking causes heart disease in part by injuring the heart vessels in ways that promote the buildup of plaque. The carbon monoxide in cigarette smoke also contributes to heart disease by blocking absorption of oxygen into the blood.

involuntary smoking   Inhaling environmental tobacco or secondhand smoke.

Joe Camel   A cartoon character reintroduced in 1988 by R. J. Reynolds Tobacco to promote Camel cigarettes. The ad campaign proved successful but was harshly criticized for attracting children and youth to smoking.

liability Legal responsibility for an act or omission, as for example, when cigarette manufacturers are held responsible for the harm of their product.

Master Settlement Agreement (MSA) Following negotiations between the major tobacco companies and state attorneys general, this agreement required tobacco companies to pay states $246 billion for the costs of treating smoking-related illnesses of Medicaid patients. It also restricted advertising, marketing, and promotional activities targeted at youth.

Medicaid A public program to pay for medical care of those unable to afford it and financed largely by states with aid from the federal government.

Medicare A public program to pay for medical care of the elderly and financed largely by the federal government.

Nicotiana tabacum One of some 60 species of plants within the *Nicotiana* genus that is most commonly used by Europeans and Americans for smoking and chewing products.

nicotine A chemical compound found in tobacco plants and tobacco smoke that can be absorbed through the body's cell membrane walls. Poisonous in large amounts, the chemical in small amounts is both stimulating and relaxing in ways that make it addictive.

nicotine replacement therapy The use of gum, patches, inhalers, and nasal sprays to moderate the withdrawal symptoms caused by smoking cessation. The products used in the therapy provide the body with its need for nicotine while avoiding the harm of cigarette tar and gases. Ideally the therapy allows former smokers to slowly reduce their nicotine consumption until the withdrawal symptoms become minor.

passive smoking Inhaling environmental tobacco or secondhand smoke.

pipe A tube of varying lengths connected to a bowl of various sizes in which specially prepared and often flavored tobacco is packed, lit, and smoked. Unlike cigarettes, pipe smoke is seldom fully inhaled, but nicotine from the smoke can, though less efficiently than in the lungs, be absorbed in the mouth.

plug A popular type of chewing tobacco.

point-of-purchase advertisement An advertisement displayed at retail outlets where products are sold. Despite laws banning cigarette advertisements from television and radio, companies have until recently been able to advertise to youth through store displays.

public health A science devoted to protection of the health of members of a community and population through preventive medicine and sanitary living conditions. It differs from clinical medicine that is based on the observation, diagnosis, and treatment of individual patients and has much relevance to the health effects in communities and populations of cigarette use.

punitive damages Damages awarded above and beyond compensatory damages to punish a negligent party for wanton, reckless, or malicious acts or omissions.

relative risk ratio A measure of the health effects of smoking that shows the number of smokers who die from a particular disease for each non-smoker who dies of the disease. For example, a relative risk ratio of 22 indicates that for every male nonsmoker who dies of lung cancer, 22 male smokers die.

roll-your-own (hand-rolled) cigarettes Cigarettes made by pouring a small amount of finely grained tobacco onto a small paper, rolling the paper and tobacco into a tube, and licking the paper to seal the tube.

"safe" cigarette Products that reduce the tar, nicotine, secondhand smoke, and additives of cigarettes, and that aim to make cigarettes safer to smoke. Experts on both sides of the issues agree, however, that all tobacco products are inherently unsafe, even if some products are less unsafe than others.

secondhand smoke Environmental tobacco smoke.

smokeless tobacco Tobacco in the form of snuff or chew that does not require smoking or inhalation but nonetheless delivers nicotine to the body.

smuggling Process of secretly moving large amounts of products across borders, without paying import or export duties and taxes. As taxes on cigarettes increase the problem of smuggling becomes more serious. European nations have accused U.S. tobacco companies of helping to smuggle cigarettes into Europe to avoid taxes and sell them at cheaper prices. Domestically some state officials are concerned about cigarettes bought without taxes on Native American lands and over the Internet.

snuff A form of powdered and (usually) flavored smokeless tobacco that is placed between the lower gum and lip, or (mostly in the past) sniffed into the nose.

stillbirth A fetus dead at birth, an outcome that occurs more often among mothers who smoked during pregnancy than those who did not smoke.

Students Helping Others Understand Tobacco (SHOUT) An intensive and long-term program designed to reduce smoking among youth.

tar A general term that encompasses particles contained in the residue or by-product of the burning of tobacco and are inhaled with tobacco smoke. It is a major source of the harmful effects of tobacco use on health but also a major source of tobacco flavor.

tar derby A term used to describe the competition among cigarette manufacturers over sales of low-tar cigarettes that occurred in the 1950s when evidence of the harm of smoking for health began to emerge. The low tar and health claims made on behalf of cigarettes became so confusing that the Federal Trade Commission took over the testing for cigarette tar.

Tobacco Industry Research Council (TIRC) An organization formed by U.S. tobacco companies in 1954 to counter the negative publicity about cigarettes with its own studies, press releases, and information on smoking.

Tobacco Institute (TI) A trade organization in Washington, D.C., that was funded by tobacco firms and promoted the interests of the tobacco industry.

tort A wrongful act or breach of contract that may warrant payment to the wronged party of monetary damages.

trust A combination of firms or corporations formed by legal arrangement particularly for the purpose of reducing competition. The American Tobacco Company formed a trust among the major cigarette manufacturers in 1890.

Turkish tobacco A type of tobacco from Turkey with a mild fragrance that comprised a popular type of imported cigarette in the 19th century. Cigarettes grew in popularity when tobacco companies blended it with American tobacco and sold the new blends at lower prices than the imported cigarettes.

warranty An assurance or guarantee of legal standing, as for example, in the claims of tobacco companies that their products were safe and not addictive. A warranty may be expressed or implied.

white burley tobacco A popular American tobacco first developed in Ohio in 1866 that could absorb additives better and had higher nicotine content than other tobacco products.

withdrawal The syndrome of painful physical and psychological symptoms that comes from the discontinuation of an addictive substance.

Women's Christian Temperance Union (WCTU) An organization founded in 1874 that advocated total abstinence from alcohol and opposed related behaviors such as smoking.

World Health Organization (WHO) An agency of the United Nations devoted to helping people throughout the world obtain the highest possible level of health. It has in recent years made special efforts to stop the global spread of cigarette use.

PART II

GUIDE TO FURTHER RESEARCH

CHAPTER 6

HOW TO RESEARCH
THE TOBACCO INDUSTRY
AND SMOKING

Beginning researchers face a number of challenges in studying the tobacco industry and smoking. First, they can become easily overwhelmed by the amount of information available on the topic. Used in Europe for 500 years and in North America for an even longer period, tobacco has spread further in recent decades to become one of the world's most widely used products. The numbers seem astounding: Across the world, close to 1 billion men and 250 million women are smokers, and they consume 15 billion cigarettes a day. Given the wide use and serious harm of cigarettes, the embattled multinational tobacco industry has similarly received much attention, being subject to antismoking legislation, litigation, and international treaties.

The importance of global tobacco use and the damage it causes have made it one of the most researched products in the world. It has relevance to issues of health, medicine, law, chemistry, biochemistry, politics, public policy, social life, psychology, economics, business, advertising, and education. No wonder the amount of available information is so vast. It spans traditional academic fields, specialized areas of research, national borders, and historical periods. Without some guidance, those new to these issues may find it difficult to comprehend the diverse information they uncover.

Second, the literature on the tobacco industry and smoking often reflects strong moral views and opinions. Once debates centered on the possible harm of smoking for health, but those debates have been settled—even the tobacco companies today admit that smoking brings risks. Debates over the addictiveness of nicotine have also largely died down as scientific evidence has shown strong similarities between use of cigarettes and addictive drugs such as cocaine and heroin. Some scholars deny such addictiveness, but they remain a minority. Instead the debates today center on the conflict between the freedom of individuals to choose their own lifestyle—however self-destructive—and the goals of public health to reduce sickness and premature death in the population. On the former side stand smokers and those devoted to political philosophies of liberty and individual choice. On the latter side stand the government and physicians who believe that society should do all it can outside of banning tobacco use to eliminate the activity. Some antismoking advocates see smoking as immoral, smokers as victimized, and cigarette makers as villains. In terms of public opinion most people side with the public health advocates and view smoking with distaste, but few would deny smokers the choice to continue their habit. Congress reveals a similar split in views, with antismoking advocates unable to pass legislation over the resistance of those committed to freedom of choice and supportive of business interests. In any case, writings on the tobacco industry and smoking do not always make these underlying views explicit, and researchers need to be aware of them.

Third, research on the tobacco industry and smoking often includes technically difficult matter. Some of the writings focus on the chemistry of cigarettes, smoke, and nicotine, and therefore go beyond the understanding of most nonscientists. Only slightly less problematic, the widespread use of statistical methods in tobacco-related research, even research addressing issues of general importance to the public, can be daunting. In understanding the harm of smoking for health, the evidence comes not from clinical observations of physicians and nurses; rather it comes from the statistical comparison of the health and mortality of smokers and nonsmokers. Similarly, in understanding the psychological and social patterns of smoking, the facts come from statistical analysis of group behaviors. Even efforts to understand the effects of public policies—taxes, advertising restrictions, smoking-prevention programs—rely on statistical techniques to separate real influences from false ones. Issues of randomness of samples, validity of measurements, and appropriateness of statistical techniques that come into play relate more to the skills of specialists than of general researchers. Readers of studies thus run across intimidating terms such as *relative risk ratios, statistical significance*, and *confidence intervals*.

How can researchers overcome these challenges? Here are some general suggestions, followed by more specific advice about where to find material.

TIPS FOR RESEARCHING THE TOBACCO INDUSTRY AND SMOKING

Here are some general suggestions:

- **Define the topic carefully.** To avoid being overwhelmed by the vast amount of material on the tobacco industry and smoking, beginning researchers need to decide in specific terms what aspects of the larger topic they want to examine. The annotated bibliography in Chapter 7 divides writings into six categories: 1) history and background, 2) health and medical aspects, 3) social and psychological aspects, 4) the tobacco business and litigation, 5) tobacco control, and 6) self-help. However, even these categories likely need to be narrowed down. If interested in the history of tobacco, researchers should then decide if they want to focus more specifically on the use of tobacco in the Americas before Columbus, the spread of tobacco through Europe, changes in preferences for tobacco types (snuff, pipes, cigars, chew), the growth of the cigarette industry, the spreading popularity of cigarettes in the early 20th century, the early use of advertising, the development of successful tobacco companies, or the emerging scientific consensus on the harm of tobacco use. With so many choices, making the research manageable requires care and precision in identifying the issue to study.

- **Consider the underlying viewpoints.** If understanding the various viewpoints and their implications for tobacco control can help researchers make sense of the diverse literature, it helps to consult works representing these various underlying viewpoints. A researcher should take care not to rely on a single article or book, particularly one that represents one side of the debates over the tobacco industry and smoking. Being familiar with the debates and how various studies fit in the spectrum of beliefs can help researchers put information into perspective.

- **Rely on studies in the best journals.** Because smoking research is common in a variety of disciplines, and each academic discipline has dozens of journals for published research, one can only rarely master all this work. In general, however, the most prestigious journals in a discipline publish the best studies—those with the most important discoveries, the strongest scientific methodologies, and the greatest influence on the scientific field. Three top journals publish particularly important work on the medical and social aspects of smoking: the *New England Journal of Medicine*, *Journal of the American Medical Association* (*JAMA*), and *American Journal of Public Health*. The first two are the nation's most prestigious medical journals, and articles related to smoking make up only a small part of any issue. Still the articles that do get published there receive much attention. The *American Journal of Public Health* publishes more on smoking than most other journals. The articles cover topics related to the health consequences of smoking, psychological and social factors influencing smoking, efforts of the tobacco industry to promote smoking, and ways to prevent and control smoking. Although important and valuable articles appear elsewhere, researchers can benefit from beginning their search of the scientific literature with these journals.

- **Focus on conclusions and limitations.** Few will want, even if they are able, to wade through the complex details of the methodology and statistical procedures in research articles. Most published articles will have met a minimum standard for scientific quality—particularly articles in the top journals. Otherwise they would be weeded out in the scientific review process and not published. Readers can therefore most efficiently concentrate on the conclusions. Articles contain a one- or two-sentence summary of the conclusion in the abstract (a one-paragraph overview that precedes the article). The abstract contains crucial information in a compact form. In addition most articles include a few paragraphs at the end on the limitations of the study and the qualifications of the conclusions. These paragraphs can be important as well. No study is perfect and knowing the weaknesses can help one in understanding its importance.

- **Be cautious of newspaper, magazine, television, and radio reports on research.** These media sources may exaggerate the importance of a study in trying to attract the interest of readers. They sometimes report early results based on press conferences rather than on articles published in top journals that have gone through the review process. The *New York Times* remains an exception to this statement: The weekly Science section often includes health stories with considerable detail and commentary from experts. However, shorter pieces on new findings in most newspapers, magazines, television reports, and radio stories need to be examined with care. If less valuable for obtaining information on research, these sources of news provide much useful reporting on events involving litigation, public policies, and trends in tobacco use. Stories typically do well to explain legal issues in clear terms, highlight their general importance, and get information to readers quickly.

- **Become familiar with some basic statistical terms.** Research articles and their abstracts often refer to "relative risk ratios." These measure the health risks of smoking (or any other drug, behavior, group membership, or medical procedure) by comparing the number of smokers who die from a particular disease for each nonsmoker who dies from the disease. A relative risk ratio of 11, for example, would mean in this context that for every nonsmoker who dies of lung cancer during a particular time span, 11 smokers die. Studies also often refer to "statistical significance." The term does not mean a statistic is necessarily important but suggests that a relationship or coefficient found in a sample (between, say, smoking and lung cancer) likely exists in the larger population. Statistical significance depends greatly on the size of the sample as well as on the strength of the relationship. Similarly a "confidence interval" refers to a range of values for a coefficient that likely contain the true value of the coefficient in the population. Although such terms appear

152

complex, these basic definitions can ease the process of understanding research on smoking.

GETTING STARTED: HOW TO FIND HELPFUL SOURCES

BOOKS

A few recent books provide good starting points for those doing research on the tobacco industry and smoking. Tara Parker-Pope's *Cigarettes: Anatomy of an Industry from Seed to Smoke* (New York: New Press, 2001) presents a readable overview of several facets of the tobacco industry and cigarette use. Her book includes many insightful facts and helpful references but not the overwhelming detail of some other general volumes. For a more technical and comprehensive overview of tobacco research, see the 800-page edited volume *Tobacco: Science, Policy, and Public Health* (Oxford: Oxford University Press, 2004). Focusing on the main topics and key conclusions of the chapters rather than on the enormous amount of detail will give insight into the current focus of scientific research. Perusing John Goodman's encyclopedia, *Tobacco in History and Culture* (Detroit: Charles Scribner's Sons, 2005), also yields a broad overview of the topic.

For more information on the history of smoking and the tobacco industry, Eric Burns's *The Smoke of the Gods* (Philadelphia: Temple University Press, 2007) offers much detail on the spread of tobacco use and is written in a style that will appeal to general readers and beginning researchers. Robert Sobel also offers a readable history in *They Satisfy: The Cigarette in American Life* (Garden City, N.Y.: Anchor Press, 1978). This book concentrates on cigarette use in the United States and says much about tobacco companies and their brands. It ends, however, with the 1970s—before many tobacco control efforts began. An impressive and thorough history of the battle between tobacco companies and antitobacco forces can be found in Alan Kluger's *Ashes to Ashes: America's Hundred-Year Cigarette War, the Public Health, and the Unabashed Triumph of Philip Morris* (New York: Alfred A. Knopf, 1996). It does not include the litigation success against the tobacco industry in the 1990s but covers just about everything on the battle up to then. Another highly praised (and more recent) history by Allan M. Brandt, *The Cigarette Century: The Rise, Fall, and Deadly Persistence of the Product That Defined America* (New York: Basic Books, 2007), focuses on efforts of tobacco companies to mislead the public about the safety of their product.

For those most interested in the health and social aspects of smoking, the various reports issued by the Office of the Surgeon General are helpful. The reports are comprehensive, and the text often assumes technical

153

knowledge. However, each volume provides nontechnical summaries and conclusions in each chapter and makes concrete policy recommendations. Readers can gain much from these summaries and then select specific parts of the longer text to examine in more detail. The text also typically includes many useful charts and graphs. Since the first report in 1964 has become outdated, a useful starting volume is the 2004 report, *The Health Consequences of Smoking: A Report of the Surgeon General* (Atlanta, Ga.: U.S. Public Health Service, National Center for Chronic Disease Prevention and Health Promotion, 2004). It provides a comprehensive review of the evidence on the harm of smoking and the public beliefs about the harm of smoking. The 2001 report, *Women and Smoking*, gives special attention to women and makes up for more extensive attention to men in the past. Even so, with 500-some pages it covers most topics related to smoking of both sexes and contains up-to-date information. For those interested in tobacco control efforts, the 2000 volume, *Regulating Tobacco*, is a comprehensive and recent source of information. Still other reports on involuntary smoking, addiction, youth, and racial groups that are listed in the bibliography represent valuable resources.

Among writings concerned with smokers' rights, Jacob Sullum's *For Your Own Good: The Anti-Smoking Crusade and the Tyranny of Public Health* (New York: Free Press, 1998), calmly presents the case of those opposed to many current tobacco control efforts.

The bibliography in the following chapter provides many suggestions for additional books to consult, and researchers can search for more books in library catalogs, bookstore lists, and databases. Remember, however, that in these searches broad keywords such as *tobacco, smoking,* and *cigarettes* will return an enormous number of hits; more specific and detailed keywords will work better. In any case, a large selection of books can be found through electronic bookstores such as Amazon.com (http://www.amazon.com) and Barnes and Noble's web site (http://www.barnesandnoble.com). The listings sometimes helpfully include summaries and reviews of the books, as well as the comments of individual readers. Besides using a public or university library for a catalog search, researchers can find references using the comprehensive listings of the Library of Congress (http://www.loc.gov). This huge database includes subject headings on a variety of topics related to tobacco and smoking (which again requires care in selecting keywords for a search).

ARTICLES

Two types of articles may be useful for those researching the tobacco industry and smoking: articles published in scientific journals that include original research and articles published in magazines and newspapers that target general audiences.

First, for access to scientific articles one might begin with a search of the top medical and public health journals: the *New England Journal of Medicine* (http://www.nejm.org), *JAMA* (http://jama.ama-assn.org), and the *American Journal of Public Health* (http://www.ajph.org). The Internet home pages of these journals allow users to search for and identify the most relevant articles. The searches almost always return the abstract with the bibliographic citation. For those wanting to avoid the details of the scientific method, the abstract provides a helpful summary of the key findings. Many of the editorials, letters, and brief reports available online in these journals can also prove useful. To explore the article text more fully, it is possible for subscribers (and sometimes nonsubscribers) to view the full article online; if not available online in its full form, an article can be found in the journals at university and medical school libraries.

One other journal deserves special mention. *Morbidity and Mortality Weekly Report (MMWR)*, published by the Centers for Disease Control and Prevention (CDC), provides much descriptive information on smoking and smoking-related health conditions. Moreover the journal articles are available online (http://www.cdc.gov/mmwr). Unlike the other journals, *MMWR* does not focus on development of new ideas and tests of hypotheses, but it does report reliable and useful figures in a way most readers can understand. The figures come from the best available data sets on smoking and can be easily used in reports.

Several databases of scientific articles on health, medicine, and social science can, with appropriate care, be used for searches on the tobacco industry and smoking. In general the larger the database, the narrower the search terms should be. Terms such as *tobacco*, *smoking*, and *cigarettes* may work well when searching a single journal but are too broad when searching databases made up of a large number of journals. With this caution in mind, several reference sources prove most helpful. PubMed (http://www.ncbi.nlm.nih.gov/PubMed), a free resource available to the public as part of the National Library of Medicine and sponsored by the National Institutes of Health, contains more than 12 million citations dating back to the mid-1960s. It includes an important medical database, MEDLINE, and tends to list many hard science references, such as physiology, biochemistry, and neuroscience. For those interested in such research rather than in research on the use and prevention of tobacco, PubMed may be ideal. Otherwise, OCLC First Search gives users access to dozens of databases, including Social Sciences Full Text, which focuses more on social than medical aspects of smoking. However, OCLC First Search is available only through subscribing libraries.

Second, for access to less technical articles targeted to a general audience, those doing research on the tobacco industry and smoking can use several databases. The above-mentioned OCLC First Search contains an electronic version of Reader's Guide that lists articles in *Time, Newsweek, Business Week*, and a large number of other magazines. Again, however, users generally need access to a subscribing library for this database. InfoTrac (http://infotrac.thompsonlearning.com) also compiles articles for general interest audiences and sometimes includes an abstract with the citation or an abstract and a full text article. It, too, requires library privileges. Ingenta Library Gateway (http://www.ingenta.com) includes 24 million citations and allows searches within specific subject areas, such as medicine and social science. Searching Ingenta is free and many citations can be accessed without charge, but other citations require a subscription.

Newspaper articles can provide useful information on court cases, legislation, business changes, and current events related to tobacco. The *New York Times, The Washington Post*, and the *Wall Street Journal* are particularly useful. Libraries usually subscribe to databases that include these newspapers. For example, users can have access to abstracts and full articles through First Search (select the LexisNexis Academic or ProQuest database within First Search).

RESEARCH ON THE INTERNET

Although the Internet represents an extraordinary resource in terms of the wealth of information available to researchers, combing through all the web sites listed by searches can consume much time. Moreover the information obtained is not always reliable and unbiased. Researchers can proceed in several ways.

Popular and general search engines such as Google (http://www.google.com), Yahoo! (http://www.yahoo.com), AltaVista (http://www.altavista.com), Excite (http://www.excite.com), Lycos (http://www.lycos.com), MSN (http://www.msn.com), Ask (http://www.ask.com), and many others can identify web sites that contain information on the tobacco industry and smoking. Effectively using these search engines requires the thoughtful selection of narrow search terms. Nonetheless, taking the time to work through hundreds of web sites found by using general terms can sometimes lead to an unexpected and intriguing discovery.

A more efficient way to proceed involves searching directories relevant to the tobacco industry and smoking. In Yahoo! directories, under "Recreation & Sports > Hobbies > Smoking," one can find web sites and information on antismoking organizations, cigars, Joe Camel, secondhand smoke, and teen smoking; under "Health > Diseases and Conditions > All Diseases and Conditions > Smoking addictions," one can find information on smoking cessation and cessation support groups. In Google (http://www.google.com) relevant directories include "Health > Addictions > Substance abuse > Smoking" and "Health > Support Groups > Smoking cessation." Other directories besides those of Yahoo! and Google are available as well. The directory indexes have some advantages over general searches. They do not attempt to compile every link but evaluate a link for usefulness and quality before including it in the directory. This selectivity can save time and frustration, even if it may miss some sites a researcher would find useful. In addition the directories organize the links by topic and thus avoid the disorganized listing obtained from a general search. Use of the directories does not, however, eliminate the need to use the links carefully and critically.

Several web sites devoted specifically to tobacco provide useful starting points for researchers. Tobacco.org (http://www.tobacco.org) contains the latest tobacco headlines, an archive of news briefs, quotes about smoking, an information page, tobacco documents, book releases, and graphs (subscribers can obtain additional information). Given its extensive information the web site can best be used with the search command. The Tobacco Reference Guide (http://www.globalink.org/tobacco/trg), compiled by David Moyer, presents a collection of materials from a variety of public sources. The online tobacco encyclopedia *TobaccoPedia* (http://tobaccopedia.org) is supported by the International Union Against Cancer (UICC) and includes entries relating to a wide range of topics.

For information relating to tobacco control and antismoking efforts it helps to consult the web sites of several organizations. Action on Smoking and Health (ASH) advertises its web page as "Everything for People Concerned about Smoking and Nonsmokers' Rights, Smoking Statistics, Quitting Smoking, Smoking Risks, and Other Smoking Information" (http://ash. org). As it claims, the site contains an assortment of antismoking information. The Campaign for Tobacco Free Kids (http://www.tobaccofreekids. org) offers resources for helping to reduce youth smoking. The Office of Smoking and Health (http://www.cdc.gov/tobacco), a unit within the CDC and the U.S. Department of Health and Human Services, leads and coordinates efforts to prevent tobacco use among youth, promote smoking cessation, protect nonsmokers from secondhand smoke, and eliminate tobacco-related health disparities. The office's web site contains resources for reaching these goals.

For those wanting to know more about the worldwide spread of tobacco, the second edition of *The Tobacco Atlas* (http://www.cancer.org/docroot/AA/content/AA_2_5_9x_Tobacco_Atlas.asp) contains full-color maps and graphics. Tables in the appendices list the raw data used to create the maps and graphics. Like most other sources, this one has the goal of reducing tobacco use and the harm it causes. The World Health Organization provides information on the goals and plans for implementation of the Framework Convention on Tobacco Control on a web page for the treaty (http://www.who.int/tobacco/framework/en).

Fewer sites support tobacco use than oppose it, but Forces (Fight Ordinances and Restrictions to Control and Eliminate Smoking) International (http://www.forces.org) presents arguments in favor of smokers' rights and includes links to other web sites with like-minded views. Web sites of tobacco companies (British American Tobacco, Philip Morris, R. J. Reynolds) defend their decision to continue producing and selling cigarettes but include much information on limiting tobacco use by young people. Two trade journals, *Tobacco Journal International* (http://www.tobaccojournal.com) and *Tobacco Reporter* (http://www.tobaccoreporter.com) present news stories that reflect the concerns and interests of those in the tobacco industry. Yahoo! profiles each of the major tobacco companies as part of its Finance Industry Center (http://biz.yahoo.com/ic/profile/tobaco_1203.html).

COURT CASES

Litigation against the tobacco industry has mushroomed in the last few years because of the admission by tobacco companies in the Master Settlement Agreement of past wrongdoing, the availability of internal tobacco company documents to demonstrate their past misrepresentation, and some large awards against tobacco companies. Information on the suits, jury decisions, awards, appeals, and final judgments can be found through searches of newspapers, tobacco web sites (Tobacco.org), and general web sites (by using Google, Yahoo!, or other search engines). More specific lists of cases and links of documents are provided by the Tobacco Control Resources Center (http://www.tobacco.neu.edu/litigation/cases/index.htm) and by Find Law (http://news.findlaw.com/legalnews/lit/tobacco/index.html). To obtain the written decisions in cases, electronic law libraries such as Westlaw (http://www.westlaw.com) and Lexis-Nexis (http://www.lexisnexis.com) include court opinions but require a subscription. Opinions of the Supreme Court relevant to tobacco issues can be obtained from the Legal Information Institute (http://www.law.cornell.edu). To read an overview of the history of tobacco litigation and a review of the most important cases, see the Surgeon General's 2000 report on regulating tobacco, which includes a long chapter on legal action to control tobacco.

CHAPTER 7

ANNOTATED BIBLIOGRAPHY

The following bibliography contains six major sections:

- history and background,
- health and medical aspects,
- social and psychological aspects,
- tobacco business and litigation,
- tobacco control, and
- self-help.

Within each of these sections the citations are divided into subsections for books, articles, and Web documents. The topics and citation types cover a vast amount of material and although the bibliography cannot be fully comprehensive, it includes a representative mix of materials on the tobacco industry and smoking. The sections to follow thus list technical and nontechnical works, historical and contemporary sources, and research and opinion pieces. (See Chapter 6 for an overview on how to most effectively use the diverse materials.) The sections cover history, science, and research but also include self-help selections on how to quit smoking and sources of information useful to those interested in becoming involved in tobacco control activities.

HISTORY AND BACKGROUND

BOOKS

Brandt, Allan M. *The Cigarette Century: The Rise, Fall, and Deadly Persistence of the Product That Defined America*. New York: Basic Books, 2007. A Harvard medical historian addresses the puzzle of continued tobacco use despite clear scientific evidence of its harm and eventual widespread acceptance of this harm. He traces much of the problem to false information spread by the tobacco industry about the safety of the product. More than this, the book offers a detailed and illuminating history of cigarettes in the 20th century, one that has received considerable praise from reviewers.

Burnham, John C. *Bad Habits: Drinking, Smoking, Taking Drugs, Gambling, Sexual Misbehavior, and Swearing in American History.* New York: New York University Press, 1993. This study places the acceptance of smoking within a framework of broader social changes that led to permissiveness toward a wider variety of "bad habits." Smoking and other misbehaviors overcame strong and organized opposition in the first part of the 20th century to become common in American society.

Burns, Eric. *The Smoke of the Gods: A Social History of Tobacco.* Philadelphia: Temple University, 2007. This history begins with use of tobacco to accompany prayer in Mayan rituals and ends with a chapter on the release of the 1964 Surgeon General's report on the harm of smoking. It describes people, events, and anecdotes throughout history, the failures of movements to ban cigarettes, and the outrageous claims made by cigarette advertisements. The clear and straightforward writing offers numerous examples that help make the history real.

Cox, Howard. *The Global Cigarette: Origins and Evolution of British American Tobacco, 1880–1945.* New York: Oxford University Press, 2000. This history examines efforts of the British American Tobacco Company to pursue markets in colonies across the world. These early efforts would set the groundwork for the later success of multinational cigarette manufacturers in promoting their products in developing nations and begin the process toward internationalization by the cigarette industry.

Elliot, Rosemary. *Women and Smoking Since 1890.* New York: Routledge, 2007. Written by a researcher at the University of Glasgow, this book has a more academic orientation than the book by Segrave and gives more attention to Britain than the United States. It connects the adoption of smoking by women to changes in modern gender roles and identities and thus gives more attention to broad social trends than other histories of tobacco use.

Fahs, John. *Cigarette Confidential: The Unfiltered Truth about the Ultimate American Addiction.* New York: Berkley Books, 1996. The author, an investigative reporter, examines the pleasures and pains of nicotine addiction, the costs of the addiction, the actions of the tobacco industry, and the scenes behind the cigarette wars.

Forey, Barbara, et al. *International Smoking Statistics: A Collection of Historical Data from 30 Economically Developed Countries.* 2d ed. Oxford, U.K.: Oxford University Press, 2002. This comprehensive reference work is filled with data on trends in smoking and cigarette consumption and will interest researchers and those wanting to know more about differences across nations in the use of tobacco.

Gately, Iain. *Tobacco: The Story of How Tobacco Seduced the World.* New York: Grove Press, 2001. Beginning with the first use of tobacco by Native peoples in the Americas and ending with the spread of tobacco throughout the world, this book asks why tobacco has and continues to have such a hold on humankind, why it has been accepted in so many cultures across the world, and why its use has persisted well after it has been revealed as a killer. In answering the questions the author gives particular attention to the habit in premodern societies.

Gilman, Sander L., and Zhou Xun, eds. *Smoke: A Global History of Smoking.* London: Reaktion Books, 2004. Each chapter examines the culture of smoking in a different society, and the book overall compares diverse places and times such as Central America, Victorian England, sub-Saharan Africa, India, Japan, and Imperial China. The cross-society comparisons illustrate the varied and changing meanings of smoking. Viewed sometimes as a part of ritual, as a cure for sickness, as an indicator of sophistication, and as a source of pleasure, tobacco use has become an important part of nearly all societies exposed to it.

Goodman, Jordan, ed. *Tobacco in History and Culture: An Encyclopedia.* Detroit: Charles Scribner's Sons, 2005. Divided into two volumes, each with more than 700 pages, this encyclopedia contains an impressive amount for information on a variety of tobacco-related topics. Written by experts, each entry discusses the topic in detail, usually with clear and accessible writing. Like any encyclopedia, the separate entries mean the volumes lack an integrative framework but make it easy to find information on specialized topics.

———. *Tobacco in History: The Cultures of Dependence.* London: Routledge, 1993. Written more for scholars than the public, this study posits that acceptance of tobacco must be understood as part of the history of the product. It focuses on the dependence of producers as well as consumers on tobacco and gives special attention to cultivation and production in premodern as well as modern societies.

Gottsegen, Jack. *Tobacco: A Study of Its Consumption in the United States.* New York: Pittman, 1940. Filled with facts and statistics, this book presents a scientific and data-oriented approach to the history of tobacco use in the United States. It gives much attention to changing fashions in the preferences for snuff, chew, pipes, cigars, and cigarettes and offers many historical examples of the changing fashions.

Hilton, Matthew. *Smoking in British Popular Culture, 1800–2000.* Manchester, U.K.: Manchester University Press, 2000. Although focused on Britain rather than the United States, this historical study describes changes in the cultural acceptability of smoking. The author argues that the rise of smoking has related to strengthening beliefs about the importance of individuality and independence and later to new understandings of masculinity and femininity.

Hirschfelder, Arlene B. *Encyclopedia of Smoking and Tobacco.* Phoenix, Ariz.: Oryx Press, 1999. This encyclopedia is comprehensive in its listings and a useful reference source. However, its reliance on the alphabetical ordering of items means it lacks a coherent framework to organize the vast material on smoking and tobacco.

Howard, Red. *Cigars.* New York: MetroBooks, 1997. This history of cigars offers a guide to choosing, preparing, and enjoying cigars and includes photographs, examples of advertisements, and fine art reproductions.

Hughes, Jason. *Learning to Smoke: Tobacco Use in the West.* Chicago: University of Chicago Press, 2003. Most literature on smoking takes a biological or pharmacological approach that views cigarettes as a nicotine-delivery system. To supplement this approach the author argues that across histories and societies, individuals have interpreted the meaning of these physical cues differently, and that social context is crucial to understanding smoking.

Klein, Richard. *Cigarettes Are Sublime.* Durham, N.C.: Duke University Press, 1993. Stimulated by the difficulties he faced in quitting, the author presents a literary-based review of what makes cigarettes so satisfying. He also criticizes current antismoking campaigns as excessive and puritanical.

Kluger, Alan. *Ashes to Ashes: America's Hundred-Year Cigarette War, the Public Health, and the Unabashed Triumph of Philip Morris.* New York: Alfred A. Knopf, 1996. An impressively detailed history of the tobacco industry and the attempts to control it in the United States over the last century, this volume is unique in the comprehensiveness of the story it tells. It relies on interviews with hundreds of people, thoroughly covers relevant documents, and gives special attention to the growth of the Philip Morris tobacco company.

Kulikoff, Allan. *Tobacco and Slaves: The Development of Southern Cultures in the Chesapeake, 1680–1800.* Chapel Hill: University of North Carolina Press, 1986. This history describes the development of the tobacco economy in eastern Maryland and Virginia from the late 1600s to 1880 and the development of slave-based cultures among whites and blacks associated with the tobacco economy.

Lock, S., L. A. Reynolds, and E. M. Tansey, eds. *Ashes to Ashes: The History of Smoking and Health.* Atlanta, Ga.: Rodopi, 1998. Articles in the volume address issues concerning the history of tobacco advertising, antitobacco movements, tobacco in art and literature, and the emergence of policies to control tobacco.

Mackenzie, Compton. *Sublime Tobacco.* New York: Macmillan, 1958. A smoker who started at age four, the author offers a prologue about his own smoking life before describing historical events that led to the spread of tobacco. Of special historical interest is the epilogue, which deals with the benefits tobacco has brought to humanity and provides a perspective on the product quite different from the one that dominates today.

Norris, James D. *Advertising and the Transformation of American Society, 1865–1920.* Westport, Conn.: Greenwood Press, 1990. This history of the emergence of advertising appropriately gives prominent attention to cigarettes—a product whose growth coincided with the widespread use of various forms of advertising.

Ragsdale, Bruce A. *A Planters' Republic: The Search for Economic Independence in Revolutionary Virginia.* Madison: University of Wisconsin, 1996. The author argues that the desire for economic independence more than the desire for political liberty led to the war for independence. With tobacco the primary product, concern about the British economic regulation led the planter class in Virginia to support revolution.

Reynolds, Patrick, and Tom Shachtman. *Gilded Leaf: Triumph, Tragedy, and Tobacco: Three Generations of the R. J. Reynolds Family and Fortune.* Boston: Little, Brown, 1989. A descendant of R. J. Reynolds and a writer tell a story of family wealth and misfortune. Despite his famous relatives, Patrick Reynolds has become an antismoking activist.

Rogozinski, Jan. *Smokeless Tobacco in the Western World: 1550–1950.* Westport, Conn.: Greenwood Press, 1990. In contrast to most books on tobacco this one gives attention to smokeless tobacco and to differences across nations of Europe in the use and regulation of smokeless products

Segrave, Kerry. *Women and Smoking in America, 1880–1950.* Jefferson, N.C.: McFarland, 2005. The author divides the spread of cigarette smoking by women into four periods. From 1880 to 1908, smoking was limited in the United States to upper-class women using the product in their homes and at parties. From 1908 to 1919, women began to smoke in some public places such as restaurants, but these actions remained a source of controversy. From 1919 to 1927, young educated women at universities began to take up the habit, but most people viewed smoking on the street by women as shocking and sometimes even deserving arrest. From 1927 to 1950, advertising directed toward women contributed to the widespread acceptance of female smoking. This book describes these changes clearly and gives numerous examples to support its claims.

Siegel, Frederick F. *The Roots of Southern Distinctiveness: Tobacco and Society in Danville, Virginia, 1780–1865.* Chapel Hill: University of North Carolina Press, 1987. Danville, Virginia, and the surrounding area became a thriving center of tobacco marketing and manufacturing. In describing the entrepreneurs, planters, and slaveholders in the vicinity, this history reveals how the culture mixed traits of southern agriculture and slavery with northern business traits of entrepreneurship.

Sobel, Robert. *They Satisfy: The Cigarette in American Life*. Garden City, N.Y.: Anchor Press, 1978. Focusing on the tobacco industry, cigarette advertising, and smoking fashions in the United States up to the 1970s, this history gives much detail about tobacco brands, prices, companies, sales, and marketing. It also offers brief biographies of leading tobacco executives and their opponents and stories about the use of cigarettes in U.S. history.

Tate, Cassandra. *Cigarette Wars: The Triumph of the "Little White Slaver."* Oxford, U.K.: Oxford University Press, 1999. A historical study from the end of the 19th century to the Great Depression, this book describes the early anticigarette movement and its relationship in the United States to the Progressive Era—a period of protest against smoking, drinking, and other habits. It gives particular attention to legal and social restrictions on smoking a century ago and to the cultural trends that overcame the restrictions.

Tennant, Richard. *The American Cigarette Industry*. New Haven, Conn.: Yale University, 1950. Focused largely on economics, this technical study provides much information on the business during the early part of the 20th century but has become dated with the new information accruing about smoking and cigarettes.

Tenner, Edward. *Why Things Bite Back: Technology and the Revenge of Unintended Consequences*. New York: Knopf, 1996. In arguing that technological breakthroughs often have serious unexpected results, the author provides many examples and gives attention to how innovations involving the creation of low-tar cigarettes have encouraged smoking.

Tilly, Nannie May. *The R. J. Reynolds Tobacco Company*. Chapel Hill: University of North Carolina Press, 1985. Covering the history of the company from 1875 to 1963, this book discusses labor relations, advertising, and competition for sales with other tobacco companies.

Wagner, Susan. *Cigarette Country: Tobacco in American History and Politics*. New York: Praeger Publishers, 1971. Beginning with the use of tobacco by Native peoples in the present-day Mexican state of Chiapas, this book traces the history of tobacco up to the 1960s.

Whelan, Elizabeth. *A Smoking Gun: How the Tobacco Industry Gets Away with Murder*. Philadelphia: George F. Stickley, 1984. Vigorously antitobacco, this book offers a clear if opinionated history of tobacco use and industry efforts to promote its products. It treats the tobacco industry as a villain in its battle with scientists, public health experts, and policy makers. The book is dated in terms of current public policies but suggested the use of many strategies to control tobacco that later were adopted.

Winter, Joseph C., ed. *Tobacco Use by Native North Americans: Sacred Smoke and Silent Killer*. Norman: University of Oklahoma Press, 2000. Native Americans continue to view tobacco—when used properly—as a sacred product that has played an important role in their history. The chapters in the edited volume cover the history of tobacco use by American Indians, the contribution of smoking to myth and tradition, and current problems of Native Americans stemming from modern use of cigarettes.

ARTICLES

Centers for Disease Control and Prevention. "Morbidity and Mortality Weekly Report: State-Specific Prevalence of Current Cigarette Smoking Among Adults and the Proportion of Adults Who Work in a Smoke-Free Environment—United States, 1999." *JAMA*, vol. 284, December 13, 2000, p. 2,865. States vary widely in the level of cigarette use, with 31.5 percent of residents of Nevada smoking and 13.9 percent of residents of Utah smoking. States also vary in exposure of their residents to second-hand smoke at work: 61.3 percent of indoor workers in Mississippi reported a workplace policy on smoking and 82.0 percent in Washington, D.C. reported such policies.

Cutler, Abigail. "The Ashtray of History." *Atlantic Monthly*, vol. 299, no. 1, January/February 2007, p. 37. As background to the recent spread of smoking bans across the world (including such places as France, Cuba, and Hong Kong), this article describes smoke-free movements of the past. The bans from 1642 to 1942 rarely proved permanent, however

Dinan, John, and Jac C. Heckelman. "The Anti-Tobacco Movement in the Progressive Era: A Case Study of Direct Democracy in Oregon." *Explorations in Economic History*, vol. 42, no. 4, October 2005, pp. 529–546. Only once in U.S history did a statewide smoking ban go up for popular vote. This study of the social movement to ban tobacco in Oregon in 1930 finds the greatest support for the ban in counties with high percentages of evangelical Protestants, women, and rural residents. The case study illustrates the resistance to smoking in the early decades of the 20th century.

Fenster, Julie M. "Hazardous to Your Health: 1964 Surgeon General's Report on Smoking." *American Heritage*, vol. 57, no. 5, October 2006, pp. 62–63. A special issue on 1964 in this magazine of popular history devotes an article to an event of enormous historical importance: The publication by the U.S. government's chief medical official of a report summarizing evidence of the harm of smoking for health and calling for smokers to quit and young people to not start. The article tells of the people behind the report and the evidence they used to make their case. It calls the report "one of those triumphs of science . . . [that] was eventually successful in persuading people not to smoke."

Gardner, Martha N., and Allan M. Brandt. "'The Doctor's Choice Is America's Choice': The Physician in U.S. Cigarette Advertisements, 1930–1953." *American Journal of Public Health*, vol. 96, no. 2, February 2006, pp. 222–232. Not only did the majority of physicians smoke in the 1930s and 1940s, but tobacco companies placed them in ads to imply the safety of cigarettes. This article traces the growth of physician-based ads during these years and their demise in the 1950s when evidence of the harm of cigarettes made such ads unconvincing, even preposterous.

Rozin, Paul. "The Process of Moralization." *Psychological Science*, vol. 10, May 1999, pp. 218–221. The author, a psychologist at the University of Pennsylvania, describes the process that translates antismoking preferences into views of cigarette use as an immoral act. Moralization shows not just in the dislike of cigarette smoking but also in the outrage of nonsmokers when confronted by undesired cigarette smoke, in the crusading views of antismoking advocates, and in the association of smoking with weakness.

Saad, Lydia. "A Half-Century of Polling on Tobacco: Most Don't Like Smoking but Tolerate It." *Public Perspective*, vol. 9, August/September 1998, pp. 1–4. Summarizes polling results on government regulation of smoking, the right to smoke, awareness of hazards, tobacco use, and teen smoking over the period 1954–96. The trends over time reveal more negative public opinions on smoking but continued support for the right to smoke.

Wynder, Ernest L. "Tobacco and Health: A Review of the History and Suggestions for Public Policy." *Public Health Reports*, vol. 103, January/February 1988, pp. 8–18. One of the first physicians to scientifically demonstrate a link between smoking and lung cancer reviews the early evidence of the link and the slow steps toward widespread acceptance of the harm of tobacco use on health. He notes that progress in preventing tobacco use has come even more slowly than the understanding of its harm.

WEB DOCUMENTS

Borio, Gene. "The Tobacco Timeline." Tobacco.org. Available online. URL: http://www.tobacco.org/resources/history/Tobacco_History.html. Downloaded in April 2008. With an impressively long and detailed timeline, this web site offers a history of world tobacco use. It consists of eight chapters, the first on discovery, which begins with the sacred use of the tobacco pipe and the growth of tobacco in the Americas as far back as 6000 B.C. The last chapter on the New Millennium ends with entries on smoking bans that go into effect in 2008. The chapters between contain a wealth of information on the spread and decline of tobacco and the actions of tobacco companies over the last century.

Breed, Larry. "Breed's Collection of Tobacco History Sites." Available online. URL: http://smokingsides.com/docs/hist.html. Updated on July 2, 2002. This web site lists many (often hard to find) documents on tobacco use by Native Americans before Columbus traveled to the new world. The guide includes more specialized documents than most researchers will need, but particularly interesting are topics such as tobacco use and shamanism in South America and cross-cultural comparisons of tobacco use in tribal societies. For more recent centuries, it lists books published in the 19th century on the effects of tobacco and displays some old tobacco ads.

Moyer, David. "The Tobacco Reference Guide." UICC Globalink. Available online. URL: http://www.globalink.org/tobacco/trg. Downloaded in April 2008. This Web-based book, available for use without copyright restrictions, has 45 chapters that compile information on a wide variety of topics, including one on the history of tobacco. Other chapters list deaths of celebrities from smoking-related causes, review the history and facts on women and smoking, and discuss the problem of tobacco use in movies. By compiling the information in a single location, David Moyer, a physician in Oakland, California, provides a helpful resource for researchers.

National Commission on Marihuana and Drug Abuse. "History of Tobacco Regulation." Schaffer Library of Drug Policy. Available online. URL: http://www.druglibrary.org/schaffer/LIBRARY/studies/nc/nc2b.htm. Downloaded in April 2008. Perhaps surprisingly, tobacco has always been subject to regulation. This report describes efforts to prohibit the planting of tobacco in New England in 1629, the imposition of federal taxes on tobacco sales by Alexander Hamilton in the late 18th century, and state bans on cigarette use in the late 19th and early 20th century. It also describes more recent regulations such as bans on tobacco advertising.

Tobacco.org. "Tobacco News and Information." Available online. URL: http://www.tobacco.org. Downloaded in February 2003. For nonsubscribers this service provides recent tobacco headlines, an archive of news briefs, quotes about smoking, an information page, tobacco documents, book releases, and graphs; subscribers can copy stories and obtain new ones via e-mail.

UICC Globalink. "*TobaccoPedia:* The Online Tobacco Encyclopedia." Available online. URL: http://tobaccopedia.org. Downloaded in February 2003. The online tobacco encyclopedia supported by the International Union against Cancer (UICC) includes entries relating to health effects of active and passive smoking, chemistry of addiction, smoking cessation, and tobacco control.

HEALTH AND MEDICAL ASPECTS

BOOKS

Bock, Gregory, and Jamie Goode, eds. *Understanding Nicotine and Tobacco Addiction.* Hoboken, N.J.: John Wiley & Sons, 2006. Those wanting a more scientific understanding of the addictive properties of nicotine and tobacco will find in this edited volume to be useful. To take advantage of the scientific discoveries and knowledge, however, readers must feel comfortable with references to "receptor functions," "dopamine-based reward," and "pharmogenetics."

Boyle, Peter, Nigel Gray, Jack Henningfield, John Seffrin, and Witold Zatonski, eds. *Tobacco: Science, Policy, and Public Health*. Oxford: Oxford University Press, 2004. At nearly 800 pages, this comprehensive volume of 44 chapters covers a huge number of topics. Summarizing knowledge of the harm of tobacco use for cancer, respiratory disease, heart disease, and other diseases get the most attention. In addition, chapters review research on the addictive properties of nicotine and the dependence of smokers on tobacco. Perhaps most interesting are the chapters at the end of the book on policies that work and don't work. Each chapter considers policies such as legislation, global treaties, litigation, and smoking bans.

Frenk, Hanan, and Reuven Dar. *A Critique of Nicotine Addiction*. Boston: Kluwer Academic Publishers, 2000. Based on a review of articles and books on the subject the authors criticize claims that nicotine is an addictive drug. The book offers a minority view on this issue, one that the Surgeon General and most public health experts dispute.

Gold, Mark S. *Drugs of Abuse*. Vol. 4, *Tobacco*. New York: Plenum, 1995. Covering the history of tobacco, the effects of nicotine on the brain and the body, psychiatric aspects of tobacco use, and treatment programs, the author emphasizes medical and physical aspects of addiction.

Gori, Gio Batta. *Virtually Safe Cigarettes: Reviving an Opportunity Once Tragically Rejected*. Amsterdam: IOS Press, 2000. In the face of the failure to end use of cigarettes, despite clear evidence of the harm of the product, this book argues that developing a safe cigarette could save thousands of lives and discusses issues in creating and marketing such a product.

Haustein, Knut-Olaf. *Tobacco or Health: Physiological and Social Damages Caused by Tobacco Smoking*. Berlin: Springer, 2003. This translation of a German work covers in some 464 pages the history of tobacco, tobacco components and additives, the health effects of smoking, smoking and pregnancy, passive smoking, nicotine dependence, preventing smoking, and the tobacco industry and advertising.

Koven, Edward L. *Smoking: The Story Behind the Haze*. New York: Nova Science Publishers, 1996. The most interesting chapter of this book describes the smoking habits of famous people, such as Lucille Ball, Leonard Bernstein, Gary Cooper, Waylon Jennings, Michael Landon, and Lyndon Johnson, and how the habit led to early death or health problems. Another unique chapter includes cartoons about the harm of tobacco.

Kozlowski, Lynn T., Jack E. Henningfield, and Janet Brigham. *Cigarettes, Nicotine, and Health: A Biobehavioral Approach*. Thousand Oaks, Calif.: Sage Publications, 2001. The biobehavioral approach focuses on the physical effects and addictiveness of nicotine. The chapters cover the history of nicotine use, the effects of nicotine on the body, smoking as nicotine addiction, the relation of smoking to drinking and drug use, and helping smokers quit.

Krogh, David. *Smoking: The Artificial Passion.* New York: W. H. Freeman, 1991. In addressing the question of why people smoke, this well-written summary of the scientific literature discusses the biological and psychological research on nicotine use. The research finds that smoking creates positive feelings of both stimulation and relaxation, which make it difficult to quit the habit. The author notes that it is more than physical dependence that keeps smokers puffing away—smoking becomes associated with positive social feelings as well.

Napier, Kristine M., et al., eds. *Cigarettes—What the Warning Label Doesn't Tell You: The First Comprehensive Guide to the Health Consequences of Smoking.* New York: American Council on Science and Health, 1996. Each chapter addresses the health effects of smoking from the viewpoint of a different medical specialty. The harm involves not only lung cancer and heart disease but also diabetes, cataracts, psoriasis, and impotence.

National Cancer Institute, National Institutes of Health. *Cigars: Health Effects and Trends.* Smoking and Tobacco Control Monograph 9. Washington, D.C.: U.S. Department of Health and Human Services, 1998. A comprehensive volume on how cigars, although less likely to cause lung cancer and heart disease than cigarettes, nonetheless have risks for oral and esophageal cancer similar to those for cigarettes. It also describes the upward trend in cigar use.

———. *The FTC Cigarette Test Method for Determining Tar, Nicotine, and Carbon Monoxide Yields of U.S. Cigarettes: Report of the NCI Expert Committee.* Smoking and Tobacco Control Monograph 7. Washington, D.C.: U.S. Department of Health and Human Services, 1996. More than others in the series, this volume focuses on technical issues of chemical composition and measurement.

———. *Respiratory Health Effects of Passive Smoking: Lung Cancer and Other Disorders. The Report of the U.S. Environmental Protection Agency.* Smoking and Tobacco Control Monograph 4. Washington, D.C.: U.S. Department of Health and Human Services, 1993. Like the earlier report of the Surgeon General on involuntary smoking, this report from the Environmental Protection Agency (EPA) describes the evidence of the harm of environmental tobacco smoke on health and the need for clean indoor air policies.

———. *Risks Associated with Smoking Cigarettes with Low Machine-Measured Yields of Tar and Nicotine.* Smoking and Tobacco Control Monograph 13. Washington, D.C.: U.S. Department of Health and Human Services, 2001. This volume describes the design of low-tar and low-nicotine cigarettes, their effects on health and disease, the public understanding of the risks of these productions, and efforts of tobacco companies to market them. It concludes that the risks of these cigarettes for health problems remain high.

Peto, Richard, et al. *Mortality from Smoking in Developed Countries, 1950–2000: Indirect Estimates from National Vital Statistics.* Oxford, U.K.: Oxford University Press, 1994. Data for each country include the number and proportion of deaths due to smoking over the last half of the 20th century. Although filled with numbers and tables and based on some complex calculations, the book presents a summary of the information in the first chapters that readers will find helpful.

Piasecki, Melissa, and Paul A. Newhouse, eds. *Nicotine in Psychiatry: Psychopathology and Emerging Therapeutics.* Washington, D.C.: American Psychiatric Press, 2000. Designed for practicing clinicians rather than general readers, the book provides scientific information on the neurological and biological bases of the effects of nicotine, the association between smoking and mental illness, and the effectiveness of clinical programs to reduce smoking.

Rippe, James M., ed. *Lifestyle Medicine.* Malden, Mass.: Blackwell Science, 1999. In emphasizing the important connections between positive lifestyle behaviors and clinical medicine, this volume discusses how a smoke-free lifestyle can contribute to better health.

Schaler, Jeffrey A. *Addiction Is a Choice.* Chicago: Open Court Publishers, 2000. The author disputes the common notion that smoking is an addiction and that addicts cannot help themselves. While recognizing the difficulty of quitting, the author believes people have the choice to stop and presents research on addiction to support his points.

Sonder, Ben. *Dangerous Legacy: The Babies of Drug-Taking Parents.* New York: Watts, 1994. Including tobacco along with cocaine, crack, opiates, alcohol, and marijuana in its purview, the book describes the short-term and sometimes long-term effects of drug use by parents on the well-being of their infants and children.

Stratton, Kathleen, et al., eds. *Clearing the Air: Assessing the Science Base for Tobacco Harm Reduction.* Washington, D.C.: National Academy Press, 2001. The Institute of Medicine evaluates the methods used to claim that certain products reduce the harmful health effects of smoking and the addiction to cigarette nicotine. The products evaluated include pharmaceuticals, medical devices, and modified tobacco products.

Terry, Luther L. "The Surgeon General's First Report on Smoking and Health." In *The Cigarette Underworld: A Front Line Report on the War Against Your Lungs,* edited by Alan Blum. Secaucus, N.J.: Lyle Stuart, 1985. The same surgeon general responsible for the famous 1964 report on the harm of cigarette smoking gives his recollections about the production of the report and its reception.

Annotated Bibliography

U.S. Department of Health and Human Services. *The Health Consequences of Involuntary Exposure to Tobacco Smoke: A Report of the Surgeon General.* Washington, D.C: U.S. Department of Health and Human Services, Public Health Service, Office of the Surgeon General, 2006. Also available online. URL: http://permanent.access.gpo.gov/lps71463/FullReportChapters. Downloaded in April 2008. This comprehensive volume covers a wide variety of topics related to secondhand smoke: toxicology, prevalence, effects on reproduction and fetal development, respiratory effects on children, cancer among adults, cardiovascular diseases, and control strategies. Given these dangers, the volume makes a case for expansion of bans on smoking in public places.

———. *The Health Consequences of Smoking: Nicotine Addiction. A Report of the Surgeon General.* Washington, D.C.: U.S. Department of Health and Human Services, 1988. This volume lays out in detail the evidence that smoking is more addictive than heroin or cocaine. The information on pharmacology makes the material less accessible than other reports of the Surgeon General, but the introduction clearly summarizes the basis for making claims about addictiveness of nicotine.

———. *The Health Consequences of Smoking: A Report of the Surgeon General.* Atlanta, Ga.: U.S. Public Health Service, National Center for Chronic Disease Prevention and Health Promotion, 2004. Also available online. URL: http://www.cdc.gov/tobacco/data_statistics/sgr/sgr_2004/index.htm. Downloaded in April 2008. In updating previous reports on the same topic, including the first one in 1964, this report lists the many diseases and health problems caused by active smoking. It concludes that smoking harms nearly every organ of the body and that smoking cigarettes with low tar and nicotine does little to moderate this harm. Diseases newly identified as caused by smoking include abdominal aortic aneurysms, acute myeloid leukemia, cataracts, cervical cancer, kidney cancer, pancreatic cancer, pneumonia, periodontitis, and stomach cancer. Although few need convincing, the voluminous evidence makes it hard to deny the dangers of smoking.

———. *Secondhand Smoke: What It Means To You.* Washington, D.C.: U.S. Dept. of Health and Human Services, Centers for Disease Control and Prevention, 2006. Also available online. URL: http://permanent.access.gpo.gov/lps71465/secondhandsmoke.pdf. Downloaded in April 2008. This 11-page brochure aims to convince people that even a little secondhand smoke is dangerous. The slogan on the second page summarizes the main points: "Secondhand Smoke: It hurts you. It doesn't take much. It doesn't take long." In presenting data on the harm of secondhand smoke, the brochure highlights the risks to fetuses, infants, and children from the smoke of parents and other relatives.

———. *Women and Smoking: A Report of the Surgeon General.* Washington, D.C.: U.S. Department of Health and Human Services, 2001. This comprehensive volume of more than 500 pages details the special health risks faced by women smokers, the efforts of tobacco companies to attract women smokers with advertising, and the ways to help prevent smoking among women. More generally it provides an up-to-date overview of the knowledge about the causes and consequences of smoking.

Watson, Ronald R., and Mark L. Witten, eds. *Environmental Tobacco Smoke.* Boca Raton, Fla.: CRC Press, 2001. For clinicians and researchers wanting an up-to-date overview of research on environmental tobacco smoking, this volume focuses on the harm of cigarette smoke on nonsmoking pregnant women, newborns, youth, adults, and the elderly, and the association of exposure to secondhand smoke with asthma, heart disease, cancer, problems of the immune system, and DNA damage.

ARTICLES

Atrens, Dale M. "Nicotine as an Addictive Substance: A Critical Examination of the Basic Concepts and Empirical Evidence." *Journal of Drug Issues* 31 (spring 2001): 325–394. Despite a general consensus about the addictiveness of nicotine, some scientists remain skeptical. This article reviews the reasons for the skepticism, argues that addiction has been too broadly defined to be meaningful, and concludes that the empirical evidence for the addictiveness of tobacco remains lacking.

Baker, Frank, et al. "Health Risks Associated with Cigar Smoking." *JAMA* 284 (August 9, 2000): 735–740. Summarizing the results of a 1998 conference of the American Cancer Society, the article finds consensus that smoking cigars instead of cigarettes does not reduce the risks of nicotine addiction, that inhaling of cigar smoke makes the risks of death similar to those for cigarette smoking, that cigars contain higher concentrations of toxic and carcinogenic chemicals than cigarettes, and that cigar smoking causes cancer of the lung.

Barnes, Deborah E., and Lisa A. Bero. "Why Review Articles on the Health Effects of Passive Smoking Reach Different Conclusions." *JAMA* 279 (May 20, 1998): 1,566–1,570. Of 106 articles that evaluated the evidence on passive smoking, 37 percent concluded that it was not harmful, but 74 percent of these articles were written by authors with tobacco industry affiliation. Given the strong association between affiliation and conclusions of the studies, the authors recommend that articles disclose conflicts of interest.

Centers for Disease Control and Prevention. "Morbidity and Mortality Weekly Report: Annual Smoking-Attributable Mortality, Years of Potential Life Lost, and Economic Costs—United States, 1995–1999." *JAMA* 287 (May 8, 2002): 2,355–2,358. Estimates indicate that during 1995–99 smoking caused approximately 440,000 premature deaths each year in the

United States, and that these deaths and the associated sickness that pre-ceded them caused approximately $157 billion in annual health-related economic losses.

———. "Morbidity and Mortality Weekly Report: Costs of Smoking Among Active Duty U.S. Air Force Personnel—United States, 1997." *JAMA* 283 (June 28, 2000): 3,190–3,196. This study compares lost work time (including smoke breaks, days spent in the hospital, and time spent in outpatient clinics) of smokers and of nonsmokers. With 25 percent of male and 27 percent of female personnel being current smokers, the habit costs the air force an estimated $107.2 million a year.

Chasan-Taber, Lisa, and Meir Stampfer. "Oral Contraceptives and Myocar-dial Infarction—the Search for the Smoking Gun." *New England Journal of Medicine* 345 (December 20, 2001): 1,841–1,842. This editorial reviews the evidence that smoking combined with the use of oral contraceptives by women greatly increase the risk of heart attacks. These findings em-phasize the importance of reducing smoking among young women.

"Cigarettes: The Lung Cancer Risk Lingers." *Harvard Health Letter* 30, no. 9 (July 2005): 6. The death of Peter Jennings in 2005 from lung cancer, even though he had quit smoking some 20 years earlier, offers a reminder that the harm of tobacco smoking persists. Quitting reduces the risk of lung cancer but not to the level of those who never smoked. The article also notes that former smokers may be more vulnerable to the harm of secondhand smoke, likely because smoking does lasting DNA damage to lung cells.

Cruickshanks, Karen J. "Cigarette Smoking and Hearing Loss: The Epide-miology of Hearing Loss Study." *JAMA* 279 (June 3, 1998): 1,715–1,719. To illustrate the diverse harm of smoking, this article shows that smokers are more likely to experience hearing loss than nonsmokers.

Doll, Richard, et al. "Mortality in Relation to Smoking: 40 Years' Observa-tions on Male British Doctors." *British Medical Journal* 309 (October 8, 1994): 901–911. In assessing the hazards associated with tobacco, an analysis of data over 40 years on British doctors (a study group that eliminates the influence of occupation and education since all doctors have high-prestige jobs and high education) demonstrates that smokers have risks of dying that are two to three times higher than nonsmokers.

Eisner, Mark D., et al. "Measurement of Environmental Tobacco Smoke Exposure Among Adults with Asthma." *Environmental Health Perspectives* 109 (August 2001): 809–814. Problems of asthma have increased in the U.S. population, and evidence suggests that exposure to secondhand smoke can adversely affect adults with asthma. The study, which provided nicotine badge monitors to measure exposure to environmental tobacco smoke, finds that subjects most exposed to the smoke had high risks of respiratory problems.

Eisner, Mark D., Alexander K. Smith, and Paul D. Blanc. "Bartenders' Respiratory Health after Establishment of Smoke-Free Bars and Taverns." *JAMA* 280 (December 9, 1988): 1,909–1,914. Interviewing bartenders before and after a smoking ban in San Francisco restaurants and bars, the authors assess respiratory irritation and infection. Their findings indicate that the establishment of smoke-free bars and taverns was associated with a rapid improvement of respiratory health.

Ernst, Armin, and Joseph D. Zibrak. "Carbon Monoxide Poisoning." *New England Journal of Medicine* 339 (November 26, 1998): 1,603–1,608. Tobacco smoke is an important source of carbon monoxide, a colorless, odorless, and nonirritating toxic gas. This article describes the physiological harm of carbon monoxide but focuses less on tobacco smoke than on poisoning from other sources.

Ernst, Monique, Eric T. Moolchan, and Miqun L. Robinson. "Behavioral and Neural Consequences of Prenatal Exposure to Nicotine." *Journal of the American Academy of Child and Adolescent Psychiatry* 40 (June 2001): 630–641. A review of the evidence on the consequences of smoking for pregnant women finds that prenatal exposure of the fetus of nicotine leads to problems of brain development and to higher risks of psychiatric problems and substance abuse later in life.

Ferber, Dan. "Research on Secondhand Smoke Questioned." *Science* 306 (November 19, 2004): 1,274. Debates over the potential harm of secondhand smoke involve scientists as well as public officials. As described in this science magazine, a recent report from the University of Geneva questions three decades of research by a scientist associated with the tobacco maker Philip Morris. The report disputes findings of the scientist that secondhand smoke does little harm to nonsmokers. To the contrary, other research on animals done by Philip Morris found that secondhand smoke did extensive damage to health. However, the company kept the research quiet while publicly arguing that secondhand smoke was safe. Both the scientist and the parent company of Philip Morris, Altria, deny the accusations.

Fichtenberg, Caroline M., and Stanton A. Glantz. "Association of the California Tobacco Control Program with Declines in Cigarette Consumption and Mortality from Heart Disease." *New England Journal of Medicine* 343 (December 14, 2000): 1,772–1,777. A voter-enacted initiative to use additional taxes to fund antitobacco programs in 1989 accelerated the decline in cigarette consumption in California. This study shows that the program also reduced the death rate from heart disease, which is associated with smoking, but this effect was diminished in 1992 when the program funding was cut back.

Hackshaw, A. K., M. R. Law, and N. J. Wald. "The Accumulated Evidence on Lung Cancer and Environmental Tobacco Smoke." *British Medical*

Journal 315 (October 18, 1997): 280–288. A review of numerous studies of environmental tobacco smoke leads the authors to estimate that lung cancer rates among nonsmoking women whose husbands smoke are 24 percent higher than for nonsmoking women whose husbands do not smoke.

Hu, Frank B., et al. "Diet, Lifestyle, and the Risk of Type 2 Diabetes Mellitus in Women." *New England Journal of Medicine* 345 (September 13, 2001): 790–797. Along with lack of exercise, poor diet, and abstinence from alcohol, current cigarette smoking appears associated with an increased risk of diabetes.

————. "Trends in the Incidence of Coronary Heart Disease and Changes in Diet and Lifestyle in Women." *New England Journal of Medicine* 343 (August 24, 2000): 530–537. This study finds that reductions in smoking among a sample of 85,941 women ages 34 to 59 produced a 13 percent decline in the incidence of coronary heart disease.

Istre, Gregory R., et al. "Deaths and Injuries from House Fires." *New England Journal of Medicine* 344 (June 21, 2001): 1,911–1,916. Fires started by smoking result in a higher injury rate than fires unrelated to smoking. Although most deaths from smoking involve disease, some involve injuries stemming from smoking-related fires.

Johnson, Jeffrey G. "Association Between Cigarette Smoking and Anxiety Disorders During Adolescence and Early Adulthood." *JAMA* 284 (November 8, 2000): 2,348–2,351. Smokers seem to suffer disproportionately from anxiety disorders, but it is less clear if high anxiety causes smoking or if smoking causes anxiety disorders. The study finds that cigarette smoking may increase the risk of certain anxiety disorders during late adolescence and early adulthood.

Juster, Harlan R., Brett R. Loomis, and Theresa M. Hinman. "Declines in Hospital Admissions for Acute Myocardial Infarction in New York State After Implementation of a Comprehensive Smoking Ban." *American Journal of Public Health* 97, no. 11 (November 2007): 2,035–2,039. Evidence of the health benefits of smoking bans comes from this study in New York State. It finds that declining admissions to hospitals for a common form of heart attack occurred after a comprehensive smoking ban. Controlling for other influences on admissions for myocardial infarctions, the smoking ban appears to account for an 8 percent decline. The authors conclude that "comprehensive smoking bans constitute a simple, effective intervention to substantially improve the public's health."

Lesser, Karen, et al. "Smoking and Mental Illness: A Population-Based Prevalence Study." *JAMA* 284 (November 22/29, 2000): 2,606–2,610. Although many studies report higher rates of smoking of persons with mental illness than persons in the general population, this article offers one of the few national studies of the relationship. The results indicate that persons with mental illness are twice as likely to smoke as other persons but also make substantial efforts to quit.

Lyon, Lindsay. "The Hazard in Hookah Smoke." *U.S. News & World Report*, January 28–February 4, 2008, pp. 60–61. Smoking with hookahs, tall water pipes used for centuries in the Middle East, has spread to campuses and become popular among young people. The article disputes common beliefs that hookah smoke does less harm than cigarette smoke. In fact, hookah smoking is a major health risk.

Mascola, Maria A., Helen van Vunakis, and Ira B. Tager. "Exposure of Young Infants to Environmental Tobacco Smoke: Breast-Feeding Among Smoking Mothers." *American Journal of Public Health* 88 (June 1998): 893–896. Finds that breast-fed infants of mothers who smoke had much higher exposure to nicotine than bottle-fed infants and suggests that breast-feeding more than environmental tobacco smoke affects infants of smoking mothers.

Otsuka, Ryo, et al. "Acute Effects of Passive Smoking on the Coronary Circulation in Healthy Young Adults." *JAMA* 286 (July 25, 2001): 436–441. To demonstrate that passive smoking reduces the flow of blood to the heart an experiment compares smoking and nonsmoking subjects before and after a 30-minute exposure to environmental tobacco smoke. The findings suggest that even a little secondhand smoke can negatively affect the body.

Payne, Sarah. "'Smoke Like a Man, Die Like a Man'? A Review of the Relationship between Gender, Sex, and Lung Cancer." *Social Science and Medicine* 53 (October 2001): 1,067–1,080. Differences in biologically based hormones and social smoking behaviors of men and women result in different risks of lung cancer. A review of evidence in this article indicates that women smokers have a higher risk of getting lung cancer than male smokers.

Petit-Zeman, Sophie. "Smoke Gets in Your Mind." *New Scientist* (April 13, 2002): 30–32. Although it is clear that mental illness leads to smoking, there is also emerging evidence, according to this article, that smoking may cause mental illness.

Peto, J. "Cancer Epidemiology in the Last Century and the Next Decade." *Nature* 411 (May 17, 2001): 390–396. In describing the trends and patterns of cancer across the world the author notes that the most important discovery in the history of cancer epidemiology is the carcinogenic effect of tobacco.

Seppa, N. "Cutting Back Helps, But Even a Cigarette or Two a Day Carries Risks." *Science News* 168, no. 14 (October 1, 2005): 213. This article reports on two scientific studies of the benefits of quitting smoking. In one study, heavy smokers who cut in half the number of cigarette they smoked and reduced their lung cancer risk by one-quarter. However, quitting altogether lowered the risk more dramatically. In another study, smoking only one or two cigarettes a day significantly increased the risks of lung cancer compared with not smoking at all.

Stayner, Leslie, James Bena, and Annie J. Sasco. "Lung Cancer Risk and Workplace Exposure to Environmental Tobacco Smoke." *American Journal of Public Health* 97, no. 3 (March 2007): 545–551. A review of 22 research studies finds that workers exposed to environmental tobacco smoke experienced a 24 percent increase in lung cancer risk, and that workers exposed to high levels of environmental tobacco smoke experienced a 101 percent increase. The authors use the results to call for more bans on smoking in workplaces.

Talwar, Namrita. "Taking the World Up in Smoke: A Tobacco Peril." *UN Chronicle* 41, no. 2 (June/August 2004): 67–68. This article summarizes the threat to world health of the global spread of tobacco. By most accounts, tobacco use will continue to grow. Higher incomes in developing nations allow larger parts of the world population to purchase cigarettes. With the decline in production of tobacco in the United States, tobacco growing has become a profitable crop elsewhere, making for cheaper and easier access to the main ingredient of cigarettes. The author and the United Nations more generally call for stronger tobacco control policies across the world.

Thun, Michael J., et al. "Alcohol Consumption and Mortality Among Middle-Aged and Elderly U.S. Adults." *New England Journal of Medicine* 337 (December 11, 1997): 1,705–1,714. Although focused largely on alcohol consumption, this study provides interesting facts on tobacco use. It shows that moderate alcohol consumption slightly reduces overall mortality, but the effect is far smaller than that of smoking, which doubles the risk of death.

———. "Excess Mortality among Cigarette Smokers: Changes in a 20-Year Interval." *American Journal of Public Health* 85 (September 1995): 1,223–1,230. Premature mortality, which is defined as the difference between death rates of smokers and nonsmokers, doubled in women and continued unabated in men from the 1960s to the 1980s. Smoking thus continues to impact health, even after cigarette consumption began to fall in the 1960s.

Voelker, Rebecca. "Smoke Carcinogen Affects Fetus." *JAMA* 280 (September 23/30, 1998): 1,041. The article briefly reviews a study out of the University of Minnesota Cancer Center that offers the first direct evidence of the transmittal of a cancer-causing chemical to the fetus when a pregnant women smokes. The study finds that the cancer-causing chemical shows up in the urine of infants of smoking mothers.

WEB DOCUMENTS

American Cancer Society. "Questions About Smoking, Tobacco, and Health." Available online. URL: http://www.cancer.org/docroot/PED/content/PED_10_2x_Questions_About_Smoking_Tobacco_and_Health. asp. Updated on October 23, 2007. Is there a safe way to smoke cigarettes? What in cigarette smoke is harmful? How does cigarette smoke affect the lungs? How does smoking affect pregnant women and their babies? The experts at the American Cancer Society clearly and informatively answer these and other questions on this web site.

American Lung Association. "Secondhand Smoke Fact Sheet." Available online. URL: http://www.lungusa.org/site/pp.asp?c=dvLUK9O0E&b=35422. Updated in June 2007. According to this web site, secondhand or environmental tobacco smoke contains hazardous chemicals and has been classified as a carcinogen. Estimates suggest that secondhand smoke causes about 3,400 lung cancer deaths and 46,000 heart disease deaths each year. Although such figures require some guesswork, they suggest the value of keeping children and workers away from the smoke of others.

Centers for Disease Control and Prevention. "Surgeon General's Reports." Available online. "URL: http://www.cdc.gov/tobacco/data_statistics/sgr/index.htm. Downloaded in April 2008. This site lists the titles and publication dates for each of the 27 Surgeon General's reports since 1964 on smoking and tobacco and allows several of the reports to be downloaded.

———. "Health Consequences of Smoking on the Human Body." Available online. URL: http://www.cdc.gov/tobacco/data_statistics/sgr/sgr_2004/sgranimation/flash/index.html. Updated in May 2004. Using Adobe Flash Player, this web site depicts how smoke harms most every organ in the body. A brief explanation describes the harm in words, but the impressive visuals make the web site special.

National Cancer Institute. "Cancer Topics." Available online. URL: http://www.cancer.gov/cancertopics. Downloaded in April 2008. The web site designed for the public includes information on types of cancer, treatment of cancer, coping with cancer, screening and testing for cancer, and, most relevant tobacco use, prevention of cancer.

———. "Statistics." Available online. URL: http://www.nci.nih.gov/statistics. Downloaded in February 2008. This page provides statistics, maps, and graphs on cancer prevalence, mortality, and prognosis; a guide to understanding statistics; and a list of data sources of cancer.

National Institute on Drug Abuse. "Tobacco Addiction." Available online. URL: http://www.drugabuse.gov/PDF/RRTobacco.pdf. Updated in July 2006. Those wanting less scientific information on addiction than provided by Bock and Goode in *Understanding Nicotine and Tobacco Addiction* can consult this brochure. Without going into the details, the brochure notes that genes predispose people to tobacco addiction and make some smoking cessation treatments more effective than others.

U.S. Department of Health and Human Services. "Body FX—Tobacco." Available online. URL: http://www.girlpower.gov/girlarea/bodyfx/tobacco. htm. Downloaded in February 2003. A government-sponsored web site for girls up to age 13, it describes the harms of nicotine and tobacco to health.

World Bank Group. "The Health Consequences of Smoking." Economics of Tobacco Control. Available online. URL: http://www1.worldbank. org/tobacco/book/html/chapter2.htm. Downloaded in April 2008. This web site gives particular attention to the health consequences of smoking in the developing world. Rather than repeating known facts on the risks of smoking to individuals, it instead describes the risks to societies of the spread of smoking among its population. The long delay between exposure to cigarette smoke and death means the widespread adoption of smoking in a nation will lead to death and disability in decades to come. Such problems make smoking a worldwide public health problem.

SOCIAL AND PSYCHOLOGICAL ASPECTS

BOOKS

Bachman, Jerald G., et al. *The Decline of Substance Use in Young Adulthood: Changes in Social Activities, Roles, and Beliefs.* Mahwah, N.J.: Lawrence Erlbaum Associates, 2002. Building on their previous book, the authors examine how changes in social activities, religious experiences, and individual attitudes affect substance use as youth grow into adulthood. Although it examines many forms of substance abuse, the book gives major attention to cigarette smoking.

Barth, Ilene. *The Smoking Life.* Columbus, Mich.: Genesis Press, 1997. Filled with interesting historical facts, stories, and pictures, this book resembles a coffee-table book that one would want to sample more than read straight through. Its stories and facts, however, reflect the importance of cigarettes on life in modern America and elsewhere.

Edwards, Peggy. *Evening the Odds: Adolescent Women, Tobacco, and Physical Activity.* Ottawa, Canada: Canadian Association for the Advancement of Women and Sport and Physical Activity, 1996. A feminist analysis of smoking and lack of physical activity suggests the need to improve the social circumstances of young women that leads to both problems. Exercise can meet women's needs while at the same time offering a healthy and enjoyable alternative to smoking.

Tobacco Industry and Smoking

Eysenck, Hans J. *Smoking, Health, and Personality.* Piscataway, N.J.: Transaction Publishers, 2000. The author, an accomplished and respected psychologist with unique views about smoking, argues in this reissue of a 1965 book that evidence of the harm of smoking is potentially flawed and that personality factors better predict heart disease and cancer than smoking. Along with an introduction by Stuart Brody that reviews Eysenck's work, the book provides an unusual and intriguing view of smoking.

Ferrence, Roberta G. *Deadly Fashion: The Rise and Fall of Cigarette Smoking in North America.* New York: Garland Publishing, 1989. The author views the spread of cigarettes throughout the U.S. and Canadian populations as similar to the diffusion of innovative ideas, techniques, products, and behaviors. The diffusion perspective helps make sense of the early adoption of cigarettes by some groups such as high-status men and the late adoption of cigarettes by other groups such as low-status women.

Gladwell, Malcolm. *The Tipping Point: How Little Things Can Make a Big Difference.* Boston: Little, Brown, 2000. This book views the spread of ideas, products, and messages as similar to the epidemic spread of diseases and searches for what leads to the critical mass or tipping point needed to generate the epidemic. In arguing that tipping points are reached through minor changes in the environment and the action of a small number of people, the author applies his ideas to teen smoking in one chapter.

Gottfredson, Michael R., and Travis Hirschi. *A General Theory of Crime.* Stanford, Calif.: Stanford University Press, 1990. The authors argue that smoking shares a similarity with criminal behavior: Each involves the sacrifice of long-term benefits (such as avoiding health problems, trouble in school, and prison time) in favor of short-term pleasures and immediate impulses (such as enjoyment of smoking, profit from theft, and the high of excess drugs and alcohol). Smoking does not cause crime but is associated with it.

Grossman, Michael, and Chee-Ruey Hsieh, eds. *Economic Analysis of Substance Use and Abuse: The Experience of Developed Countries and Lessons for Developing Countries.* Northhampton, Mass.: Elgar, 2001. Chapters on cigarette use focus on questions of current concern to economists such as whether addicted smokers act rationally in their use of tobacco, whether smokers are too optimistic in perceptions of their health, whether the presence of children affects men's use of cigarettes, and whether smoking costs much in lost labor productivity.

Jeanrenaud, Claude, and Nils Soguel, eds. *Valuing the Cost of Smoking: Assessment Methods, Risk Perception, and Policy Options.* Boston: Kluwer, 1999. Using an economic approach to smoking that aims to determine the financial burden faced by smokers and by nonsmokers who pay for the social costs of the habit, the chapters review the various ways to place an

180

economic value on the health costs of smoking and use economic perspectives to understand the decision to smoke.

Kilbourne, Jean. *Deadly Persuasion: Why Women and Girls Must Fight the Addictive Power of Advertising.* New York: Free Press, 1999. Because advertisers make addictive behaviors involving tobacco, alcohol, sex, and food appear not only normal but as solutions to personal problems, the author is greatly concerned about the degree to which advertisers influence the lives of American women and girls.

Lloyd, Barbara, et al. *Smoking in Adolescence: Images and Identities.* London: Routledge, 1998. In interviewing adolescents rather than adults to see their point of view about smoking, these British researchers find that teens see smokers as fun loving and nonconformist and see cigarettes as fashionable and image enhancing. The authors use these insights about the meanings smoking has for teens to make recommendations for policy.

Mackay, Judith, Michael Eriksen, and Omar Shafey. *The Tobacco Atlas.* 2nd ed. Geneva: World Health Organization, 2006. Also available online. URL: http://www.cancer.org/docroot/AA/content/AA_2_5_9x_Tobacco_Atlas.asp. Downloaded in April 2008. Each section of the atlas uses full-color maps and graphics to describe the prevalence of tobacco use, tobacco growing, and tobacco control efforts across the world. Although filled with statistics, this book is clear and interesting. It shows readers where tobacco has most recently spread and where it most threatens the future health of the world.

National Cancer Institute, National Institutes of Health. *Changing Adolescent Smoking Prevalence: Where It Is and Why.* Smoking and Tobacco Control Monograph 14. Washington, D.C.: U.S. Department of Health and Human Services, 2001. Updating the 1994 Surgeon General's report on youth smoking, the chapters cover trends in youth smoking and the programs to limit the initiation and continuation of smoking among adolescents.

———. *Smokeless Tobacco or Health: An International Perspective.* Smoking and Tobacco Control Monograph 2. Washington, D.C.: U.S. Department of Health and Human Services, 1993. Many view smokeless tobacco as a safe alternative to cigarettes. This volume disputes this view by emphasizing the harm to health of smokeless tobacco and the need for control of the product. It also examines use of the product across the world as well as in the United States.

Robinson, Robert G., Charyn D. Sutton, Denise A. James, and Carole Tracy Orleans. *Pathways to Freedom: Winning the Fight Against Tobacco.* U.S. Department of Health and Human Services, Centers for Disease Control and Prevention, 2006. Also available online. URL: http://www.cdc.gov/tobacco/quit_smoking/how_to_quit/00_pdfs/pathways.pdf. Downloaded in April 2006. The authors hope to help African-American smokers and communities to improve their health by quitting smoking. The title emphasizes the goals of freedom from addiction and poor health. Along with discussion of the harm of smoking and individual strategies to quit, the 44-page booklet has a section on organizing communities to fight the tobacco industry.

Singer, Merrill. *Drugging the Poor: Legal and Illegal Drugs and Social Inequality*. Long Grove, Ill.: Waveland Press, 2008. Singer highlights the similarity in the distribution of illegal drugs such as cocaine and heroine with the distribution of legal drugs such as tobacco and alcohol. He argues that both types of drugs represent a form of capitalism that brings business profits and victimizes the poor. By providing forms of self-medication against discrimination, poverty, and inequality, both types of drugs find buyers in poor communities. While extreme in its criticism of a legal product like tobacco, the book does more than most to discuss inequality and the implications for deprived communities of tobacco use.

Sloan, Frank A., Jan Ostermann, Christopher Conover, Donald H. Taylor Jr., and Gabriel Picone. *The Price of Smoking*. Cambridge, Mass.: MIT Press, 2004. After accounting for health care expenses and lost wages, the health economist authors calculate that a pack of cigarettes costs nearly $40. Smokers bear most of this cost ($33), but the rest of society ($5) and the family ($1) also pay. However, the authors also estimate the costs to society of smoking and find that, because smokers die younger than nonsmokers, they present fewer costs to Medicare and Social Security. The book addresses important, complex, and controversial issues.

Slovic, Paul, ed. *Smoking: Risk, Perception, and Policy*. Thousand Oaks, Calif.: Sage Publications, 2001. This volume uses data from telephone interviews to examine perceptions of the risks of smoking. Its theme, that young smokers do not fully understand the health risks of the habit and underestimate the difficulty of quitting, suggests the need for policies to do more to educate young people about these risks.

Tollison, Robert D., and Richard E. Wagner. *The Economics of Smoking*. Boston: Kluwer Academic Publishing Group, 1992. Unlike nearly all academic literature on the topic, this book treats the relationship between smoking and health with skepticism. It argues that if the harm of smoking is born by the smokers themselves, then no public policy is necessary. Their arguments bring a classic economic perspective to bear on the issue of smoking and public policy.

U.S. Department of Health and Human Services. *Tobacco Use Among U.S. Racial/Ethnic Minority Groups: African Americans, American Indians and Alaskan Natives, Asian Americans and Pacific Islanders, and Hispanics: A Report of the Surgeon General*. Washington, D.C.: U.S. Department of Health and Human Services, 1998. This report provides a single, comprehensive source of data on how each of four racial/ethnic groups use tobacco, suffer the physical effects of tobacco use, have psychosocial and social factors associated with use of tobacco, and can benefit from strategies to reduce their tobacco use. The attention to diversity in this volume complements other volumes that take a more general perspective on tobacco use and control.

Viscusi, W. Kip. *Smoking: Making the Risky Decision*. New York: Oxford University Press, 1992. The book summarizes the results of a survey that asked smokers and nonsmokers to estimate the harm of smoking for the added risk of death, the likelihood of dying from a smoking-related cause, and the years of life lost. The findings demonstrate that both groups overstate the risks identified by the scientific literature and that smokers recognize the serious health risks they face.

Waldron, Ingrid. "Contributions of Changing Gender Differences in Behavior and Social Roles to Changing Gender Differences in Mortality." In *Men's Health and Illness: Gender, Power, and the Body*, edited by Donald Sabo and David Frederick Gordon. Thousands Oaks, Calif.: Sage Publications, 1995. The author argues that smoking rates among women in modern societies—which have come to approach those of men—reflect some traditional concerns, such as staying slim, as well as new freedom to act in ways that men have acted.

World Health Organization. *Tobacco or Health: A Global Status Report*. Geneva: World Health Organization, 1997. The first several chapters summarize the worldwide trends in smoking and smoking-related mortality, but the volume is most useful for the detailed country-by-country compilation of smoking statistics and antismoking policies. It also provides a summary of current global tobacco control efforts.

Zuckerman, Marvin. *Sensation Seeking and Risky Behavior*. Washington, D.C.: American Psychological Association, 2007. The value of this book comes from the effort to link smoking with other risky behaviors such as drug use, alcohol abuse, crime, reckless driving, and dangerous sex. All involve some form of sensation seeking that, at the extreme, can harm health. The focus on individual personality characteristics and needs complements other approaches that focus on tobacco industry practices as sources of the attraction to smoking.

ARTICLES

Acevedo-Garcia, Dolores, Jocelyn Pan, and Hee-Jin Jun. "The Effect of Immigrant Generation on Smoking." *Social Science and Medicine* 61, no. 6 (September 2005): 1,223–1,242. Immigrants to the United States, typically less educated and lower status than the general U.S. population, serve as an exception to the general tendency of disadvantaged groups to smoke. Consistent with this claim, the authors find that children of U.S.-born parents smoke more than children of foreign-born parents. The authors conclude that assimilation of immigrants tends to increase smoking.

Adler, Jerry. "The Working-Class Smoker." *Newsweek*, March 31, 2008, p. 16. Also available online. URL: http://www.newsweek.com/id/128568. Downloaded in April 2008. The author gives concrete examples of the trend toward concentration of smoking among less educated and lower income groups. Adler cites figures that 35 percent of Americans with a ninth- to 11th-grade education smoked, while only 7 percent of those with a graduate degree smoked. Members of disadvantaged groups sometimes seem to use cigarettes as a source of defiance, to show that, despite their economic troubles, they can do as they please in their personal habits.

Ahluwalia, Jasjit, et al. "Sustained-Release Bupropion for Smoking Cessation in African Americans." *JAMA* 288 (July 24/31, 2002): 468–474. Since African Americans suffer disproportional harm to their health from smoking, medical research needs to do more to understand how to reduce their smoking rates. This study finds that an antidepressant, bupropion, promoted smoking cessation among a sample of 600 African-American adults who smoked 10 or more cigarettes a day.

Anda, Robert F. "Adverse Childhood Experiences and Smoking During Adolescence and Adulthood." *JAMA* 282 (November 3, 1999): 1,652–1,658. Using a sample of 9,215 adult members of a health maintenance organization (HMO) in San Diego, the study measures the extent of adverse experiences during childhood (for example, physical, emotional, or sexual abuse; a battered mother; parental separation or divorce; and the presence of substance abuse, mental illness, or incarceration of parents). These adverse experiences were strongly associated with smoking.

Becker, Gary M., and Michael Grossman. "An Empirical Analysis of Cigarette Addiction." *American Economic Review* 84 (June 1994): 396–418. This empirical study partly supports the rational addiction theory of Nobel Prize–winning economist Gary Becker, by finding that current cigarette consumption is affected by past and future cigarette price changes. The results indicate that cigarette smoking is addictive but still responsive to prices.

Benowitz, Neal L., et al. "Slower Metabolism and Reduced Intake of Nicotine from Cigarette Smoking in Chinese-Americans." *Journal of National Cancer Institute* 94 (January 16, 2002): 108–115. This study finds that Chinese Americans take in less nicotine per cigarette and metabolize it more slowly than do Latinos or whites, which could help explain why Chinese Americans have lower rates of lung cancer than do other groups. The findings may help members of different ethnic groups in developing strategies of quitting.

Bobo, Janet Kay, and Corinne Husten. "Sociocultural Influences on Smoking and Drinking." *Alcohol Research and Health* 24, no. 4 (2000): 225–232.

Consistent with arguments that smoking reflects a more generally deviant lifestyle, this review of the evidence finds a strong relationship between alcohol use and tobacco use.

Buckley, William F. "You Live with It." *National Review*, December 31, 2007, pp. 54–55. The esteemed founder of the conservative magazine *National Review* favors the liberty of tobacco companies to advertise their product in the free marketplace. People should have the opportunity, he believes, to make choices about their own pleasures and pains. Yet he also admits his ambivalence about this position. As a former smoker who suffers from emphysema, he also recognizes the damage wrought by the product. (Buckley died February 27, 2008, shortly after this article appeared.)

Chiarella, Tom. "Learning to Smoke." *Esquire*, March 2008, pp. 156–161, 194–195. The author did something quite rare these days—start to smoke at age 46—and then did something quite common—try to quit smoking. The story reported in the article is a harrowing one. He suffers physically and socially in learning to smoke, and then suffers during and after the process of quitting. The article gives fascinating insight into the encounters he faces in making friends with other smokers and dealing with the hostility of nonsmokers.

Cochran, Susan D., Vickie M. Mays, and Deborah Bowen. "Cancer-Related Risk Indicators and Preventive Screening Behaviors Among Lesbian and Bisexual Women." *American Journal of Public Health* 91 (April 2001): 591–597. This study uses seven separate surveys of 11,876 lesbian/bisexual women, a difficult group to study with surveys, to identify the prevalence of cancer risk factors. It confirms that lesbian/bisexual women have higher rates of tobacco use than heterosexual women.

Colby John P., Jr., Arnold S. Linsky, and Murray A. Straus. "Social Stress and State-to-State Differences in Smoking and Smoking-Related Mortality in the United States." *Social Science and Medicine*, vol. 38, no. 2, January 1994, pp. 373–381. An analysis of the 50 American states demonstrates that those with high rates of stress—divorces, business failures, natural disasters—also have high rates of cigarette use and lung cancer. The results suggest that populations under stress tend to engage in behavior that ultimately harms their health.

Curtis, Patricia. "Gambling with Their Lives: Young Women and Smoking." *Reader's Digest*, January 2008, pp. 140–145. Despite knowledge of the harm of smoking, many young women take up the habit. This article suggests these women are influenced by glamorous images of smokers in ads and movies and by the implied association of smoking with thinness and beauty. Some young women smoke only on weekends at bars and parties, thinking they will not become addicted. They later find out how hard it is to stop and risk damaging their health at a young age.

DuLong, Jessica. "Snuffing Out the Butts." *Advocate*, March 16, 2004, pp. 30–31. According to figures reported in the article, smoking among gays and lesbians is about 75 percent higher than the general population. The author suggests that the health risks of smoking have in the past been overshadowed among gays and lesbians by issues of HIV prevention. With the risks of smoking now receiving more attention, efforts are being made to persuade gays and lesbians to stop smoking.

DuRant, Robert H., Ellen S. Rome, and Michael Rich. "Tobacco and Alcohol Use Behaviors Portrayed in Music Videos: A Content Analysis." *American Journal of Public Health* 87 (July 1997): 1,131–1,135. About one-quarter of MTV videos portray tobacco use, and even modest levels of viewing of videos results in substantial exposure to glamorized depictions of smoking.

Ebrahim, Shahul H. "Trends in Pregnancy-Related Smoking Rates in the United States, 1987–1996." *JAMA* 283 (January 19, 2000): 361–366. Smoking has declined among pregnant women, but this study finds that the decline results largely from an overall drop in smoking among young people, rather than from women smokers giving up the habit upon pregnancy. As well as helping to prevent young women from starting to smoke, physicians need to make special efforts to help pregnant smokers to stop.

Evert, Sherry A., Rae L. Schnuth, and Joanne L. Tribble. "Tobacco and Alcohol Use in Top-Grossing American Films." *Journal of Community Health* 23 (August 1998): 317–324. In examining the top 10 moneymaking films for each year from 1985 to 1995, the authors find most films had references that supported tobacco use, and few had references to discourage use.

Gilmore, Anna, Joceline Pomerleau, and Martin McKee. "Prevalence of Smoking in 8 SP Countries of the Former Soviet Union: Results From the Living Conditions, Lifestyles and Health Study." *American Journal of Public Health* 94, no. 12 (December 2004): 2,177–2,187. Smoking rates among men in countries of the former Soviet Union are among the highest in the world—ranging from 43 to 65 percent. This article compares the prevalence across eight of the countries.

Graham, Hilary. "Cigarette Smoking: A Light on Gender and Class Inequality in Britain?" *Journal of Social Policy* 24, no. 4 (1995): 509–527. Based on interviews with low-income mothers in Britain, the author finds that those women with the heaviest caring responsibilities and lowest income were most likely to smoke. The findings suggest that deprived women use cigarette smoking as a way to help cope with their difficult circumstances.

Howard-Pitney, Beth, and Marilyn A. Winkleby. "Chewing Tobacco: Who Uses and Who Quits? Findings from NHANES III, 1988–1994." *American Journal of Public Health* 92 (February 2002): 250–256. The results of a national survey indicate that rural, lower-income black and white men had the highest regular use of chewing tobacco. Rural high-income men had the second-highest regular use, and southern men had the lowest quit rate. Unlike cigarettes, which are adopted in adolescence, chewing tobacco commonly starts in adulthood.

Jessor, Richard, Mark S. Turbin, and Frances M. Costa. "Protective Factors in Adolescent Health Behavior." *Journal of Personality and Social Psychology* 75, no. 3 (September 1998): 788–800. This study of 1,493 high school students shows that a positive orientation toward school, friendship with conventional peers, and church attendance increase health-enhancing behaviors and reduce harmful habits such as smoking.

Jha, Prabhat, et al. "Estimates of Global and Regional Smoking Prevalence in 1995, by Age and Sex." *American Journal of Public Health* 92 (June 2002): 1,002–1,006. The tables reveal that 1995 smoking percentages are highest in East Asia and eastern Europe and lowest in sub-Saharan Africa.

Kenkel, Donald S. "Health Behavior, Health Knowledge, and Schooling." *Journal of Political Economy* 99, no. 2 (1991): 287–305. Why does education lead persons to smoke less? This study demonstrates that something more than increased knowledge of the harm of cigarette smoking is involved and educational campaigns alone will not be sufficient to reduce smoking.

Kiefe, Catarina I., O. Dale Williams, and Cora E. Lewis. "Ten-Year Changes in Smoking among Young Adults: Are Racial Differences Explained by Socioeconomic Factors in the CARDIA Study?" *American Journal of Public Health* 91 (February 2001): 213–218. Although smoking has declined less among African Americans than whites, this study finds that most of the difference is due to disparities in socioeconomic status. The concentration of smoking among lower socioeconomic groups and the lower socioeconomic status of African Americans explain the widening race gap in smoking.

Long, Rob. "Branding Cigs with 'R': Smoking in Movies." *National Review*, June 11, 2007, pp. 23–24. Public health officials have strongly criticized film directors and studios for unnecessary use of cigarettes in movies. They claim that youth tend to identify with the behavior of leading and attractive actors, including smoking. This article reports on a proposal by the Motional Picture Association of American to rate a movie R if it includes smoking (unless critical to the character or period). However, the author believes such a change will have little impact because movies do little to cause youth to take up smoking. Rather they reflect the views already existing among the young that smoking is cool.

Marsh, Bill. "A Growing Cloud over the Planet." *New York Times Upfront*, March 31, 2008, pp. 28. Also available online. URL: http://query.nytimes.com/gst/fullpage.html?res=9A01E1DF153CF937A15751C0A96E9C8B63.

The first two sentences of this article nicely highlight the extent of the global problem of tobacco use: "Nearly half of the world's 1.3 billion smokers live in China, India and Indonesia, the three largest consumers of tobacco products. In China alone, more people smoke than live in the United States." Tobacco deaths worldwide have consequently reached 5.4 million a year. This short article starkly presents these and other facts about global tobacco use.

Mendez, David, Kenneth E. Warner, and Paul N. Courant. "Has Smoking Cessation Ceased? Expected Trends in the Prevalence of Smoking in the United States." *American Journal of Epidemiology* 148, no. 3 (1998): 249–258. Since data for the 1990s suggest that youth smoking initiation rates have increased and that the decline in smoking has stalled, many worry that the downward trends of the past will not continue. This study predicts to the contrary that smoking of adults will at minimum decline from its current levels of 25 percent to about 15–16 percent in the next 50 years.

Michell, Lynn, and Amanda Amos. "Girls, Pecking Order and Smoking." *Social Science and Medicine* 44, no. 12 (1997): 1,861–1,869. Although many studies suggest that social insecurities increase the likelihood of smoking, this review of the evidence concludes that smokers have higher self-esteem than nonsmokers. Girls in Scotland who have high status in peer groups and who project an image of self-esteem were viewed as most likely to smoke. The sample is specialized, but the findings are intriguing.

Mills, Sherry L. "Tobacco and Health Disparities." *American Journal of Public Health* 94, no. 2 (February 2004): 173. This article summarizes the findings of the National Conference on Tobacco and Health Disparities. The persistence of smoking among more disadvantaged social groups has concerned public health officials and scholars, who offer recommendations for addressing the problem. The recommendations aim to help communities that bear an undue share of tobacco-related diseases and premature deaths.

Molarius, Anu, et al. "Trends in Cigarette Smoking in 36 Populations from the Early 1980s to the Mid-1990s: Findings from the WHO MONICA Project." *American Journal of Public Health* 91 (2001): 206–212. A comprehensive comparison of smoking across numerous nations finds that smoking among men decreased significantly in 44 percent of the populations, changed little in most others, and increased in Beijing, China. For women, smoking increased more commonly than for men, particularly in nations where female smoking started at low levels.

Morabia, Alfredo, et al. "Ages at Initiation of Cigarette Smoking and Quit Attempts among Women: A Generation Effect." *American Journal of Public Health* 92 (January 2002): 71–74. The article concludes that young female smokers have a higher propensity to quit smoking compared with older women and suggests that efforts to encourage young smokers to quit can successfully supplement efforts to prevent nonsmokers from starting to smoke.

Orlando, Maria, Phyllis L. Ellickson, and Kimberly Jinnett. "The Temporal Relationship between Emotional Distress and Cigarette Smoking During Adolescence and Young Adulthood." *Journal of Consulting and Clinical Psychology* 69 (December 2001): 959–970. This statistical study offers an insightful perspective on stress and smoking. It finds that emotional distress in 10th graders led to smoking in 12th grade, and that smoking in 12th grade led to emotional distress in young adulthood. In short, stress initially leads to cigarette use, but then cigarette use exacerbates the stress.

Pampel, Fred C. "Cigarette Use and the Narrowing Sex Differential in Mortality." *Population and Development Review* 28 (March 2002): 77–104. Comparisons across nations reveal that the decline in the female advantage in length of life results largely from the increased smoking rates among women relative to men.

———. "Socioeconomic Distinction, Cultural Tastes, and Cigarette Smoking." *Social Science Quarterly* 87, no. 1 (March 2006): 19–35. This article suggests that social groups use cigarettes as a kind of symbol that identifies their cultural tastes and sets them apart from other groups. Consistent with this view, it finds that smoking relates to musical likes and dislikes. Preferences for classical music are associated with lower smoking, while preferences for bluegrass, jazz, and heavy metal music are associated with higher smoking. These kinds of differences in cultural tastes help explain lower rates of smoking among higher than lower classes.

———. "Tobacco Use in Sub-Sahara Africa: Estimates from the Demographic Health Surveys." *Social Science and Medicine* 66, no. 8 (2008): 1,772–1,783. This study gives figures on smoking prevalence in a region of the world that typically lacks data. It is also a region with historically low levels of smoking but one primed for increases in the future. The figures for 14 nations show moderate usage by men and low usage by women and the highest levels of smoking in east central African nations. They also show higher smoking among less-educated workers with low-skilled jobs, much as in high-income nations.

Parrott, Andrew C. "Heightened Stress and Depression Follow Cigarette Smoking." *Psychological Reports* 94, no. 1 (February 2004): 33–34. Many smokers justify their habit by saying that it helps them cope with stress and control their mood. The author of this article suggests the opposite: Nicotine addiction creates heightened feelings of stress and depression that smokers must then moderate with a cigarette. Although stopping smoking worsens this kind of stress in the short run, it leads to mood improvements in the long term.

Patton, George C., J. B. Carlin, and C. Coffey. "Depression, Anxiety, and Smoking Initiation: A Prospective Study Over 3 Years." *American Journal of Public Health* 88 (October 1998): 1,518–1,522. A study of more than 2,000 14- to 15-year-old students indicates that symptoms of depression and anxiety increase the likelihood of starting to smoke. Promoting psychological well-being may help prevent adolescent tobacco use.

Pérez-Stable, Eliseo J. "Cigarette Smoking Behavior among U.S. Latino Men and Women from Different Countries of Origin." *American Journal of Public Health* 91 (September 2001): 1,424–1,430. For men, smoking differs little among Mexican Americans, Central Americans, Puerto Ricans, Cuban Americans, South Americans, and other Latinos, but for women, Puerto Ricans have the highest rates and Central Americans the lowest rates. Interestingly, foreign-born Latinos are less likely to smoke than U.S.-born Latinos.

Pina, Hector. "The Gloom of Smoking." *Hispanic*, May 2006, pp. 20. A Norwegian study cited in this article reports on the psychological harm of smoking. According to the study, heavy smokers—those using more than 20 cigarettes a day—develop depression four times as often as those who have never smoked. Nicotine appears to affect brain chemicals in a way that modifies emotions, largely for the worse.

Plunkett, Mark, and Christina M. Mitchell. "Substance Use Rates among American Indian Adolescents: Regional Comparisons with Monitoring the Future High School Seniors." *Journal of Drug Issues* 30 (Summer 2000): 575–591. The findings reveal that Native American youth use cigarettes less than other students.

Rigotti, Nancy A., Lae Eun Lee, and Henry Wechsler. "U.S. College Students' Use of Tobacco Products: Results of a National Survey." *JAMA* 284 (August 9, 2000): 699–705. A survey of 14,138 students enrolled in 119 colleges reveals that nearly half had used a tobacco product in the last year and one-third currently used tobacco. College-age students continue to experiment with a variety of tobacco products, risk lifelong nicotine addiction with such activities, and can benefit from national efforts to monitor and prevent tobacco use.

Seffrin, John. "The Worst Pandemic in the History of the World." *Vital Speeches of the Day* 70, no. 12 (April 1, 2004): 356–360. In this speech before The Commonwealth Club in San Francisco, the CEO of the American Cancer Society and president of the International Union Against Cancer cites facts that warrant calling smoking the worst pandemic in the history of the world. He believes, however, that the Framework Convention on Tobacco Control of the World Health Organization can do much to reduce the death and disease caused by tobacco. The treaty aims to organize international as well as national action against tobacco use.

Annotated Bibliography

Shiffman, Saul, and Jean Paty. "Smoking Patterns and Dependence: Contrasting Chippers and Heavy Smokers." *Journal of Abnormal Psychology* 115, no. 3 (August 2006): 509–523. Chippers smoke only a few cigarettes a day, just on weekends, or only at parties and special events. This study examines smoking habits among 26 chippers and contrasts them with heavy smokers. It reports that chippers smoke half their cigarettes alone, indicating the habit involves more than social activity. Whether alone or with others, cigarettes help them relax, socialize, and enjoy eating and drinking alcohol. Chippers are stimulated to smoke by certain events and cues but do not have the dependence on cigarettes that heavy smokers do.

"Smoking Your Money's Worth: Views of Jerome Adda and Francesca Cornaglia." *The Wilson Quarterly* 31, no. 1 (Winter 2007): 83–84. This article summarizes the fascinating findings that two economists reported elsewhere in more technical form. Adda and Cornaglia find that the higher costs of cigarettes, the major form of tobacco control in recent years, lead smokers to compensate by smoking each cigarette more intensely. To get the same nicotine from a smaller number of more expensive cigarettes, smokers, unfortunately, draw in more of the most dangerous chemicals. These discouraging findings suggest that raises prices and taxes on cigarettes may have less benefit for public health than once thought.

Tercyak, Kenneth P., Caryn Lerman, and Janet Audrain. "Association of Attention-Deficit/Hyperactivity Disorder Symptoms with Levels of Cigarette Smoking in a Community Sample of Adolescents." *Journal of the American Academy of Child and Adolescent Psychiatry* 41 (July 2002): 799–805. A survey of more than 1,000 10th-grade students reveals that those with inattention, hyperactivity, and impulsivity symptoms are more likely to experiment with smoking and to become regular tobacco users. These psychological traits can help predict which adolescents will begin to smoke.

Unger, Jennifer B., Tess Boley Cruz, and Kurt M. Ribisl. "English Language Use as a Risk Factor for Smoking Initiation among Hispanic and Asian-American Adolescents: Evidence for Mediation by Tobacco-Related Beliefs and Social Norms." *Health Psychology* 19 (September 2000): 403–410. Research reveals that acculturation of immigrants to American culture increases smoking. In this study use of English was associated with smoking, in part because English speakers saw fewer consequences of smoking and had more friends who smoked than those who used the native language.

Vastag, Brian. "Quitting Smoking Harder for Women." *JAMA* 285 (June 20, 2001): 2,966. Reporting on a study from the National Institute on Drug Abuse, this brief article notes that nicotine replacement therapy works less well for women because they are greatly concerned about gaining weight. The study urges that smoking cessation research focus on developing methods particularly suited for women.

Williams, Geoffrey C., Elizabeth M. Cox, and Viking A. Hedberg. "Extrinsic Life Goals and Health-Risk Behaviors of Adolescents." *Journal of Applied Social Psychology* 30 (August 2000): 1,757–1,771. Examination of attitudes among adolescents discloses that smokers have stronger aspirations for wealth, fame, and image, while nonsmokers have stronger aspirations for growth, relationships, and community ties.

Wray, Linda A., et al. "The Impact of Heart Attack on Smoking Cessation among Middle-Aged Adults." *Journal of Health and Social Behavior* 39 (December 1998): 271–293. This study extends research showing that education reduces smoking in general by examining smoking among those who have experienced a heart attack. Those heart attack victims with high education were more likely to give up smoking than those with low education.

Yang, Gonghuan. "Smoking in China: Findings of the 1996 National Prevalence Survey." *JAMA* 282 (October 6, 1999): 1,247–1,253. China stands today as the world's largest producer and consumer of cigarettes and appears to be experiencing a tobacco epidemic. The statistics from this study indicate the seriousness of the situation: 63 percent of men in China smoke (compared to about 25 percent in the United States). While only 3.8 percent of women in China smoke, the potential exists for rates to rise among females.

Zucker, Alyssa N., Zaje A. Harrell, and Kathi Miner-Rubino. "Smoking in College Women: The Role of Thinness Pressure, Media Exposure, and Critical Consciousness." *Psychology of Women Quarterly* 25 (September 2002): 233–241. Among a sample of 188 female undergraduates, smokers are more likely to believe that smoking controls weight, to feel pressures from media sources to stay thin, and to lack skepticism about tobacco advertisements. The authors suggest that antismoking programs address concerns of young women about weight control.

WEB DOCUMENTS

American Lung Association. "Smoking and Hispanics Fact Sheet." Available online. URL: http://www.lungusa.org/site/pp.asp?c=dvLUK9O0E&b=36002. Downloaded in April 2008. This web site notes that Hispanics have lower rates of smoking than other race and ethnic groups, but they are still high enough to create concern among public health officials. It lists the facts on tobacco use and differences among Cuban Americans, Mexican Americans, and Puerto Ricans.

BlackHealthCare.com. "African American and Tobacco." Available online. URL: http://www.blackhealthcare.com/BHC/Smoking/Description.asp.

Downloaded in April 2008. While African-American and white adults have similar levels of smoking, the tobacco industry appears to concentrate its billboards and outside ads in the African-American community. The industry also attempts to gain support of African Americans by sponsoring cultural events, funding community organizations, and providing scholarships. To discourage smoking, this web site summarizes the health consequences of tobacco use for African Americans, a group already with higher than average mortality rates.

Campaign for Tobacco-Free Kids. "Tobacco and Women: Global Trends." Available online. URL: http://tobaccofreekids.org/campaign/global/pdf/women.pdf. Downloaded in April 2008. Although men have been the major users of tobacco across the world, smoking among women has increased dramatically in many countries. This web site gives examples of such changes, the likely health consequences, and ways to counter global marketing of tobacco companies.

———. "Warning: Big Tobacco Targets Women and Girls." Available online. URL: http://www.tobaccofreekids.org/reports/women. Downloaded in April 2008. This antitobacco web site contains facts about smoking among women and the harmful consequences of smoking for their health. It also gives many examples of how tobacco ads and marketing are designed to appeal to women and girls. The conclusion calls for more government regulation to restrict tobacco industry efforts to attract young women to smoking.

Centers for Disease Control and Prevention. "Cigarette Smoking in 99 Metropolitan Areas—United States, 2000." Available online. URL: http://www.cdc.gov/mmwr/preview/mmwrhtml/mm5049a3.htm. Posted on December 14, 2001. These older, not-yet-updated figures show smoking is highest in the South and Midwest, and lowest in the Northeast and West.

———"Fact Sheet: Cessation." Available online. URL: http://www.cdc.gov/tobacco/data_statistics/Factsheets/cessation2.htm. Updated November 9, 2007. The fact sheet offers some interesting statistics. For example, "Among current U.S. adult smokers, 70% report that they want to quit completely. In 2006, an estimated 19.2 million (44.2%) adult smokers had stopped smoking for at least 1 day during the preceding 12 months because they were trying to quit." The sheet also notes that person-to-person methods involving individual, group, or telephone counseling are effective, as are nicotine replacement therapies such as gum, inhalers, and patches.

National Cancer Institute. "Cancer Trends Progress Report—2007 Update: Youth Smoking." Available online. URL: http://progressreport.cancer.gov/doc_detail.asp?pid=1&did=2007&chid=71&coid=702&mid=. Updated on January 7, 2008. As summarized on this web site, trends in youth smoking have fluctuated in surprising ways. They rose unexpectedly in the mid to late 1990s, fell in the years afterward, and now reveal a flattened rate of decline. The fluctuations may relate to tobacco promotional activities but otherwise puzzle researchers.

Naurath, Nicole, and Jeffrey M. Jones, "Smoking Rates Around the World—How Do Americans Compare?" Gallup News Service. Available online. URL: http://www.gallup.com/poll/28432/Smoking-Rates-Around-World-How-Americans-Compare.aspx. Posted August 17, 2007. This short article nicely summarizes world patterns of smoking. The 24 percent of Americans who reported to the Gallup poll that they smoked cigarettes in the last week falls close the average of 22 percent for 90 countries across the world. Countries with the highest smoking include Cuba (40 percent), Chile (37 percent), and Russia (37 percent). Countries with the lowest smoking include Nigeria (6 percent), El Salvador (8 percent), and Afghanistan (9 percent).

World Bank. "Global Trends in Tobacco Use." Available online. URL: http://www1.worldbank.org/tobacco/book/html/chapter1.htm. Downloaded in April 2008. The World Bank provides quick and easy access to information on patterns of smoking outside the United States. Figures compare smoking levels in each of the major regions of the world, showing that levels are highest in East Asia and eastern Europe and lowest in sub-Saharan Africa.

TOBACCO BUSINESS AND LITIGATION

BOOKS

Davis, D. Layton, and Mark T. Nielsen, eds. *Tobacco: Production, Chemistry, and Technology.* Oxford, U.K.: Blackwell Science, 1999. Contains much scientific information on parts of the tobacco industry that get much less attention than marketing and sales—growing tobacco, the chemical composition of various types of tobacco, and processing, storing, and blending tobacco.

Glantz, Stanton A., et al. *The Cigarette Papers.* Berkeley: University of California Press, 1996. This volume publishes secret internal documents from Brown & Williamson Tobacco in book form and allows readers to see what tobacco manufacturers knew about the harm of their product while they were denying that any such harm occurred.

Hammond, Ross. *Addicted to Profit: Big Tobacco's Expanding Global Reach.* Washington, D.C.: Essential Action, 1998. A critic of U.S. tobacco companies argues that they now make more profit outside than inside the United States, condemns worldwide marketing and advertising efforts that contribute to rising global smoking rates, and opposes government trade programs and export legislation that promote worldwide tobacco sales.

Heyes, Eileen. *Tobacco U.S.A.: The Industry Behind the Smokescreen.* Brookfield, Conn.: Milbrook Press, 1999. This journalistic examination of the U.S. tobacco industry contains information on current tobacco farming, government support and regulation of the industry, marketing trends, and the recent problems of Big Tobacco.

Hilts, Philip J. *Smokescreen: The Truth Behind the Tobacco Industry Cover-Up.* Reading, Mass.: Addison-Wesley, 1996. An investigative report on the efforts of the tobacco industry to hide the dangers of cigarette smoking, the book argues that cigarette manufacturers had known of the harm for a long time and had targeted teens with advertising and nicotine addiction to make sure each generation takes up the habit.

Males, Mike A. *Smoked: Why Joe Camel Is Still Smiling.* Monroe, Maine: Common Courage Press, 1999. The author argues that tobacco companies maintain their power through political contributions and lobbying and believes that efforts to stop teen smoking are counterproductive and dishonest when many adults continue to smoke.

McGowan, Richard. *Business, Politics, and Cigarettes: Multiple Levels, Multiple Agendas.* Westport, Conn.: Greenwood Press, 1995. In describing the development of the tobacco industry this book gives special attention to its relationship with public policies. It explores the effects advertising regulation, smoking bans, and excise taxes have on cigarette sales but in so doing relies on complex statistical procedures.

Miller, Karen S. *The Voice of Business.* Chapel Hill: University of North Carolina Press, 1999. A study of the role of public relations in business, this book describes the practices used by the tobacco industry to promote cigarette use and protect itself from regulation.

Mollenkamp, Carrick, et al. *The People vs. Big Tobacco: How the States Took on the Cigarette Giants.* Princeton, N.J.: Bloomberg Press, 1998. This work chronicles the negotiations between the major tobacco companies and an alliance of antismoking interests that led to the 1997 settlement (ultimately revised in 1998 to create the Master Settlement Agreement). As reporters for Bloomberg News, the authors helped break the story about the negotiations.

Nuttall, Floyd H. *Memoirs in a Country Churchyard: A Tobaccoman's Plea: Clean Up Tobacco Row!* Lawrenceville, Va.: Brunswick Publishers, 1996. A man who worked 40 years in the tobacco industry as an expert on blending and flavoring tobacco describes changes in the industry from the 1930s to the 1970s. These memoirs supply a detailed look at the tobacco industry during times of increasing government attacks and negative publicity and present the author's views on the need for a cigarette that is less harmful to nonsmokers.

Orey, Michael. *Assuming the Risk: The Mavericks, the Lawyers, and the Whis-tle-Blowers Who Beat Big Tobacco.* Boston: Little, Brown, 1999. Beginning with the true-life drama about the case of Nathan Horton, a black carpenter with emphysema and lung cancer who sued American Tobacco for damages, the book traces the efforts in the state of Mississippi to bring a lawsuit against the entire industry.

Parker-Pope, Tara. *Cigarettes: Anatomy of an Industry from Seed to Smoke.* New York: New Press, 2001. A readable overview of the tobacco industry and smoking that covers much ground in relatively few pages. Filled with stories, interesting statistics, and up-to-date material, it provides a good starting point for those doing research on this topic.

Pringle, Peter. *Cornered: Big Tobacco at the Bar of Justice.* New York: Holt, 1998. As with several other books (by such authors as Mollenkamp, Orey, Zegart), this one tells the story of the initial settlement between tobacco companies and state attorneys general suing to recoup Medicaid costs for treating smoking-related illnesses. Although the settlement that the book describes is later replaced by another, the background to the initial agreement proves useful in understanding the motives and actions of both sides of the negotiations.

Rabinoff, Michael. *Ending the Tobacco Holocaust: How Big Tobacco Affects Our Health, Pocketbook and Political Freedom—And What We Can Do About It.* Santa Rosa, Calif.: Elite Books, 2006. The psychiatrist author aims to make this exposé of the tobacco industry of interest to both nonsmokers and smokers. It aims to motivate smokers to quit and nonsmokers to become active in antitobacco efforts. While the tobacco industry deserves the most blame for its marketing, deceitful advertising, and lobbying for favorable legislation, movie makers and celebrities also come under criticism for making cigarette use look cool and influencing young people to take up the habit.

Rosenbaum, David I., ed. *Market Dominance: How Firms Gain, Hold, or Lose It and the Impact on Economic Performance.* Westport, Conn.: Praeger Publishers, 1998. This collection of essays on companies that attained dominance in their market includes a chapter on American Tobacco, which monopolized cigarette production and sales for several decades from the late 1800s to the early 1900s and remained a dominant company during the rest of the 20th century.

Snell, Clete. *Peddling Poison: The Tobacco Industry and Kids.* Westport, Conn.: Praeger, 2005. As reflected in the title, the tobacco industry serves in the villain in this book on youth smoking. The author criticizes the efforts of tobacco companies to attract youth smokers and reviews claims of the U.S. Food and Drug Administration that the companies used deceptive methods to gain young new smokers. To protect youth against the dangers of tobacco, he recommends not only placing regulations on tobacco but also funding more tobacco-prevention programs at the state and local level.

Sobel, Robert. *When Giants Stumble: Classic Business Blunders and How to Avoid Them.* Paramus, N.J.: Prentice-Hall, 1999. An analysis of 15 major business catastrophes in post–World War II America, this book includes a chapter on the events and pivotal mistakes of corporate leaders resulting in the problems of the tobacco industry.

Thibodeau, Michael, and Jana Martin. *Smoke Gets in Your Eyes: A Fine Blend of Cigarette Packaging, Branding and Design.* New York: Abbeville Press, 2000. In presenting pictures of the designs of cigarette packages, this book offers a history of how cigarettes have been promoted over the years, what factors led to a successful brand, and why some symbols became particularly popular. It covers well-known campaigns for Camel and Marlboro cigarettes, but also many less successful campaigns for now-unknown cigarette brands.

Thompson, Argus V., ed. *The Tobacco Industry: Wheezing or Breezing.* New York: Nova Science Publishers, 2002. A chapter on the economic performance of the U.S. tobacco companies in domestic and world markets reviews the business side of the industry. Other chapters examine litigation against and regulation of the tobacco industry.

Twitchell, James B. *Twenty Ads That Shook the World: The Century's Most Groundbreaking Advertising and How It Changed Us All.* New York: Crown Publishers, 2000. Among the 20 advertisers and advertising campaigns discussed in this book is the highly successful effort to promote Marlboro cigarettes.

Tye, Larry. *The Father of Spin: Edward L. Bernays and the Birth of Public Relations.* New York: Crown, 1998. Bernays's use of psychological insights to develop successful advertising campaigns for American Tobacco in the early part of the 20th century proved important in the widening acceptance of tobacco. This biography supplies much background on the man and on early public relations strategies.

Warner, Kenneth E. *Selling Smoke: Cigarette Advertising and Public Health.* Washington, D.C.: American Public Health Association, 1986. After discussing the public's understandings of the hazards of smoking, the author considers the magnitude of cigarette advertising and its effects and concludes that a ban on tobacco advertising is warranted.

Wright, John R. "Tobacco Industry PACs and the Nation's Health: A Second Opinion." In *The Interest Group Connection: Electioneering, Lobbying, and Policymaking in Washington,* edited by Paul S. Herrnson, Ronald G. Shaiko, and Clyde Wilcox. Chatham, N.J.: Chatham House Publishing, 1998. In an analysis of voting in the Senate, the author disputes claims that tobacco Political Action Committees strongly influence voting outcomes and suggests that even with high campaign contributions, tobacco policies respond largely to ideological values.

Tobacco Industry and Smoking

Zegart, Dan. *Civil Warrior: The Legal Siege on the Tobacco Industry.* New York: Delacorte Press, 2000. Written in the form of a narrative story, this book follows the civil litigation against the tobacco industry from the perspective of the trial lawyers who brought the suits, particularly Ron Motley.

ARTICLES

Alterman, Eric. "How Cigarettes Helped Victor Navasky Prove a Philosophical Truth: Cosa Nostra Syndicate." *New Yorker,* August 25–September 1, 1997, p. 58. Victor Navasky, editor of *Nation* magazine, purchased one share of R. J. Reynolds stock with friends (using the name Cosa Nostra Syndicate) in 1964. The goal was to show that self-destructive behavior, such as cigarette smoking, generates huge profits. Indeed, the sale of the stock in 1995 left them with a large return on their investment.

Anderson, Thomas M. "The Virtues of Vice Stocks." *Kiplinger's Personal Finance,* February 2008, pp. 27–31. This article notes that stocks in companies selling vices such as tobacco, alcohol, and gaming tend to do well in recessions. Given their worries during bad economic times, people have special difficulties giving up addictions and perhaps become even more attracted to them as a way to cope with their problems. Recommendations to buy vice stocks reflect the continued prosperity across the world of the tobacco industry in the face of public criticism, antismoking legislation, and continuing litigation.

Barron, Kelly. "Smoking Gun." *Forbes,* August 21, 2000, p. 54. The largest distributor of cigarettes in the United States outside of the tobacco companies themselves is McLane Co., a subsidiary of Wal-Mart Stores. The article describes the ability of the company to both avoid lawsuits and produce profits from cigarette distribution.

Biener, Lois, and Michael Siegel. "Tobacco Marketing and Adolescent Smoking: More Support for a Causal Inference." *American Journal of Public Health* 90 (May 2000): 407–411. Scientific studies have trouble proving that advertising by tobacco companies causes smoking rather than merely prodding current smokers to switch brands. This study finds that youth familiar with tobacco brands and products were more likely to adopt smoking than those not familiar. This study proves more effective than others in demonstrating that tobacco advertising leads nonsmoking youth to become smokers.

Carey, John. "Philip Morris' Latest Smoke Screen: Lobbying the FDA to Rein in Incidence of Teen Smoking." *Business Week,* July 16, 2001, p. 43. This article views efforts by one powerful tobacco company to reduce teen smoking as a gimmick designed to avoid further regulation. It criticizes the claims of Philip Morris that it now is motivated to act in the public interest rather than to maximize profits.

Carlyle, Joshua, Jeff Collin, Monique E. Muggli, and Richard D. Hurt. "British American Tobacco and Formula One Motor Racing." *BMJ* 329, no. 7,457 (July 10, 2004): 104–106. Also available online. URL: http://bmj.bmjjournals.com/cgi/content/full/329/7457/104. Downloaded in April 2008. This article illustrates how tobacco companies publicize their products when laws restrict direct advertising. It cites the use of race car logos and names to gain effective publicity for tobacco companies and illustrates the strategy with the sponsorship by British American Tobacco of a Formula One racing team.

Derthick, Martha. "Federalism and the Politics of Tobacco." *Publius* 31 (Winter 2001): 47–63. A case history of the Master Settlement Agreement that is informed by theory and research in the field of political science.

Douglas, Clifford E., Ronald M. Davis, and John K. Beasley. "Epidemiology of the Third Wave of Tobacco Litigation in the United States, 1994-2005." *Tobacco Control* 15 Supplement 4 (December 2006): iv9–iv16. According to the figures reported in this study, plaintiffs won 41 percent of the 75 cases against tobacco companies that went to verdict during the 10 years from 1994 to 2005. Seven plaintiffs received $115 million in awards. Since 2000, the number of ongoing class-action suits has declined. The authors, who take a strong antitobacco view, favor litigation as one way to block tobacco sales.

Enrich, David. "Jeffrey Wigand." *U.S. News & World Report* August 20–27, 2001, p. 70. As part of a special section on heroes, this article tells the story of Jeffrey Wigand, the former chief research scientist at Brown & Williamson Tobacco who helped government investigators, lawyers, and journalists prove that tobacco companies had set out to addict cigarette users.

Fairclough, Gordon. "As Marlboro Loses Ground, Altria Expands the Brand." *Wall Street Journal*, January 29, 2003, p. B1. Philip Morris, the U.S. tobacco unit of Altria, aims to get tobacco sales and profits up with the introduction of a new variety of Marlboro cigarettes. This article describes the goals of the new product and the strategies of tobacco companies in a strongly antismoking environment.

———. "Cheap Smokes Are Squeezing Big Tobacco." *Wall Street Journal*, November 14, 2002, p. C1. In the 1990s tobacco companies cut the prices of their major brands to complete with discount brands, but such discounting in the 2000s is harder with the need to pay huge damages to the states. Discount brands could cut into the profits of major companies, such as Philip Morris.

Fernandez, Senaida, Norval Hickman, and Elizabeth A. Klonoff. "Cigarette Advertising in Magazines for Latinas, White Women, and Men, 1998–2002: A Preliminary Investigation." *Journal of Community Health* 30, no. 2 (April 2005): 141–151. This study examines how magazine ads differ depending on whether the readers are likely to be white men, white women, or Latinas. Its findings illustrate the efforts of tobacco companies to identify and appeal to market segments with the most potential to use cigarettes.

Fonda, Daren. "Why Big Tobacco Won't Quit: Profits Up and Setbacks for Lawsuits Against Industry." *Time*, July 2, 2001, pp. 38–39. Detailing some reasons why the economic future of the tobacco industry looks positive, this article makes the point that states have become dependent on funds from the tobacco companies and ultimately on the sales of cigarettes. That plus the victories of Republicans in recent elections make the political environment in the 2000s somewhat more supportive of tobacco companies.

Foust, Dean. "The High Cost of Nicotine Withdrawal." *Business Week*, May 23, 2005, p. 40. Three of the tobacco companies that signed the Master Settlement Agreement, in which four tobacco companies pay the states billions of dollars each year to cover the cost of health care for smokers, say they deserve to get back some of their payments. They claim they are losing business to smaller cigarette companies that did not sign the agreement. States were supposed to tax these other tobacco companies so they could not undercut the prices of the four signing companies, but disputes remain over whether the states have adequately done so.

France, Mike. "Why 'Little Tobacco' Looms Larger." *Business Week*, September 14, 1998, p. 136. With the tobacco settlement, smaller tobacco companies not burdened by the cost of litigation and payments to the states may make inroads in the market share of Big Tobacco.

Freedman, Michael. "Smokin'." *Forbes*, June 18, 2007, pp. 144, 146–147. This article in a well-known business magazine tells of the success of British American Tobacco (BAT) in selling its product outside of the United States and Europe. As reported in the article, the company sold an astounding 689 billion cigarettes in 2006, mostly in Russia and Brazil.

Gilmore, A. B., and M. McKee. "Tobacco and Transition: An Overview of Industry Investments, Impact and Influence in the Former Soviet Union." *Tobacco Control* 13, no. 2 (June 2004): 136–142. The opening of the former Soviet Union to investment from foreign companies offers an opportunity to study the expansion of the tobacco industries into new markets. According to this article, transnational tobacco companies invested $2.7 billion in 10 countries of the former Soviet Union and helped block tobacco control efforts in many of them.

Gladwell, Malcolm. "The Spin Myth: Work of E. L. Bernays." *New Yorker*, July 6, 1998, pp. 66–69ff. In the 1920s Edward L. Bernays became one of the first to sell cigarettes by appealing to women's right to smoke. This article tells of his public relations scheme to send 10 women down Fifth Avenue in New York City while smoking cigarettes and demanding freedom and of other campaigns that helped promote acceptance of cigarettes.

Greenblatt, Alan. "Secondhand Spokesman: The Tobacco Industry Remains a Potent Lobbying Force, Partly by Letting Other Groups Advocate on Its Behalf." *Governing* 15 (April 2002): 38–40. According to this article, groups acting in ways that benefit the tobacco industry include restaurant associations opposed to banning tobacco in their businesses and taxpayer organizations opposed to higher taxes on consumer products. By focusing on economic issues, these organizations distract smoking debates from issues of public health.

Grimm, David. "Is Tobacco Research Turning Over a New Leaf?" *Science* 307 (January 7, 2005): 36–37. The tobacco industry continues to fund research on reduced-harm tobacco products. The goal of the research is to allow smokers to enjoy tobacco but with less harm to their health. However, critics say that tobacco companies have shown little interest in the health of smokers and that eliminating smoking rather than reducing the harm should be the goal. This article discusses debates over whether university scientists should accept tobacco-industry funding for research on reduced-harm tobacco products. The debate raises issues of academic freedom as well as tobacco control strategies.

Gruber, Jonathan. "Tobacco at the Crossroads: The Past and Future of Smoking Regulation in the United States." *Journal of Economic Perspectives* 15 (Spring 2001): 193–212. An economist reviews the history of the tobacco industry and the effects of regulations on the industry.

Headden, Susan. "The Marlboro Man Lives! Restrained at Home, Tobacco Firms Step Up Their Marketing Overseas." *U.S. News & World Report* 125, September 21, 1998, pp. 58–59. As described in this article, tobacco companies have made efforts to make up for a stagnant domestic cigarette market with intensified international marketing. Manufacturers argue that U.S. laws cannot dictate their behavior abroad and hope to use open markets in other nations to fuel continued growth in profits.

Lavelle, Marianne. "Big Tobacco Rises from the Ashes: Profits Up at Tobacco Companies Despite Costly Settlement." *U.S. News & World Report* November 13, 2000, p. 50. Despite having to make the first installment of the $246 billion payment to the states, tobacco companies have continued, at least initially, to make profits by raising prices.

Lewis, M. Jane, and Olivia Wackowski. "Dealing with an Innovative Industry: A Look at Flavored Cigarettes Promoted by Mainstream Brands." *American Journal of Public Health* 96, no. 2 (February 2006): 244–251. As a case study of tobacco marketing, this article examines the strategy of tobacco companies to introduce flavored brands of Kool, Camel, and Salem cigarettes. Though tobacco companies deny it, the flavoring appears to be targeted at youth. In advancing the public health goals of the journal and its readers, the article takes a critical view of the marketing efforts but also gives background information on tobacco industry trends.

Mintz, Morton. "Blowing Smoke Rings around the Statehouses: Philip Morris' 'Smoking Gun' Campaign to Prevent Increases in State Cigarette Taxes." *Washington Monthly*, May 1996, pp. 20–22. Since a large share of cigarette taxes comes from legislation at the state level, tobacco companies have made major lobbying efforts in each state. Their success from such efforts has led them to support states' rights in developing tobacco control legislation.

O'Connell, Vanessa. "Tobacco Gets Favorable Ruling; Declining Market Share May Let Cigarette Makers Cut Payments to the States." *Wall Street Journal*, March 29, 2006, p. B.3. Major cigarette makers in the United States say that their loss of market share to other cigarette makers should reduce the payments they must make to states under the Master Settlement Agreement. The article gives the details on what the tobacco companies stand to gain and the states stand to lose from changes in cigarette sales.

Parloff, Roger. "Is the $200 Billion Tobacco Deal Going Up in Smoke?" *Fortune*, March 7, 2005, pp. 126–128, 130, 132, 134, 136, 138, 140. The author reviews many criticisms of the Master Settlement Agreement, in which four tobacco companies agreed to pay the states billions of dollars each year to cover the cost of health care for smokers. According to the article, "The states are addicted to the money it provides. But the comically convoluted settlement is riddled with problems, and judges' patience for it is wearing thin." Indeed, claims and counterclaims about what the tobacco companies should pay have led to new court battles over tobacco sales.

Pascual, Aixa M. "LeBow Turns Over a New Leaf." *Business Week*, May 7, 2001, pp. 71–72. This profile of the CEO of the company that owns the Liggett Group, a relatively small cigarette manufacturer, explains how Bennett LeBow was the first to agree to settle with the states over their suits against the tobacco companies and is now working to have his company develop a safer cigarette with fewer carcinogens and another with no nicotine.

Pekkanen, John. "Thank You for Smoking." *Washingtonian*, December 2007, pp. 82–85, 110–114. The author denounces the American government for using international trade agreements to help tobacco companies market their cigarettes across the globe. Although the government has done much to prevent Americans from smoking, it may have helped foster the spread of tobacco use to other parts of the globe.

Pollay, Richard W. "The Last Straw? Cigarette Advertising and Realized Market Shares Among Youth and Adults, 1979–1993." *Journal of Marketing* 60, no. 2 (1996): 1–16. Analysis of data over time reveals that competition between cigarette firms works mainly to shift brand market share among the young.

Powledge, T. M. "Tobacco Pharming." *Scientific American* 285 (October 2001): 25–26. One company is attempting to use tobacco that carries the tobacco mosaic virus to create medicines and cure cancer. This article describes a genetic engineering effort that may find a more beneficial use for tobacco than smoking.

Sepe, Edward, and Stanton A. Glantz. "Bar and Club Promotions in the Alternative Press: Targeting Young Adults." *American Journal of Public Health* 92 (January 2002): 75–78. This study of tobacco advertising in alternative newspapers in San Francisco and Philadelphia finds an enormous increase in product advertisements and promotions. It appears that the tobacco industry has increased its use of bars and clubs as promotional venues and its efforts to reach the young adults who frequent these establishments.

Shamasunder, Bhavna, and Lisa Bero. "Financial Ties and Conflicts of Interest between Pharmaceutical and Tobacco Companies." *JAMA* 288 (August 14, 2002): 738–744. Tobacco industry documents reveal that tobacco companies pressured pharmaceutical companies to scale back the smoking cessation educational materials that accompany nicotine gum and to restrict the marketing of nicotine patches. The authors recommend that financial ties between the tobacco companies and pharmaceutical products be made public.

Yach, Derek, and Stella Aguinaga Bialous. "Junking Science to Promote Tobacco." *American Journal of Public Health* 91 (November 2001): 1,745–1,748. The authors dispute use of the term *junk science* by tobacco companies to discredit evidence of the harm of secondhand smoke for nonsmokers. They recommend that policymakers recognize the sources and funding of studies in reaching conclusions about appropriate public action.

WEB DOCUMENTS

Altria. "Altria Group Awards More Than $3 Million to Visual Arts and Cultural Organizations across the Country." Available online. URL: http://www.altria.com/media/press_release/03_02_pr_2004_09_09_03. asp. Posted September 9, 2004. This press release highlights the efforts of Altria, the parent company of Philip Morris, which makes Marlboro cigarettes, to create goodwill by funding the arts community. It lists a large number of exhibits at prestigious art museums and galleries across the country that receive such funding.

British American Tobacco. Available online. URL: http://www.bat.com. Downloaded in April 2003. The owner of Brown & Williamson, the third-largest cigarette maker in the United States, British American Tobacco sells Kent, Lucky Strike, and Pall Mall cigarettes. Its web site contains views on smoking and consumers, trade, health, science, and social responsibility. The page on smoking and health, for example, states clearly that the pleasures of smoking bring risks of serious disease and that many people find it difficult to quit.

Campaign for Tobacco Free Kids. "Big Tobacco: Still Addicting Kids." Available online. URL: http://www.tobaccofreekids.org/reports/addicting. Downloaded in April 2008. This site disputes claims of tobacco companies that they have ended efforts to attract kids to smoke.

———. "Tobacco Advertising Gallery." Available online. URL: http://tobaccofreekids.org/adgallery. Downloaded in April 2008. A group opposed to cigarette advertising and efforts to manipulate users into smoking illustrates the ads used by the tobacco companies. Users of the page can view ads organized by country, brand, company, and type.

Centers for Disease Control and Prevention, National Center for Chronic Disease Prevention and Health Promotion, Office on Smoking and Health. "Tobacco Brand Preferences." Available online. URL: http://purl.access.gpo.gov/GPO/LPS84747. Updated on April 27, 2007. This fact sheet tells about the kinds of cigarettes that smokers prefer. Nearly all (99 percent) of purchased cigarettes are filtered, 84 percent are classified as light or ultra-light (defined as containing 1–15 milligrams of tar), and about 27 percent are mentholated. Marlboro remains far and away the most popular brand: It has 40 percent of the market share. Newport (8.9 percent), Camel (6.6 percent), Doral (4.4 percent), Basic (3.8 percent), Winston (3.5 percent), and Kool (3.2 percent) follow in popularity.

Court Library. "Court TV Casefiles: *Carter v. Williamson* (8/96)." Court TV. Available online. URL: http://www.courttv.com/casefiles/verdicts/carter.html. Downloaded in April 2008. The case file summarizes the legal issues and verdict of the case that successfully used grounds of fraud and misrepresentation to obtain damages from tobacco companies in a jury trial. Although overturned on a technicality, the case represented a major victory for antismoking forces.

Everything 2. "Master Settlement Agreement." Available online. URL: http://everything2.com/e2node/Master%2520Settlement%2520Agreement. Downloaded in April 2008. Those wanting a clear summary of the Master Settlement Agreement without all the legal details in the full text can consult this web site.

Frontline. "Inside the Tobacco Deal." PBS Online. Available online. URL: http://www.pbs.org/wgbh/pages/frontline/shows/settlement. Downloaded in April 2008. Based on a PBS documentary on the settlement between the states and Big Tobacco companies, the web site provides biographies and interviews with the main participants, a timeline of major events, and background information on the deal. Because the documentary covers events only up to April 1998, it lacks information on the final outcome of the negotiations.

Lorillard Tobacco Company. Available online. URL: http//www.lorillard. com. Downloaded in April 2008. The fourth-largest and oldest cigarette manufacturer in the United States stresses its corporate responsibility and desire to cooperate with rather than confront antismoking forces. One part of its web site lists its efforts to prevent youth smoking.

National Association of Attorneys General. "Multistate Settlement with the Tobacco Industry." Available online. URL: http://news.findlaw.com/ hdocs/docs/tobacco/multistate_settlement.html. Downloaded in April 2008. This agreement requires the four signing tobacco companies to pay billions of dollars each to all but a few states in return for dismissal of suits brought by the attorneys general. The document contained here provides the legal details of this hugely important agreement. The settlement has not ended legal battles between the tobacco companies and states, but it represented a watershed point in the history of the tobacco industry.

Philip Morris USA. Available online. URL: http://www.philipmorrisusa. com. Downloaded in February 2003. The largest cigarette manufacturer in the United States and one of the largest companies in the world, Philip Morris is best known for its Marlboro cigarettes. Its web site includes commentary on smoking and health, reducing underage smoking, quitting tobacco use, the Master Settlement Agreement, and stopping the importation of counterfeit cigarettes.

RetailMerchandiser. "Smokers Welcome." Available online. URL: http:// www.retail-merchandiser.com/index.php?option=com_content&task=vie w&id=13738. Downloaded in April 2008. This site tells the story of a company named Smoker Friendly that has responded to the negative treatment of smokers by developing stores that do more than sell cigarettes at low prices. They also attempt to make their stores a pleasant place for smokers to visit. As the president of the company, Terry Gallagher, Jr., says, "Smoker Friendly is a place where consumers looking to buy cigarettes and other tobacco products can come and be treated with respect and not feel like second-class citizens—as they are so often made to feel these days." The success of the company reflects the continued demand for cigarettes among a minority of the population.

R. J. Reynolds Tobacco Company. Available online. URL: http://www.rjrt. com. Downloaded in April 2008. The second-largest tobacco maker in the United States sells Camel, Doral, Winston, and Kool cigarettes. Its marketing of Camel cigarettes with the Joe Camel cartoon character has come under particular criticism in the past. The web site has material on its views of health and smoking, law and regulation, and adult choices and links to government material on the health effects of smoking.

TJI: *Tobacco Journal International.* Available online. URL: http://www.
tobaccojournal.com. Downloaded in April, 2008. The leading trade journal for the global tobacco industry includes articles on topics of interest
to tobacco executives and workers. A subscription is required to read the
articles, but the site's list of recent titles summarizes the latest news and
trends. A recent issue, for example, describes court cases, production
trends, and new bans on smoking in all or parts of Latvia, the United
Arab Emirates, Canada, and Australia. Unlike nearly all popular magazines, the web site gives insight into the concerns and views of the tobacco industry.

Tobacco Control Archives, a collection in GALEN: UCSF Digital Library.
Available online. URL: http://www.library.ucsf.edu/tobacco. Downloaded
in April 2008. The University of California at San Francisco has assem-
bled millions of documents obtained from tobacco companies. The documents contain scientific studies done by Brown & Williamson to
understand the addictive nature of tobacco, background information
from R. J. Reynolds on the Joe Camel advertising campaign, efforts to
fight clean air initiatives in California, papers from British American Tobacco, and complaints filed by various government organizations against
tobacco companies. The information is overwhelming, but skimming
through a few of the documents can illustrate the past actions of tobacco
companies.

Tobacco-Free Kids Action Fund. "Campaign Contributions by Tobacco
Interests Quarterly Report: January 2003." URL: http://www.tobacco
freekids.org/reports/contributions. Downloaded in April 2008. This page
shows that the tobacco industry contributed nearly $1 million to Political
Action Committees for federal candidates in the 2007–2008 election
cycle. Documents on the specific companies making contributions and
the candidates receiving them can also be found here.

Tobacco Products Liability Project TPTP, a division of the Public Health
Advocacy Institute. Available online. URL: http://www.tobacco.neu.edu/
index.html. Downloaded in April 2008. This compendium of court documents and presses releases on recent cases can help researchers track litigation against tobacco companies.

Tobacco Reporter. Available online. URL: http://www.tobaccoreporter.com.
Downloaded in April 2008. A trade journal out of Raleigh, North Carolina, *Tobacco Reporter* publishes stories of special interest to the those in the
tobacco industry (much like *Tobacco Journal International*). The titles of
the stories listed on magazine's web site summarize recent events and
trends that can help in keeping up with changes in the tobacco industry.

Willemsen, Marc C., and Boudewijn de Blij. "Tobacco Advertising." UICC
Tobacco Control Factsheets. Available online. URL: http://factsheets.
globalink.org/en/advertising.shtml. Downloaded in April 2008. This fact

sheet examines the evidence that advertising stimulates tobacco sales and concludes that a ban on advertising is needed for countries to reduce tobacco use.

Yahoo! Finance Industry Center—Tobacco. "Tobacco Industry Profile." Available online. URL: http://biz.yahoo.com/ic/profile/tobaco_1203. html. Downloaded in April 2008. Focused on the business aspects of the tobacco industry, this web site describes the challenges companies face and the strategies they use to maintain profitability. As the site says, "Despite the health problems, lawsuits, and rising prices associated with cigarettes, there's still something seductive about tobacco—the profits." Links on the page briefly describe major companies that dominant the American market: Altria (formerly Philip Morris Companies), Reynolds American, Loews subsidiary Lorillard Tobacco Company (part of Carolina Group), and Vector Group's Liggett unit. Links also describe foreign companies such as British American Tobacco, Japan Tobacco, Gallaher Group, Altadis, Imperial Tobacco Group, and Swedish Match AB.

TOBACCO CONTROL

Books

Abbott, Ann Augustine, ed. *Alcohol, Tobacco, and Other Drugs: Challenging Myths, Assessing Theories, Individualizing Interventions.* Washington, D.C.: NASW Press, 2000. This volume compiles articles by social work educators for social work practitioners on addiction, its consequences, its treatments, and its prevention.

Abrams, David, et al. *The Tobacco Dependence Treatment Handbook: A Guide to Best Practices.* New York: Guilford Press, 2003. The chapters contain up-to-date information for clinicians on the assessment, planning, and evaluation of treatment strategies for tobacco dependence. The recommendations are based on scientific research and experiences of practitioners.

Bonnie, Richard J., Kathleen Stratton, and Robert B. Wallace, eds. *Ending the Tobacco Problem: A Blueprint for the Nation.* Washington, D.C.: The National Academies Press. Also available online. URL: http://www.nap. edu/catalog.php?record_id=11795. Downloaded in April 2008. Despite considerable progress in reducing smoking, nearly a quarter of the American population still uses cigarettes—to the great detriment of the nation's health. How might the country address the persistence of this public health problem? The contributors first review the history of smoking, the motivations for use of cigarettes, and past policy efforts. They next offer a blueprint for change. The blueprint calls for strengthening current tobacco control efforts at the state and local levels, developing a new legal framework at the federal level to allow for more aggressive regulation of tobacco, and supporting innovative research on tobacco control.

Centers for Disease Control and Prevention. *Best Practices for Comprehensive Tobacco Control Programs—August 1999*. Atlanta, Ga.: U.S. Department of Health and Human Services, Centers for Disease Control and Prevention, Office of Smoking and Health, 1999. This book describes the best practices for tobacco control in nine areas: community programs, disease prevention programs, schools, enforcement, statewide, countermarketing, cessation, surveillance, and administration.

Chapman, Simon. *Public Health Advocacy and Tobacco Control: Making Smoking History*. Malden, Mass.: Blackwell, 2007. A professor of public health at the University of Sydney and a longtime antitobacco advocate, Simon Chapman presents his views on effective and ineffective strategies for tobacco control. His ideas include developing community-based efforts to "denormalize" smoking. A large section of the book labeled "An A-Z of Strategy" covers terms ranging from action alerts to whistle-blowers.

Derthick, Martha. *Up in Smoke: From Legislation to Litigation in Tobacco Politics*. 2nd ed. Washington, D.C.: CQ Press, 2005. Arguing that litigation does not work as well as legislation in designing tobacco control policies, this book argues that when lawsuits in the 1990s came to replace ordinary politics and legislation, it changed public policy for the worse. To support this claim, the second edition presents recent evidence that litigation resulting in the Master Settlement Agreement and payment of billions by tobacco companies to states has done little to improve public health. Derthick says that "the states were more interested in raising revenue than in improving tobacco control, that the enrichment of wealthy tort lawyers violated the legal profession's ethics, and that the agreement, ironically, spawned the rise of small, upstart cigarette manufacturers able to undersell the major companies."

Fibkins, William L. *What Schools Should Do to Help Kids Stop Smoking*. Larchmont, N.Y.: Eye on Education, 2000. This book identifies what programs work best to prevent kids from smoking and how teachers and administrators can implement the programs. It presents examples of successful efforts at both the school and state level.

Forst, Marin L., ed. *Planning and Implementing Effective Tobacco Education and Prevention Programs*. Springfield, Ill.: Charles C. Thomas, 1999. The chapters describe experiences with a variety of programs for tobacco education and prevention in Native American, African-American, Hispanic, Asian and Pacific Islander, and gay and lesbian communities. A summary chapter evaluates the effects of the various tobacco control programs.

Glantz, Stanton, and Edith D. Balbach. *Tobacco Wars: Inside the California Battles*. Berkeley: University of California Press, 2000. In tracing the history of tobacco control efforts in California, these antitobacco advocates provide a detailed description of the politics behind tobacco change and the efforts of the tobacco industry to prevent such change. The authors argue that elected officials regularly and repeatedly ignored the wishes of the voters for tobacco control and supported instead the interests of the tobacco industry.

Goel, Rajeev K., and Michael Nelson. *Global Efforts to Combat Smoking— An Economic Evaluation of Smoking Control Policies*. London: Ashgate Publishing, 2008. This book evaluates the effectiveness of two types of tobacco control policies, one involving higher prices and taxes, the other involving restrictions on sales, advertising, places to smoke, and packaging. Of special value is the fact that the book uses evidence not only from the United States but also from places around the world where smoking is on the rise.

Jacobson, Peter D., et al. *Combating Teen Smoking: Research and Policy Strategies*. Ann Arbor: University of Michigan Press, 2001. This comprehensive volume reviews the political context of smoking policy, trends in youth smoking, and use of the mass media, tax increases, and regulation as forms of tobacco control. It concludes that antismoking mass media campaigns and regulation of cigarettes would be effective but that a comprehensive set of interventions would do most to reduce teen smoking.

Jha, Prabat, and Frank J. Chaloupka, eds. *Tobacco Control in Developing Countries*. New York: Oxford University Press, 2000. With smoking on the increase in developing countries across the world, public health programs must concentrate on tobacco control in nations outside North America and Europe. This volume, which offers an economic framework for tobacco control, provides much information on the most effective interventions for developing countries and highlights both the importance and potential of such interventions.

Kessler, David. *A Question of Intent: A Great American Battle with a Deadly Industry*. New York: Public Affairs, 2001. The former director of the Food and Drug Administration writes about his efforts and those of the agency to regulate tobacco. The book shows the difficulties and complexities of government policy making in general and of fighting the tobacco industry specifically. In the end, the regulatory effort failed.

Leichter, Howard M. *Free to Be Foolish: Politics and Health Promotion in the United States and Great Britain*. Princeton, N.J.: Princeton University Press, 1991. The United States and Great Britain take different public health approaches to protecting individuals against their own risky lifestyles and against use of cigarettes in particular. In describing these differences the book offers a case study of comparative public policy.

Lichter, S. Robert, and Stanley Rothman. *Environmental Cancer—A Political Disease?* New Haven, Conn.: Yale University Press, 1999. Surveys of cancer scientists and analysis of the content of media reports suggest that environmental activists, media representatives, and sympathetic politicians overstate the risk of environmental agents, including environmental tobacco smoke, as causes of cancer. The views of the scientists and the scientific studies differ from those presented to the public by nonscientists concerned about the environment.

Oakley, Don. *Slow Burn: The Great American Antismoking Scam (And Why It Will Fail)*. Roswell, Ga.: Eyrie Press, 1999. Criticizing the nation's (sometimes hysterical, according to the book) three-decade crusade against smoking, the author concludes that much of the evidence of the harm of cigarettes and secondhand smoke is overstated. He views the crusade as a threat to personal freedom and responsibility.

Oaks, Laury. *Smoking and Pregnancy: The Politics of Fetal Protection*. New Brunswick, N.J.: Rutgers University Press, 2001. Using interviews with 46 women and 27 health professionals and antitobacco advocates, and a range of written sources, the author examines how concerns about the effects on fetuses of smoking by pregnant women became a crucial public policy concern and could erode the reproductive rights of women.

Pertschuk, Michael. *Smoke in Their Eyes: Lessons in Movement Leadership from the Tobacco Wars*. Nashville, Tenn.: Vanderbilt University Press, 2001. A longtime antitobacco advocate offers an inside view of the failed efforts of Congress to pass a tobacco control bill. He points not only to the power of tobacco industry lobbying to block legislation but also to internal conflicts in the antismoking movement as contributing to the lost opportunity of Congress to regulate cigarettes.

Rabin, Robert L., and Stephen D. Sugarman, eds. *Regulating Tobacco*. Oxford, U.K.: Oxford University Press, 2001. Articles in this volume consider the effectiveness of various means to control tobacco use such as raising taxes on tobacco, using tort litigation, and implementing clean indoor air restrictions. The volume gives special attention to the politics of tobacco control in European nations as well as in the United States.

Ranney, Leah, Cathy Melvin, Linda Lux, Erin McClain, Laura Morgan, and Kathleen N. Lohr. *Tobacco Use: Prevention, Cessation, and Control*. Rockville, Md.: Agency for Healthcare Research and Quality, 2006. Also available online. URL: http://www.ahrq.gov/downloads/pub/evidence/pdf/tobaccouse/tobuse.pdf. Posted in June 2006. Based on review of the gigantic literature on preventing nonsmokers from starting to smoke and helping smokers to stop, this volume presents an up-to-date view on what works. The recommendations offered by the report include the following: self-help strategies alone are generally ineffective in helping to quit but may work in combination with counseling and psychotherapy, and school-based prevention have short-term but not long-term effects in smoking prevention.

Reid, Roddey. *Globalizing Tobacco Control: Anti-Smoking Campaigns in California, France, and Japan.* Bloomington, Ind.: Indiana University Press, 2005. Despite the spread of antismoking norms across the world, campaigns to control tobacco have taken different forms in different places. They differ because of varied national histories, forms of democratic governments, marketing strategies of tobacco companies, and programs of public health agencies. Although the book will most interest academics and scholars, its comparison of California, one of the U.S. states with the most extensive antismoking programs, with France and Japan offers a useful perspective on varied approaches to tobacco policy.

Schaler, Jeffrey A., and Magada E. Schaler, eds. *Smoking: Who Has the Right?* Amherst, N.Y.: Prometheus Books, 1998. Expert contributors present diverse viewpoints on the title's question, considering issues of personal responsibility and public health. The book allows readers to form their own conclusions about the right to smoke versus the public health goal of a tobacco-free society.

Seidman, Daniel F., and Lirio S. Covey. *Helping the Hard-Core Smoker: A Clinician's Guide.* Mahwah, N.J.: Lawrence Erlbaum, 1999. Given that the decline in smoking rates has slowed and that success rates in quitting are low, the contributions to this volume, edited by clinical psychologists at Columbia University, explain why current approaches are often inadequate and how to best help today's highly nicotine-dependent smokers. It is useful for physicians, psychiatrists, nurses, psychologists, counselors, and other clinicians.

Shames, Lisa. *Tobacco Settlement: States' Allocations of Payments from Tobacco Companies for Fiscal Years 2000 Through 2005: Testimony before the Committee on Health, Education, Labor, and Pensions, U.S. Senate.* Washington, D.C.: U.S. Government Accountability Office, 2007. Also available online. URL: http://frwebgate.access.gpo.gov/cgi-bin/getdoc.cgi?dbname =gao&docid=f:d07534t.pdf. Posted February 27, 2007. The 1998 Master Settlement Agreement required the four signing tobacco companies to make yearly payments to 46 states as reimbursement for tobacco-related health care costs. It imposed no restrictions on how the states could spend the money, however. This testimony from the Acting Director of Natural Resources and Environment of the U.S. General Accountability Office reports that, of the $52.6 billion received from 2000 through 2005, about 30 percent went to health care, while about 41 percent went to paying for budget shortfalls, infrastructure, debt relief, and general-purpose expenses. Only 3.5 percent went to tobacco control.

Shaw, David. *The Pleasure Police: How Bluenose Busybodies and Lily-Livered Alarmists Are Taking All the Fun Out of Life.* New York: Doubleday, 1996. The author argues that if used with moderation and common sense, tobacco, alcohol, sex, and food bring much pleasure to life. We would be happier, according to the author, if we stopped worrying so much about these things and if public health advocates left people alone to enjoy themselves.

Studlar, Donley T. *Tobacco Control: Comparative Politics in the United States and Canada*. Orchard Park, N.Y.: Broadview Press, 2002. This study of comparative politics describes differences in the development of regulation and taxation policies used to control tobacco in the United States and Canada. It relates general differences in political institutions and policy-making procedures to specific differences in tobacco control policies.

Sullum, Jacob. *For Your Own Good: The Anti-Smoking Crusade and the Tyranny of Public Health*. New York: Free Press, 1998. While recognizing the harm of smoking for health, the author argues that antismoking advocates have reached the point where they are now attempting to impose their preferences against cigarettes on another group that has freely chosen to enjoy the product. This book offers a reasoned defense of the view that government antismoking efforts wrongly threaten the freedom of individuals and businesses.

U.S. Congress, Senate Committee on the Judiciary. *Raising Tobacco Prices: New Opportunities for the Black Market? Hearings before the Committee on the Judiciary, United States Senate, One Hundred Fifth Congress, Second Session*. Washington, D.C.: U.S. Government Printing Office, 1999. The hearings examine the likely effect of legislation proposing to increase the price of tobacco products on the tobacco industry and opportunities for black market cigarette sales.

U.S. Congress, Senate Committee on Labor and Human Resources. *Tobacco Settlement: Public Health or Public Harm? Hearings of the Committee on Labor and Human Resources, United States Senate, One Hundred Fifth Congress, First Session*. Washington, D.C.: U.S. Government Printing Office, 1997. The hearings are concerned with the scope of the settlement, the administration's position on the settlement, and public health aspects of the settlement.

U.S. Department of Health and Human Services. *Healthy People 2010*. Washington, D.C.: U.S. Department of Health and Human Services, 2000. Some consider the government goals for reducing smoking by 2010 to be overly ambitious and unlikely to be realized, but the goals play a major role in current public health efforts.

———. *Preventing Tobacco Use Among Young People. A Report of the Surgeon General*. Washington, D.C.: U.S. Department of Health and Human Services, 1994. This volume provides an overview of the research on trends and causes of youth smoking, and the successes and failures of policies designed to reduce youth smoking. It makes the case that preventing youth from starting to smoke, despite advertising and promotions encouraging them to do so, will help deal with the public health problem of cigarette use in the future.

————. *Reducing the Health Consequences of Smoking: 25 Years of Progress. A Report of the Surgeon General.* Washington, D.C.: U.S. Department of Health and Human Services, 1989. This volume provides an overview of the new evidence to emerge about the harm of smoking since the 1964 Surgeon General's report, and the progress made in reducing the use of cigarettes and the health problems they cause.

————. *Regulating Tobacco Use. A Report of the Surgeon General.* Washington, D.C.: U.S. Department of Health and Human Services, 2000. After describing the historical efforts to reduce smoking in the United States, this volume reviews the scientific evidence on the effectiveness of several ways to reduce cigarette smoking: education efforts, programs to help smokers quit, government regulation, litigation strategies, economic approaches, and comprehensive programs. An essential guide to understanding current tobacco control endeavors.

————. *Smoking Cessation: Clinical Practice Guideline.* Washington, D.C.: U.S. Department of Health and Human Services, 1996. This short but technical volume based on a review of the scientific literature contains strategies and recommendations designed to assist clinicians, smoking cessation specialists, and health-care administrators in helping smokers stop their habit.

U.S. House of Representatives. *Can Tobacco Cure Smoking? A Review of Tobacco Harm Reduction: Hearing Before the Subcommittee on Commerce, Trade, and Consumer Protection of the Committee on Energy and Commerce, House of Representatives, One Hundred Eighth Congress, First Session, June 3, 2003.* Washington, D.C.: U.S. Government Printing Office, 2003. Also available online. URL: http://frwebgate.access.gpo.gov/cgi-bin/getdoc.cgi?dbname=108_house_hearings&docid=f:87489.pdf. Downloaded in April 2008. This hearing debates the controversial proposition that smokers who cannot quit would benefit from smoking less hazardous cigarettes. For example, one witness states that smokeless tobacco is 98 percent safer than cigarettes and represents a potential substitute. Others disagree, arguing that no form of tobacco use is safe and advocating the elimination of tobacco use altogether. The hearing has a balanced list of witnesses and includes a statement from Philip Morris.

U.S. Senate. *The Need for FDA Regulation of Tobacco: Hearing Before the Committee on Health, Education, Labor, and Pensions, United States Senate, One Hundred Tenth Congress, First Session on Examining S. 625, To Protect the Public Health by Providing the Food and Drug Administration with Certain Authority to Regulate Tobacco Products, February 27, 2007.* Washington, D.C.: U.S. Government Printing Office. Many senators and witnesses at this hearing believe that effective tobacco control requires regulation of the product by the government, specifically the U.S. Food and Drug Administration (FDA), which regulates other addictive substances. Many public health officials, antitobacco advocates, and researchers say that tobacco companies continue to mislead the public with false claims about tobacco and to market their product to children. Only government regulation can place controls on tobacco sales and marketing. Most witnesses therefore support the proposed bill to give regulatory control over tobacco to the FDA. Other witnesses oppose the legislation. A representative of the convenience-store industry favors state regulation over federal regulation, and several witnesses oppose regulation in favor of banning tobacco products altogether. The arguments made for and against the legislation give insight into debates over tobacco control.

Viscusi, W. Kip. *Smoke-Filled Rooms: A Postmortem on the Tobacco Deal.* Chicago: University of Chicago Press, 2002. A prominent critic of public health policy toward smoking, the author argues that smokers pay more in taxes than nonsmokers but consume fewer government benefits because they die earlier. In this book Viscusi criticizes the Master Settlement Agreement between the states and tobacco companies on economic grounds, arguing that the legislative branch more than the judicial branch can efficiently deal with the problem of tobacco use.

Wolfson, Mark. *The Fight Against Big Tobacco: The Movement, the State, and the Public's Health.* New York: Adline De Gruyter, 2001. Focusing on Minnesota's tobacco control activities, the author tells the history of the antismoking movement. He emphasizes the connections between the government and antitobacco movements, and links tobacco control efforts to theories about social movements more generally.

World Bank. *Curbing the Epidemic: Governments and the Economics of Tobacco Control.* Washington, D.C.: World Bank, 1999. In addressing the economic aspects of tobacco control from an international perspective, this short book concludes that raising taxes on tobacco can save millions of lives. From a review of existing evidence it also suggests that comprehensive bans on cigarette advertising and promotions can similarly reduce deaths worldwide. It thus encourages leaders and public health officials in developing nations to take action against tobacco use in their countries.

World Health Organization. *Building Blocks for Tobacco Control: A Handbook.* Geneva: World Health Organization, 2004. Also available online. URL: http://www.who.int/tobacco/resources/publications/tobaccocontrol_handbook/en/. Downloaded in April 2008. The Tobacco Free Initiative of the World Health Organization aims to help nations across the world develop the capacity to control smoking in their populations. This volume aids in that goal by describing legislation, media campaigns, and economic interventions that can help citizens avoid or stop smoking. The attention to parts of the world other than the United States and western

Annotated Bibliography

Europe gives the book a global focus, and the numerous and clearly written examples of lessons learned nicely summarize the consensus on effective tobacco control.

ARTICLES

Bauer, Ursula E., et al. "Changes in Youth Cigarette Use and Intentions Following Implementation of a Tobacco Control Program: Findings from the Florida Youth Tobacco Survey, 1998–2000." *JAMA* 284 (August 9, 2000): 723–728. According to results of surveys of high school students at the start and end of the two-year Florida Pilot Program on Tobacco Control, tobacco use decreased in each year of the program. The results suggest that comprehensive statewide programs effectively prevent and reduce youth tobacco use.

Bayer, Ronald, et al. "Tobacco Advertising in the United States: A Proposal for a Constitutionally Acceptable Form of Regulation." *JAMA* 287 (June 12, 2002) 2,990–2,995. The Supreme Court has struck down public health regulation of advertising as a violation of the First Amendment guaranteeing free speech. To continue regulating tobacco without violating free speech rights, the authors recommend taxing tobacco advertisements and promotion and requiring use of half the space in an advertisement for health warnings.

Bigland, Anthony, and Ted K. Taylor. "Why Have We Been More Successful in Reducing Tobacco Use Than Violent Crime?" *American Journal of Community Psychology* 28 (June 2000): 269–302. The authors hold up tobacco control efforts as a successful model for reducing unwanted behavior. As public health advocates have been able to convey the harm of the tobacco problem, to understand the causes of tobacco use, and to develop tobacco reduction programs, so might they use similar strategies to reduce violent crime.

Blumenstyk, Goldie. "Taking Cash from Tobacco Will Cost Researchers." *Chronicle of Higher Education* 50, no. 24 (Febrary 20, 2004): A1. Available online. URL: http://chronicle.com/weekly/v50/i24/24a00101.htm. Downloaded in April 2008. The American Cancer Society has decided to stop funding scientists who also get research funding from tobacco companies. According to this article, advocates view the decision as a courageous moral stand against the agenda of tobacco companies to distort scientific research, while critics say that evaluating results not by their scientific quality but by the source of research funds sets a dangerous precedent. Some universities have faced another negative consequence of accepting tobacco funding—vigorous protest from faculty and alumni.

Calfee, John E. "Why the War on Tobacco Will Fail." *Weekly Standard,* July 20, 1998, pp. 23–26. Taking a critical view of tobacco control efforts, this

215

article argues that higher tobacco taxes make governments dependent on revenues generated by tobacco sales and on continued cigarette smoking among citizens.

Collier, Christopher Percy. "Europe Is Trying to Kick the Habit: Public Smoking Bans." *Arthur Frommer's Budget Travel*, April 2007, pp. 50–51. Europe has followed some American states in banning smoking in public places, but unlike the United States, laws there generally apply to the whole nation. Ireland first implemented a general ban and other nations have followed. This article presents a map of smoking restrictions in European countries and gives some tips on finding smoke-free hotels.

David, Sean. "International Tobacco Control: A Focus Group Study of U.S. Anti-Tobacco Activists." *Journal of Public Health Policy* 22, no. 4 (2002): 415–428. Interviews of 1,500 antismoking activists provide insights on their views about tobacco marketing and regulation and progress toward changing public opinion on tobacco issues.

"Faith Leaders Press DeLay on Tobacco." *The Christian Century* 122, no. 25 (December 13, 2005): 16. Regular churchgoers with strong commitment to their religion have low cigarette use. This article tells of how interfaith groups have pressed Republicans to drop their opposition to stronger federal tobacco controls. More regulation fits the personal preferences of most churchgoers but also reflects their moral views that tobacco companies wrongly target teens with tobacco marketing and promotions. The contradictory impulses among religious conservatives to support business on the one hand and protect youth from addictive substances on the other hand make for interesting alliances in the area of tobacco control.

Farkas, Arthur, et al. "Association between Household and Workplace Smoking Restrictions and Adolescent Smoking." *JAMA* 284 (August 9, 2000): 717–722. Based on data from national surveys, this study finds that adolescents living in smoke-free homes and working in smoke-free workplaces were less likely to smoke than those living in homes and working in places without smoking restrictions. Policies affecting work and home environments can thus do much to prevent smoking among youth and adults.

Fiori, Michael C., et al. "A Clinical Practice Guideline for Treating Tobacco Use and Dependence: A U.S. Public Health Service Report." *JAMA* 283, (June 28, 2000): 3,244–3,254. This article summarizes a longer publication released by the Public Health Service on recommendations for clinical interventions to treat tobacco use and dependence. Among other conclusions the report finds that although brief treatment can be effective, longer-term treatment brings better results, and various types of counseling and social support prove especially effective.

Fiori, Michael C., Dorothy K. Hatsukami, and Timothy B. Baker. "Effective Tobacco Dependence Treatment." *JAMA* 288 (October 9, 2002): 110–113.

Annotated Bibliography

Physician-delivered interventions can effectively and inexpensively help smokers quit. To supplement comprehensive programs at the national, state, and local level to treat tobacco dependence, physicians should, according to the authors, do all they can to counsel every tobacco user about the risks of smoking, the benefits of stopping, and how to quit.

Gilpin, Elizabeth A., Arthur J. Farkas, and Sherry L. Emery. "Clean Indoor Air: Advances in California, 1990–99." *American Journal of Public Health* 92 (May 2002): 785–791. A review of surveys on the experiences of individuals with secondhand smoke in workplaces and homes shows considerable progress toward clean indoor air in California. For example, indoor workers reporting smoke-free workplaces increased from 35.0 percent in 1990 to 93.4 percent in 1999.

Gostin, Lawrence O. "Corporate Speech and the Constitution: The Deregulation of Tobacco Advertising." *American Journal of Public Health* 92 (March 2002): 352–355. Noting that the Supreme Court, by invalidating Massachusetts regulations to reduce underage smoking, has sided with business rights to advertise hazardous products, the author argues that the high value of population health should trump the low value of corporate free speech.

Gross, Cary P., et al. "State Expenditures for Tobacco-Control Programs and the Tobacco Settlement." *New England Journal of Medicine* 347 (October 3, 2002): 1,080–1,086. This evaluation of the state expenditures of funds received for tobacco control from the Master Settlement Agreement in 1998 finds that only a small proportion of the funds are being used as specified by the agreement. In fact, states with higher smoking tend to spend less of the funds on tobacco control than states with lower smoking.

Ibrahim, Jennifer K., and Stanton A Glantz. "The Rise and Fall of Tobacco Control Media Campaigns, 1967–2006." *American Journal of Public Health* 97, no. 8 (August 2007): 1,383–1,396. The authors review the strategies used by tobacco companies to limit the influence of anti-tobacco media campaigns. In response to such campaigns in Arizona, California, Florida, Massachusetts, Minnesota, and Oregon, the tobacco industry tried to limit the target audience and the content of the messages, reduce or eliminate the funding, and pursue litigation against the sponsors. The authors are highly critical of the tobacco industry and call for more vigorous action against it.

Jacobson, Peter D., and Jeffrey Wasserman. "The Implementation and Enforcement of Tobacco Control Laws: Policy Implications for Activists and the Industry." *Journal of Health Politics, Policy, and Law* 24 (June 1999): 567–598. Based on the experiences of seven states and 19 cities, the authors describe and evaluate the effectiveness of clean indoor air laws and laws restricting youth access to tobacco.

Kaplan, Robert M., Christopher F. Ake, and Sherry L. Emery. "Simulated Effect of Tobacco Tax Variation on Population Health in California." *American Journal of Public Health* 91 (February 2001): 239–244. Economic simulations reveal that higher taxes on cigarettes reduce smoking, sickness, and mortality. The authors conclude that a tobacco excise tax may be among a few policy options that will enhance a population's health status.

Katz, James E. "Tobacco Control Policies." *Society* 43, no. 3 (March/April 2006): 25–32. As discussed in this article, tobacco control policies must balance two competing goals: protect the public from harm while maintaining individual freedom. The author discusses the problem of individual rights in tobacco control and ways to establish greater controls on environmental tobacco smoke without violating these rights.

Kessler, David A., and Matthew L. Myers. "Beyond the Tobacco Settlement." *New England Journal of Medicine* 345 (August 16, 2001): 535–537. Noting that the tobacco settlement has failed to restrict advertising targeted toward youth or dilute the power of tobacco companies to attract new cigarette users, this article calls for national and state legislation to regulate tobacco and fund comprehensive smoking prevention programs.

Klonoff, Elizabeth A., Hope Landrine, and Delia Lang. "Adults Buy Cigarettes for Underage Youth." *American Journal of Public Health* 91 (July 2002): 1,138–1,139. In an interesting real-life experiment, 16 youths ages 15–17 approached 1,285 adult strangers to request that they purchase cigarettes for them. Few of the adults asked about the youth's age, and 32.1 percent bought cigarettes for the youths. Adult strangers may be a significant source of tobacco for minors.

Kluger, Jeffrey. "Hollywood's Smoke Alarm: Smoking in Motion Pictures." *Time*, April 23, 2007, pp. 59–60. The article reports on efforts of the Harvard School of Public Health and antismoking groups to prevent the exposure of young people to smoking in movies. Although smoking has declined in recent decades, use of cigarettes in movies has increased. One survey found that 75 percent of all Hollywood films and 36 percent of G- or PG-rated films contained smoking and potentially influenced children to take up the habit.

Lavelle, Marianne. "Teen Tobacco Wars: Antismoking Campaigns Funded with Tobacco Settlement Versus Cigarette Marketing." *U.S. News & World Report* February 7, 2000, pp. 14–16. This describes the plans of the Legacy Foundation, an independent organization created using $1.5 billion of the $246 billion paid by the tobacco companies under the Master Settlement Agreement, to produce hard-hitting ads that discourage teen smoking.

Ling, Pamela M., and Stanton A. Glantz. "Using Tobacco-Industry Marketing Research to Design More Effective Tobacco-Control Campaigns."

JAMA 287 (June 12, 2002): 2,983–2,989. This article recommends that antismoking ads, in using the knowledge gained by tobacco companies in marketing their products, should include people of all ages, particularly young adults rather than teens alone, should note the monetary costs of smoking, and should help make smoking socially unacceptable by emphasizing the harm of secondhand smoke.

Merrill, Ray M., June E. Stanford, and Gordon B. Lindsay. "The Relationship of Perceived Age and Sales of Tobacco and Alcohol to Underage Customers." *Journal of Community Health* 25 (October 2000): 401–410. Based on estimates of age by 49 gas station and convenience store clerks, the study finds that requesting identification of anyone perceived to be under age 27 works well in minimizing illegal tobacco sales. The results support the policies required by the Food and Drug Administration since 1997 to check IDs for anyone who appears younger than 27.

Mitka, Mike. "Picture This: Smoking Kills." *JAMA* 283 (February 23, 2000): 993. A brief report on efforts in Canada to discourage smoking with graphic images of the effects of tobacco use, such as diseased lungs and damaged hearts. Antismoking advocates believe these images will work better than current warning statements about the harm of cigarettes.

Moolchan, Eric T., Monique Ernst, and Jack Henningfield. "A Review of Tobacco Smoking in Adolescents: Treatment Implications." *Journal of the American Academy of Child and Adolescent Psychiatry* 39 (June 2000): 682–693. This article summarizes and evaluates current knowledge about the nature and determinants of adolescent smoking and how it differs from adult smoking. The authors conclude that smoking cessation treatment for adolescents has been disappointing due to low participation and high attrition.

Patrick, Steven, and Robert Marsh. "Current Tobacco Policies in U.S. Adult Male Prisons." *Social Science Journal* 38 (2000): 27–31. Prohibitions of smoking in prisons have followed trends more generally to ban smoking in public places. This article describes the trends and discusses the problems that have emerged in enforcing the bans.

Patton, Zach. "Mixed Smoke Signals." *Governing* 19, no. 3 (December 2005): 64. Also available online. URL: http://vnweb.hwwilsonweb.com/hww/results/external_link_maincontentframe.jhtml?_DARGS=/hww/results/results_common.jhtml.16. Downloaded in April 2008. This article describes the spread of local regulations to restrict smoking: "More than 2,000 communities have introduced local laws that restrict smoking, and over 40 percent of the American population is under some form of either a state or local limit." However, the many and varied local ordinances can make it hard for smokers to know where and when they can light up.

Pierce John P., and Elizabeth A. Gilpin. "Impact of Over-the-Counter Sales on Effectiveness of Pharmaceutical Aids for Smoking Cessation." *JAMA*

288 (September 11, 2002): 1,260–1,264. Surveys of Californians about smoking, efforts to quit smoking, and use of over-the-counter aids such as nicotine patches find increases from 1992 to 1999 in both efforts to quit and use of pharmaceutical aids. However, since becoming available over the counter, nicotine replacement therapies have become less effective in long-term smoking cessation.

Rigotti, Nancy A. "Treatment of Tobacco Use and Dependence." *New England Journal of Medicine* 346 (February 14, 2002): 506–512. The article provides a review of evidence supporting various strategies for physicians to help smoking patients quit their habit and makes clinical recommendations involving the use of nicotine replacement therapy, an antidepressant (bupropion), and counseling.

Ringel, Jeanne S., and William N. Evans. "Cigarette Taxes and Smoking during Pregnancy." *American Journal of Public Health* 91 (November 2001): 1,851–1,856. The study finds that high cigarette excise taxes reduce smoking rates among pregnant women.

"Saved by the Smokers." *Economist*, November 24, 2001, p. 33. Citing examples from several states, the article illustrates how funds from the tobacco settlement have been used for purposes other than the antismoking programs for which they were intended. With only about 5 percent being used for tobacco control, the funds largely go to spending on state schools, health care for the poor, and other nontobacco programs.

Spangler, John G. "Current Efforts and Gaps in U.S. Medical Schools." *JAMA* 288 (September 4, 2002): 1,102–1,109. Noting that U.S. medical schools have been found to inadequately teach tobacco intervention skills, this article reviews the instructional methods currently being taught. It concludes that innovative methods such as counseling and role playing work better than traditional efforts to tell patients of the harm of tobacco, but gaps remain in how medical education trains future physicians to use these techniques.

Voorhees, Carolyn C., Robert T. Swank, and Frances A. Stillman. "Cigarette Sales to African-American and White Minors in Low Income Areas of Baltimore." *American Journal of Public Health* 87 (April 1997): 652–654. This study provides evidence that age restrictions on sales are often not followed: Six minors ages 14–16 were sent into 83 stores in a low-income neighborhood and were able to purchase cigarettes in 85.5 percent of the stores.

Warner, Kenneth E. "Tobacco." *Foreign Policy* 130 (May/June 2002): 20–28. The author, a well-known tobacco expert, discusses the difficulty of controlling the global spread of tobacco. He recommends that countries across the world implement effective tobacco control policies such as tax increases, bans on smoking in public places, bans on all tobacco advertising and promotion, and public education initiatives.

Wilson, C. "My Friend Nicotine." *New Scientist* 172 (November 10, 2001): 28–31. The author calls government efforts to slowly reduce cigarette use through propaganda, higher taxes, and medical intervention ineffective against the strong addictive powers of nicotine. He advocates other approaches to tobacco reduction such as using less harmful forms of tobacco as a recreational drug.

Worth, Robert F. "A Smoking Ban in City's Jails Worries Correction Officers." *New York Times*, January 5, 2003, p. 27. The article describes the importance of cigarettes to prisoners and the possible trouble in maintaining control of the population that banning smoking in New York City prisons may create.

Zwarun, Lara. "Ten Years and 1 Master Settlement Agreement Later: The Nature and Frequency of Alcohol and Tobacco Promotion in Televised Sports, 2000 through 2002." *American Journal of Public Health* 96, no. 8 (August 2006): 1,492–1,497. Despite restrictions on tobacco ads on television, companies manage to make their products visible at sporting events. After observing 83 hours of televised sports programming, the author describes the techniques used to get around advertising restrictions and influence young people to smoke.

WEB DOCUMENTS

Action on Smoking and Health. "Everything for People Concerned About Smoking and Nonsmokers' Rights, Smoking Statistics, Quitting Smoking, Smoking Risks, and Other Smoking Information." Available online. URL: http://ash.org. Downloaded in April 2008. As the title suggests, this web site contains an enormous amount of information on a variety of topics, links to other antismoking organizations, news about tobacco control, and helpful actions to control tobacco use. The information supports antismoking goals of the sponsoring organization.

American Lung Association of San Diego and Imperial Counties. "Tobacco Laws and Regulations—Local." Available online. URL: http://www.lung sandiego.org/tobacco/advocate_local.asp. Downloaded in April 2008. This page describes the extensive regulations in San Diego and Imperial County, California, to limit tobacco advertising and youth access to cigarettes. The regulations may serve as a model for other cities and counties aiming to control teen smoking.

American Nonsmokers' Rights Foundation. URL: http://www.no-smoke. org. Downloaded in April 2008. The web site includes news on tobacco control efforts, summaries of recent research articles, alerts about new antitobacco action, position papers, and lists of smoke-free towns and places. It also provides information on youth smoking prevention programs and on avoiding secondhand smoke.

Centers for Disease Control and Prevention. "Save Lives, Save Money: Make Your Business Smoke-Free." Available online. URL: http://www. cdc.gov/tobacco/secondhand_smoke/00_pdfs/save_lives_save_money. pdf. Posted in June 2006. According to this 24-page report, business owners and managers can save money and help their employees by banning smoking. Smoke-free businesses save on insurance premiums, help smokers quit, improve worker safety, and protect nonsmokers from dangerous secondhand smoke. The report gives practical advice on setting up a task force, developing a formal policy, and offering to help workers quit.

————. "Smoking and Tobacco Use: Surveillance and Estimation." Available online. URL: http://quitsmoking.about.com/gi/dynamic/offsite. htm?zi=1/XJ/Ya&sdn=quitsmoking&cdn=health&tm=24&gps=238_1340_1060_424&f=10&tt=14&bt=1&bts=1&zu=http%3A//www.cdc. gov/tobacco/statehi/html_2002/state_highlights2002.htm. Downloaded in April 2008. This web site gives access to information on state tobacco control policies. Click "State Tobacco Activities Tracking and Evaluation (STATE) System," and then "Tobacco Control Highlights Report." The query system then allows one to select a state and year and get statistics on tobacco use, state antitobacco spending, and smoke-free policies.

Florida Tobacco Control Clearinghouse. Available online. URL: http:// www.ftcc.fsu.edu. Downloaded in April 2008. Funded by the Florida Department of Health, this web site provides a centralized resource center with the latest information and materials on tobacco use and its control. It lists the latest news on litigation, tax increases, and tobacco control policies, and it includes links to publications on tobacco control, the tobacco industry, and local antitobacco ordinances.

Forces International. Available online. URL: http://www.forces.org. Downloaded in April 2008. This web site supports smokers' rights and is devoted to the idea that consumers should be able to choose their own lifestyles without government interference. It aims to provide information on prosmoking views that the media and the government do not present.

Foundation for a Smokefree America. "TobaccoFree.org." Available online. URL: http://tobaccofree.org. Downloaded in April 2008. The site includes educational videos, motivational talks, tips for quitting, antismoking messages for youth and adults, and resources for finding antitobacco information.

Global Partnership for Tobacco Control. "Essential Action." Available online. URL: http://www.takingontobacco.org/index.html. Downloaded in April 2008. Focused on international tobacco control, this organization and web site aim to create ties between U.S. antitobacco groups and similar groups in Asia, Africa, Latin America, central and eastern Europe, and the former Soviet Union. To motivate collaboration of governments, communities, hospitals, schools, and faith organizations across the world, the web site includes stories on the threats of tobacco use to global health and successful strategies for combating the threat.

Public Health Law and Policy, Technical Assistance Legal Center. "What's New." Available online. URL: http://www.phi.org/talc. Downloaded in April 2008. This page summarizes model tobacco control policies for states, counties, and cities to adopt and ways to hold tobacco-free events.

Smoke Free Movies. "As Pressure Builds on MPAA and Major Studios, Hollywood Continues to Duck and Weave." URL: http://smokefreemovies. ucsf.edu/news/August-9-07-StatusReport.html. Downloaded in April 2008. This web site criticizes the major American film studios—Disney, Time Warner, Universal, Sony, Fox, and Paramount—for promoting smoking among kids with images of cigarette use in their movies. It calls for several practices to limit the impact of movies on smoking among children. Some studios have taken minor steps but much more needs to be done.

Smokers with Attitude. "The Smoking Section." Available online. URL: http://www.smokingsection.com. Downloaded in April 2008. This web site for smoker's rights includes a smokers' bookstore with many references as well as pages that dispute evidence on the health risks faced by smokers and tally the steep taxes paid by smokers when purchasing cigarettes.

U.S. Department of the Treasury. "The Economic Costs of Smoking in the United States and the Benefits of Comprehensive Tobacco Legislation." Available online. URL: http://www.ustreas.gov/press/releases/reports/ tobacco.pdf. Downloaded in February 2003. This press release presents figures showing that smoking in the United States in 1998 costs the country $130 billion in medical care, lost workdays, early death and retirement, and smoking-related fires but notes that legislation could reduce the amount by $78 billion.

U.S. General Accounting Office. "Cigarette Smuggling: Federal Law Enforcement Efforts and Seizures Increasing." Available online. URL: http://www.gao.gov/new.items/d04641.pdf. Posted in May 2004. As taxes on cigarettes increase, so does smuggling of cigarettes to avoid the taxes. The report views smuggling as a significant source of lost tax revenues and profits for organized crime that also contributes to smoking prevalence and poor health. The report recommends that Congress pass legislation to increase the penalties for smuggling and foster collaboration with other nations.

World Bank. "Economics of Tobacco Control." Available online. URL: http://www1.worldbank.org/tobacco. Downloaded in April 2008. This web site contains information about curbing tobacco use across the world, country profiles on tobacco use and policy, smoke-free workplaces, and key tobacco facts. The site is for researchers, policymakers, advocates, and others who desire to choose and implement effective tobacco control measures.

World Health Organization. "WHO Framework Convention on Tobacco Control (WHO FCTC)." Available online. URL: http://www.who.int/tobacco/framework/en. Downloaded in April 2008. The web site describes a treaty designed to foster cooperation of nations in worldwide tobacco control. It also lists the 168 nations who have signed the treaty. It's not clear yet what impact the treaty will have, but the cooperation among nations has much potential for tobacco control.

SELF-HELP

BOOKS

Brigham, Janet. *Dying to Quit: Why We Smoke and How We Stop.* Washington, D.C.: National Academy Press, 1998. More than most self-help books on smoking, this one provides much in the way of numerical information on trends and patterns but also describes why smoking is so difficult to stop and offers personal stories.

Carr, Allen. *Allen Carr's Easy Way to Stop Smoking.* Revised and updated. New York: Sterling Publishing, 2006. This popular book books has gone through several editions since its first publication in 2005 and has sold more 5 million copies. It helps smokers to eliminate the psychological reasons for using cigarettes and avoid tempting situations to smoke.

Chenoweth, Bruce. *Changing Your Mind About Smoking.* New Plymouth, Idaho: A.B. Company, 2000. This how-to guide differs from most in recommending that smokers first develop a self-image as a nonsmoker through autosuggestion before trying to quit.

Fisher, Edwin B. *American Lung Association 7 Steps to a Smoke Free Life.* New York: John Wiley & Sons, 1998. This helps smokers identify the places, times, moods, and conditions that trigger the need to smoke and offers techniques to resist the temptation.

Gronberg, Erli, and Katherine Srb. *Smokers and Quitters: What Smoking Means to People and How They Manage to Quit.* Commack, N.Y.: Kroshka Books, 1998. Collects personal stories about smoking and quitting that can help current smokers quit and nonsmokers understand smokers.

Hoffman, Elizabeth Hanson, and Christopher Douglas Hoffman. *Recovery from Smoking: Quitting with the 12 Step Process.* 2nd ed. Center City, Minn.: Hazelden Information Education, 1999. Following the model of popular 12-step programs originally developed to deal with alcoholism, the author recommends that smokers accept their powerlessness over the addiction and the need for emotional as well as physical recovery from addiction.

Kleinman, Lowell, et al. *Complete Idiot's Guide to Quitting Smoking.* Indianapolis, Ind.: Macmillan, 2000. Dr. Kleinman, a family practice physician called Dr. Quit, and his coauthors provide a description of the difficulties of smoking cessation and the steps needed to quit. The advice includes setting goals, choosing patches and medication, finding a support network, and dealing with stress and depression.

Schwebel, Robert. *How to Help Your Kids Choose to Be Tobacco-Free: A Guide for Parents of Children Ages 3 through 19.* New York: Newmarket Press, 1999. The author, a family psychologist, offers advice to parents about helping their children make wise choices about tobacco use and preparing them to meet their physical, social, and emotional needs without tobacco. He argues that antitobacco efforts of parents should begin with preschool children and continue through adolescence.

ARTICLES

"The FDA Approves New Drug for Smoking Cessation." *FDA Consumer* 40, no. 4 (July/August 2006): 1. Also available online. URL: http://www.fda.gov/fdac/features/2006/406_smoking.html. Downloaded in April 2008. The FDA approved a new drug in May 2006 to help smokers ages 18 and over to stop smoking. Called Chantix, the newly approved drug takes the form of tablets and is used for a 12-week therapy period. To ease withdrawal symptoms, it mimics the effects of nicotine on the brain; to prevent relapse, it also blocks the effects of nicotine if a person resumes smoking. Clinical trials suggest that Chantix works better than another common cessation drug on the market call bupropion (Zyban). Given the difficulty many have in quitting, medications like Chantix will become an increasingly popular way to treat nicotine addiction.

Lewis, Kristyn Kusek. "The Best Ways to Stop Smoking." *Health,* September 2007, pp. 97–98, 100. This article describes research findings that women are particularly vulnerable to the addictive effects of nicotine and harm of carcinogens in cigarette smoke. It then describes the stories of four women who quit successfully using methods such as exercise, directed visualization, and a nicotine patch.

Pearson, Patricia. "How I Prevailed vs. Ciggies." *Maclean's,* January 26, 2004, pp. 30–31. Among the suggestions for stopping smoking that this article offers, one highlights the difficulties of the change. The author suggests expanding residential programs for nicotine addiction. Much as breaking the alcohol addiction requires living in treatment facilities, breaking the nicotine addiction may require the same. Inpatient addiction treatment for smokers may become more common.

WEB DOCUMENTS

Mayo Clinic. "Nicotine Dependence Center in Minnesota." Available online. URL: http://www.mayoclinic.org/ndc-rst. Downloaded in April 2008. The prestigious Mayo Clinic offers an eight-day residential program to stop smoking that includes individual and group counseling, medications to relieve withdrawal symptoms, and physician supervision. Other less-intense and -expensive programs include group counseling, individualized outpatient programs, and telephone counseling.

National Cancer Institute. "Quitting Tobacco: Challenges, Strategies, and Benefits." Available online. URL: http://www.cancer.gov/cancertopics/tobacco/quittingtips. Downloaded in April 2008. The National Cancer Institute has published a series of 14 short fact sheets that give advice on how those quitting smoking can deal with several kinds of problems they face: cravings, irritability, depression, and urges when eating or drinking coffee and alcohol. This particular fact sheet gives practical and specific advice on how to quit, avoid relapse, and find help.

Quitnet: Quit All Together. Healthways. Available online. URL: http://www.quitnet.com. Downloaded in April 2008. For a fee, this web site provides a virtual support network to stop smoking.

QuitSmokingSupport.com. Available online. URL: http://www.quitsmokingsupport.com/intro.htm. Downloaded in April 2008. To give free support to those quitting, this web page has links to chat rooms, inspirational letters, and information on quitting products, methods of quitting, and benefits of quitting.

"Quitting Tips." The Foundation for a Smokefree America. Available online. URL: http://www.anti-smoking.org/quitting.htm. Downloaded in April 2008. This web site offers many examples of what smokers have done to quit and gives tips on how to make a quit attempt successful. For example, it suggests using deep-breathing exercises to resist urges to smoking, contacting smoking quit lines, and attending Nicotine Anonymous meetings to get personal support.

WhyQuit.com. "Motivation, Education, and Support for Cold Turkey Nicotine Cessation." Available online. URL: http://whyquit.com. Downloaded in April 2008. Provides resources to help smokers stop smoking completely without medical aids. These resources include information to motivate action, educate about the dangers of smoking, expose misleading tobacco marketing, and find support through message boards and e-mail counseling.

CHAPTER 8

ORGANIZATIONS AND AGENCIES

The organizations and agencies listed in this chapter fall into six categories:

- federal government agencies,
- business organizations and trade associations,
- research and charitable organizations,
- national advocacy groups,
- international advocacy groups, and
- state and local advocacy groups.

The categories overlap because, for example, research and charitable organizations often take advocacy positions and advocacy organizations often sponsor research. Still, most organizations fit better in one category than the other, and the classification helps organize an otherwise diverse domain. For each organization, the listing includes (when available) the web site, e-mail address, phone number, postal address, and a brief description. Rather than list their e-mail address, many organizations include a web-based form for submitting questions and comments via the Internet. In these cases, the text notes that e-mail is available via a web form.

FEDERAL GOVERNMENT AGENCIES

Bureau of Alcohol, Tobacco, Firearms, and Explosives (ATF)
URL: http://www.atf.treas.gov
E-mail: ATFMail@atf.gov
Phone: (202) 927-5000
Office of Alcohol and Tobacco

650 Massachusetts Avenue, NW
Washington, DC 20226
A law enforcement organization within the Department of the Treasury, the ATF is concerned with stopping contraband cigarette trafficking and preventing loss of tax revenues.

Centers for Disease Control and Prevention (CDC)
URL: http://www.cdc.gov
E-mail: tobaccoinfo@cdc.gov
Phone: (800) 311-3435
1600 Clifton Road
Atlanta, GA 30333
The principal federal agency for protecting the health and safety of Americans both at home and abroad. The CDC carries out extensive research on tobacco use and control.

Federal Election Commission (FEC)
URL: http://www.fec.gov
Phone: (800) 424-9530
999 E Street, NW
Washington, DC 20463
The FEC enforces federal election campaign laws and provides campaign finance reports and data, including contributions from tobacco companies and related political action committees.

Federal Trade Commission (FTC)
URL: http://www.ftc.gov
Phone: (202) 326-2222
600 Pennsylvania Avenue, NW
Washington, DC 20580
The FTC enforces antitrust and consumer protection laws and has been active in regulating tobacco advertising.

Food and Drug Administration (FDA)
URL: http://www.fda.gov
Phone: (888) 463-6332
5600 Fishers Lane
Rockville, MD 20857

The FDA's mission is to promote public health by reviewing clinical research and regulating food and medical products to ensure they are safe. Its attempt in the late 1990s to regulate tobacco was blocked by the Supreme Court.

National Cancer Institute (NCI)
URL: http://www.nci.nih.gov
E-mail: cancergovstaff@mail.nih.gov
Phone: (800) 422-6237
6116 Executive Boulevard
MSC 8322
Suite 3036A
Bethesda, MD 20892-8322
As the government's principal agency for cancer research and training, the NCI gives particular attention to tobacco and tobacco-related cancers.

National Center for Health Statistics (NCHS)
URL: http://www.cdc.gov/nchs
E-mail: nchsquery@cdc.gov
Phone: (301) 458-4636
3311 Toledo Road
Hyattsville, MD 20782
Part of the Centers for Disease Control and Prevention, the nation's principal health statistics agency compiles information to improve the health of Americans, including much information on tobacco use and tobacco-related health problems.

National Heart, Lung, and Blood Institute (NHLBI)
URL: http://www.nhlbi.nih.gov
E-mail: nhlbiinfo@nhlbi.nih.gov
Phone: (301) 592-8573
Room 5A52

31 Center Drive
MSC 2846
Building 31
Bethesda, MD 20892-2846
Given the influence of smoking on heart, lung, and blood vessel diseases, this institute funds research on the consequences of tobacco use and promotes tobacco control.

National Institute for Occupational Safety and Health (NIOSH)
URL: http://www.cdc.gov/niosh
E-mail: cdcinfo@cdc.gov
Phone: (202) 245-0625
95 E Street, SW
Suite 9200
Patriots Plaza Building
Washington, DC 20201
As the federal agency responsible for conducting research and making recommendations on the prevention of work-related disease and injury, the institute investigates lung disease and other problems related to workplace tobacco smoke.

National Institute of Child Health and Development (NICHD)
URL: http://www.nichd.nih.gov
E-mail: NICHDClearinghouse@mail.nih.gov
Phone: (800) 370-2943
Room 2A32
31 Center Drive
MSC 2425
Building 31
Bethesda, MD 20892-2425
The institute conducts and supports research on the reproductive, neurobiological, developmental, and behavioral processes that determine the health of adults, families, and children, including research on the effect of tobacco use by parents on the health of children.

National Institute of Environmental Health Sciences (NIEHS)
URL: http://www.niehs.nih.gov
E-mail: webcenter@niehs.nih.gov
Phone: (919) 541-3345
P.O. Box 12233
111 T.W. Alexander Drive
Research Triangle Park, NC 27709
This institute focuses on understanding how environmental factors, including cigarette and tobacco smoke, contribute, along with individual susceptibility and age, to human health and disease.

National Institute on Drug Abuse (NIDA)
URL: http://www.drugabuse.gov
E-mail: information@lists.nida.nih.gov
Phone: (301) 443-1124
6001 Executive Boulevard
Room 5213
Bethesda, MD 20892-9561
The institute sponsors research on abuse of and addiction to drugs, including nicotine; the effects of drugs on the brain and behavior; and the treatment and prevention of drug abuse and addiction.

Occupational Safety and Health Administration (OSHA)
URL: http://www.osha.gov
E-mail: web form

Phone: (800) 321-6742
U.S. Department of Labor
200 Constitution Avenue
Washington, DC 20210
With a mission to save lives, prevent injuries, and protect the health of U.S. workers, this agency is concerned with workplace clean air problems created by tobacco use.

Office of Disease Prevention and Health Promotion (ODPHP)
URL: http://odphp.osophs.dhhs.gov
Phone: (240) 453-8280
1101 Wootton Parkway
Suite LL100
Rockville, MD 20852
This office sponsors the National Health Information Center and promotes the Healthy People 2010 goals, which include reducing adult smoking to 15 percent.

Office of Safe and Drug-Free Schools (OSDFS)
URL: http://www.ed.gov/about/offices/list/osdfs
E-mail: customerservice@inet.ed.gov
Phone: (800) 872-5327
U.S. Department of Education
400 Maryland Avenue, SW
Washington, DC 20202
This office in the Department of Education administers, coordinates, and recommends policy for drug and violence prevention activities.

Office of Smoking and Health
URL: http://www.cdc.gov/tobacco
E-mail: tobaccoinfo@cdc.gov

Phone: (800) 311-3435
1600 Clifton Road
Atlanta, GA 30333
This office leads and coordinates efforts to prevent tobacco use among youth, promote smoking cessation, protect nonsmokers from secondhand smoke, and eliminate tobacco-related health disparities.

Office of the Surgeon General
URL: http://www.surgeongeneral.gov
Phone: (301) 443-4000
5600 Fishers Lane
Room 18-66
Rockville, MD 20857
With the goal of improving health and reducing illness and injury, the Surgeon General provides the public with the best scientific information, including that on the harm of tobacco use.

Substance Abuse and Mental Health Services Administration (SAMHSA)
URL: http://www.samhsa.gov
E-mail: SHIN@samhsa.hhs.gov
Phone: (877) 726-4727
1 Choke Cherry Road
Rockville, MD 20857
In working to improve the quality and availability of prevention, treatment, and rehabilitation for substance abuse and mental illness, SAMHSA makes statistics and data on smoking and tobacco use available to interested users.

U.S. Department of Agriculture (USDA)
URL: http://www.usda.gov

230

E-mail: AgSec@usda.gov
1400 Independence Avenue, SW
Washington, DC 20250
The USDA includes offices concerned with tobacco statistics, farming, prices, and trade.

U.S. Department of Health and
Human Services (HHS)
URL: http://www.hhs.gov
E-mail: web form
Phone: (202) 619-0257
200 Independence Avenue, SW
Washington, DC 20201
As the major government agency for protecting the health of Americans and providing essential ser-

vices, particularly for those less able to help themselves, the department aims to reduce the harm of tobacco use in the country.

U.S. Department of Justice
(DOJ)
URL: http://www.justice.gov
E-mail: AskDOJ@usdoj.gov
Phone: (202) 514-2000
950 Pennsylvania Avenue, NW
Washington, DC 20530-0001
The DOJ filed a high-profile suit against tobacco companies under civil racketeering laws to stop unlawful marketing practices and recover smoking-related health care costs.

BUSINESS ORGANIZATIONS AND TRADE ASSOCIATIONS

Altadis
URL: http://www.altadis.com/en
E-mail: info@altadisusa.com
Phone: 34 91 360 90 00
C/ Eloy Gonzalo, 10
28010 Madrid
Spain
One of Western Europe's largest cigarette makers, with headquarters in Spain and France, the company was purchased in 2008 by Imperial Tobacco.

Alternative Cigarettes
URL: http://www.altcigs.com
E-mail: web form
Phone: (800) 225-1838
P.O. Box 678
Buffalo, NY 14207

This business manufactures and sells nicotine-free herbal cigarettes and value-priced cigarettes.

Altria
URL: http://www.altria.com
E-mail: web form
Phone: (804) 274-2200
6601 West Broad Street
Richmond, VA 23230
The parent company of Philip Morris USA, Philip Morris International, and John Middleton cigar makers is the world's largest private tobacco company. Based largely on its most popular cigarette brand, Marlboro, the company is also number one in U.S. sales.

Tobacco Industry and Smoking

American Bar Association (ABA)
URL: http://abanet.org
E-mail: askaba@abanet.org
Phone: (800) 285-2221
321 N. Clark Street
Chicago, IL 60610
The nation's and the world's largest voluntary professional association, the ABA works to assist lawyers and judges in their work and to improve the legal system for the public. It also offers information on health-related law and litigation associated with tobacco.

British American Tobacco (BAT)
URL: http://www.bat.com
E-mail: web form
Phone: (44 207) 845 1000
Globe House
4 Temple Place
London WC2R 2PG
England
Along with 300 brands such as Kent, Lucky Strike, and Pall Mall and the world's second-largest market share, the company has a 42 percent interest in the U.S. business that came from the 2004 merger of Brown & Williamson and the R. J. Reynolds Tobacco Company.

Gallaher Group Plc
URL: http://www.gallaher-group.com
E-mail: web form
Phone: (44 1932) 372 000
Members Hill, Brooklands Road
Weybridge, Surrey KT13 0QU
England
This British-based international tobacco company was purchased by Japan Tobacco in 2007 and sells brands such as Benson & Hedges, Silk Cut, and Mayfair.

Imperial Tobacco Group
URL: http://www.imperial-tobacco.com
E-mail: itg@uk.imptob.com
Phone: (44 0117) 963 6636
P.O. Box 244
Upton Road
Bristol BS99 7UJ
England
This British company is the fourth-largest international tobacco company in the world and recently purchased Altadis.

Japan Tobacco (JT)
URL: http://www.jti.co.jp/JTI_E
E-mail: web form
2-1, Toranomon 2-chome, Minato-ku
Tokyo 105-8422
Japan
The world's third-largest tobacco company is partly owned by the Japanese government and has expanded from the Japanese market to sell Camel, Salem, and Winston brands outside the United States.

Liggett Vector Brands
URL: http://www.liggettvector brands.com
E-mail: consumer.relations@lvbrands.com
P.O. Box 490
Mebane, NC 27302
Having sold its line of traditional products of L&M, Chesterfield, and Lark in 1999 to concentrate on discount-priced and generic

232

brands and on low-tar and low-nic- otine cigarettes, the Liggett Group merged in 2005 with Vector To- bacco to create this company.

Lorillard Tobacco Company
URL: http://www.lorillard.com
Phone: (877) 703-0386
P.O. Box 21688
Greensboro, NC 27420
The third-largest and oldest ciga- rette manufacturer in the United States, it has recently been sold by its former owners, Loews Cor- poration and the Carolina Group. It makes Newport, the number- one selling menthol cigarette in the United States, and Kent, True, and Old Gold.

National Association of Convenience and Petroleum Retailing
URL: http://www.nacsonline. com
E-mail: nacs@nacsonline.com
Phone: (800) 966-6227
1600 Duke Street
Alexandria, VA 22314
This industry trade group helps set policies on cigarette sales and offers advice on how to comply with state tobacco laws.

Philip Morris USA
URL: http://www.philipmorris usa.com
E-mail: web form
Phone: (800) 343-0975
P.O. Box 26603
Richmond, VA 2326
The largest cigarette manufacturer in the United States and one of the

largest tobacco companies in the world, Philip Morris is a subsidiary of Altria and best known as the maker of Marlboro cigarettes.

Reynolds American
URL: http://www.reynolds american.com
E-mail: web form
Phone: (336) 741-7693
P.O. Box 2990
Winston-Salem, NC 27102-2990
Founded after merging Brown & Williamson with R. J. Reynolds Tobacco, the company also owns R. J. Reynolds International Products (a worldwide distributor of ciga- rettes), Conwood Company (maker of smokeless tobacco), and Santa Fe Natural Tobacco Company (maker of additive-free products).

R. J. Reynolds Tobacco Company (RJRT)
URL: http://www.rjrt.com
E-mail: web form
Phone: (336) 741-5000
P.O. Box 2959
Winston-Salem, NC 27102-2959
A subsidiary of Reynolds Ameri- can, this company is the second- largest cigarette manufacturer in the United States and makes Win- ston, Salem, Camel, and Doral cigarettes.

Santa Fe Natural Tobacco Company (SFNTC)
URL: http://www.nascigs.com
E-mail: feedback@sfntc.com
Phone: (800) 332-5595
P.O. Box 25140
Santa Fe, NM 87504

Owned by Reynolds American, this company produces cigarettes advertised as additive free, whole leaf, and unreconstituted.

Swedish Match
URL: http://www.swedishmatch.
   com
E-mail: contactus@swedishmatch.
   com
Phone: 46-8-6580200
Rosenlundsgatan 36
SE-118 85 Stockholm
Sweden
This Swedish company is the world's second-largest producer of cigars and cigarillos and makes other noncigarette tobacco products such as Red Man Chewing Tobacco.

Swisher International
URL: http://www.swisher.com
E-mail: web form
Phone: (203) 656-8000
20 Thorndal Circle

Darien, CT 06820-5421
This company dominates the little cigar market with its Swisher Sweets product and also produces smokeless tobacco.

**Tobacco Merchants Association
   (TMA)**
URL: http://www.tma.org
E-mail: tma@tma.org
Phone: (609) 275-4900
P.O. Box 8019
Princeton, NJ 08543-8019
This trade association for tobacco companies is a source of information on the worldwide tobacco industry.

UST
URL: http://www.ustinc.com
Phone: (203) 817-3000
6 High Ridge Park, Building A
Stamford, CT 06905-1323
This company is the world's leading producer and marketer of smokeless tobacco products such as Copenhagen snuff and Skoal fine cut.

RESEARCH AND CHARITABLE ORGANIZATIONS

**Adolescent Substance Abuse
   Prevention (ASAP)**
URL: http://asap.bsd.uchicago.
   edu
E-mail: asap@uchicago.edu
Phone: (773) 702-6368
Department of Psychiatry
University of Chicago Hospitals
5841 South Maryland Avenue
MC3077
Chicago, IL 60637-5416

ASAP sponsors a community service program that combats adolescent substance abuse by having medical students visit schools and introduce students to the risks and causes of smoking, drinking, and drug taking.

American Cancer Society (ACS)
URL: http://www.cancer.org
Phone: (800) 227-2345

E-mail: web form
1599 Clifton Road
Atlanta, GA 30329
With goals of eliminating cancer as a major health problem and preventing cancer through research, education, advocacy, and service, this organization supports a variety of antitobacco programs.

American Council on Science and Health (ACSH)
URL: http://www.acsh.org
E-mail: acsh@acsh.org
Phone: (866) 905-2694
1995 Broadway
Second Floor
New York, NY 10023-5860
This consumer education group is concerned with promoting scientifically sound public policies related to health and the environment. It is highly critical of tobacco companies for unscientific claims about tobacco but also criticizes some antismoking groups for exaggerating the risks of secondhand smoke.

American Heart Association
URL: http://www.americanheart. org
E-mail: web form
Phone: (800) 242-8721
7272 Greenville Avenue
Dallas, TX 75231
This association has as its goal to reduce disability and death from cardiovascular disease and, among many other activities, promotes smoke-free lifestyles and lobbies for tobacco control.

American Lung Association
URL: http://www.lungusa.org
E-mail: press_contact@lungusa. org
Phone: (800) 586-4872
61 Broadway
Sixth Floor
New York, NY 10006
The oldest voluntary health organization in the United States fights lung disease in all forms and gives special emphasis to tobacco control.

American Medical Association (AMA)
URL: http://www.ama-assn.org
E-mail: web form
Phone: (800) 621-8335
515 North State Street
Chicago, IL 60610
This organization of physicians is dedicated to improving the health of Americans and in so doing supports a variety of antismoking programs and initiatives.

American Public Health Association (APHA)
URL: http://www.apha.org
E-mail: comments@apha.org
Phone: (202) 777-2742
800 I Street, NW
Washington, DC 20001
This organization of public health professionals deals with a broad set of issues affecting personal and environmental health, including tobacco use and control.

American Society of Addiction Medicine (ASAM)
URL: http://www.asam.org
E-mail: email@asam.org

Phone: (301) 656-3920
601 N. Park Avenue
Upper Arcade #101
Chevy Chase, MD 20815
This organization aims to increase access to addiction treatment by physicians, including treatment for nicotine addiction.

**Cancer Research and
  Prevention Foundation**
URL: http://www.preventcancer.
  org
E-mail: info@preventcancer.org
Phone: (800) 227-2732
1600 Duke Street
Suite 110
Alexandria, VA 22314
The foundation supports prevention and early detection of cancer through scientific research and education, and focusing on cancers that can be prevented by lifestyle change, such as stopping cigarette use.

**National Center for Tobacco-
  Free Older Persons**
URL: http://tcsg.org/tobacco.
  htm
E-mail: tcsg@tcsg.org
Phone: (734) 665-1126
2307 Shelby Avenue
Ann Arbor, MI 48103
Part of the Center for Social Gerontology at the University of Michigan, this group emphasizes the special harm of smoking for older persons and how to reduce that harm.

**National Center on Addiction
  and Substance Abuse at
  Columbia University**

URL: http://www.casacolumbia.
  org
E-mail: web form
Phone: (212) 841-5200
633 Third Avenue
19th Floor
New York, NY 10017-6706
This research group offers information about the costs of substance abuse, ways to prevent addiction, and the need to remove the stigma of substance abuse.

**Robert Wood Johnson
  Foundation (RWJF)**
URL: http://www.rwjf.org
E-mail: web form
Phone: (877) 843-7953
P.O. Box 2316
College Road East and Route 1
Princeton, NJ 08543-2316
The foundation is devoted to improving the health and health care of Americans by promoting healthy communities and lifestyles and by reducing the harm due to the abuse of tobacco, alcohol, and illicit drugs.

**Society for Research on
  Nicotine and Tobacco
  (SRNT)**
URL: http://www.srnt.org
E-mail: info@srnt.org
Phone: (608) 443-2462
2810 Crossroads Drive
Suite 3800
Madison, WI 53718
This organization sponsors scientific meetings and publications and arranges for expert advice to policymakers and legislators on issues involving nicotine and tobacco.

NATIONAL ADVOCACY GROUPS

Action on Smoking and Health (ASH)
URL: http://ash.org
E-mail: web form
Phone: (202) 659-4310
2013 H Street, NW
Washington, DC 20006
The national antismoking and non-smokers' rights organization promotes legal action on behalf of nonsmokers.

American Legacy Foundation
URL: http://www.americanlegacy.org
E-mail: info@americanlegacy.org
Phone: (202) 454-5555
1724 Massachusetts Avenue, NW
Washington, DC 20036
Established in 1999 as a result of the Master Settlement Agreement and supported by funds from the tobacco companies, this organization is devoted to reducing youth tobacco use, decreasing exposure to secondhand smoke, increasing successful quit rates, and eliminating disparities in access to tobacco prevention and cessation.

Americans for Nonsmokers' Rights
URL: http://www.no-smoke.org
E-mail: web form
Phone: (510) 841-3032
2530 San Pablo Avenue
Suite J
Berkeley, CA 94702
This national lobbying organization dedicated to nonsmokers' rights, including protection from second-hand smoke and youth addiction, has worked in the past for legislation to ban smoking from worksites and public places.

Campaign for Tobacco-Free Kids
URL: http://www.tobaccofreekids.org
E-mail: info@tobaccofreekids.org
Phone: (202) 296-5469
1400 I Street
Suite 1200
Washington, DC 20005
Committed to protecting children from tobacco addiction and secondhand smoke, this private nonprofit organization works to inform the public about the harm of tobacco, change public policies, educate young people, and expose tobacco marketing practices that addict kids.

Children Opposed to Smoking Tobacco (COST)
URL: http://www.costkids.org
E-mail: costkids@costkids.org
Founded by a group of students who want to keep tobacco products away from children, this group offers a list of activities that young people can do to help reach this goal.

Foundation for a Smokefree America
URL: http://www.anti-smoking.org
E-mail: manager@tobaccofree.org
Phone: (310) 471-0303

P.O. Box 492028
Los Angeles, CA 90049-8028
Working toward the goal of motivating youth to stay free of tobacco and helping smokers quit, this organization sponsors local, regional, and national programs, school educational programs, and peer teaching programs.

Friends of Tobacco
URL: http://www.fujipub.com/fot
Phone: (919) 522-4769
403B East New Bern Road
Kinston, NC 28501
A grassroots organization opposed to the loss of freedom to enjoy tobacco.

**Institute for Sustainable
  Communities**
URL: http://www.iscvt.org
E-mail: isc@iscvt.org
Phone: (202) 777-7575
888 17th Street, NW
Suite 610
Washington, DC 20006
As part of its efforts to promote effective social justice leadership, achieve a just society, and foster economic equality and public health, the institute sponsors the Tobacco Control Project and the Smoking Control Advocacy Resource Center.

**National Association of
  Attorneys General (NAAG)**
URL: http://www.naag.org
E-mail: web form
Phone: (202) 326-6000
2030 M Street, NW
8th Floor
Washington, DC 20036

With state attorneys general having taken action in suing tobacco companies, this organization has become a major force in the fight for tobacco control.

**National Latino Council
  on Alcohol and Tobacco
  Prevention (NLCATP)**
URL: http://www.nlcatp.org
E-mail: lcat@nlcatp.org
Phone: (202) 265-8054
101 Avenue of the Americas
Suite 313
New York, NY 10013
This organization uses research, policy analysis, community education, training, and information dissemination to reduce the harm caused by alcohol and tobacco in the Latino community.

Nicotine Anonymous
URL: http://www.nicotine-
  anonymous.org
E-mail: info@nicotine-
  anonymous.org
Phone: (415) 750-0328
419 Main Street, PMB# 370
Huntington Beach, CA 92648
Modeled on other 12-step programs, this is a voluntary group whose members help other members live free of nicotine.

**Public Health Advocacy
  Institute (PHAI)**
URL: http://www.phaionline.
  org
Phone: (617) 373-2026
102 The Fenway
Suite 117CU
Boston, MA 02115

This legal reseach center focuses on protecting the health of the public and, with the goal of tobacco control, sponsors the Tobacco Products Liability Project.

Smokefree.net
URL: http://www.smokefree.net
E-mail: tac@smokefree.net
Phone: (202) 667-6653
1711 18th Street, NW
Washington, DC 20008
This network is designed to fight for smoke-free air by facilitating communication and information sharing between smoke-free advocates and decision makers.

Survivors and Victims of Tobacco Empowerment
URL: http://www.tobacco survivors.org
E-mail: info@tobaccosurvivors. org

Phone: (888) 886-4237
14701 US Highway 52 N
Suite A
Wadesboro, NC 28170
Survivors of tobacco-related illnesses in this network tell their painful and personal stories about the effects of tobacco.

Tobacco Technical Assistance Consortium (TTAC)
URL: http://www.ttac.org
E-mail: ttac@sph.emory.edu
Phone: (404) 712-8474
Rollins School of Public Health, Emory University
1518 Clifton Road, GCR 808
Atlanta, GA 30322
By providing technical assistance, this consortium helps states and local communities to support comprehensive tobacco control programs.

INTERNATIONAL ADVOCACY GROUPS

Essential Action: Global Partnerships for Tobacco Control
URL: http://www.takingon tobacco.org
E-mail: tobacco@essential.org
Phone: (202) 387-8030
P.O. Box 19405
Washington, DC 20036
The program pairs groups in the United States and Canada with groups in Asia, Africa, Latin America, Central and Eastern Europe, and the former Soviet Union. It then assists them in initiating and

strengthening international tobacco control activities at the grassroots level.

European Network for Smoking Prevention (ENSP)
URL: http://www.ensp.org
E-mail: info@ensp.org
Phone: (32 02) 230 65 15
144 Chaussée d'Ixelles
Brussels 1050
Belgium
In coordinating antitobacco efforts among nations of the European Union, the network makes special

efforts to support programs that span national boundaries.

Forces International
URL: http://www.forces.org
E-mail: info@forces.org
Phone: (304) 765-5394
P.O. Box 533
Sutton, WV 26601
Devoted to the idea that consumers have the freedome to choose lifestyles without government interference, this group supports smokers' rights.

Framework Convention Alliance for Tobacco Control
URL: http://www.fctc.org
E-mail: fca@fctc.org
Rue Henri-Christiné 5
Case Postale 567
CH-1211 Geneva 4
Switzerland
Made up of almost 300 organizations representing more than 100 countries around the world, the alliance works to support the signing, ratification, and effective implementation of the Framework Convention on Tobacco Control (FCTC).

Institute for Global Tobacco Control
URL: http://www.jhsph.edu/global_tobacco
E-mail: gethelp@jhsph.edu
Phone: (410) 614-5378
Johns Hopkins Bloomberg School of Public Health
627 N. Washington Street
2nd Floor
Baltimore, MD 21205

The institute has the goal of preventing death and disease from tobacco use around the world through research, education, and policy development.

International Network of Women Against Tobacco (INWAT)
URL: http://www.inwat.org
E-mail: info@inwat.org
Phone: (604) 875-2633
E311-4500 Oak Street, Box 48
Vancouver, BC
Canada V6H 3N1
With the goal of improving women's health around the world, the network addresses the problem of tobacco use among women and young girls.

International Union Against Cancer (UICC)
URL: http://www.uicc.org
Phone: (41 22) 809 1811
62 route de Frontenex
1207 Geneva
Switzerland
A global organization with 291 cancer-fighting organizations in 87 countries as members, this union promotes awareness and responsibility for the growing global cancer burden and the need for worldwide tobacco control.

Tobacco Free Initiative (TFI)
URL: http://tobacco.who.int
E-mail: tfi@who.int
Phone: (41 22) 791 2126
World Health Organization
20 Avenue Appia 20 1211
CH-1211 Geneva 27
Switzerland

This project of the World Health Organization works for worldwide tobacco control with publications, press releases, web news, and anti-tobacco information.

World Bank Group
URL: http://www.worldbank.org
E-mail: pic@worldbank.org
Phone: (202) 473-1000
1818 H Street, NW
Washington, DC 20433
Although largely focused on helping nations fight poverty, the World Bank also works in partnership with the World Health Organization on issues of tobacco control.

World Health Organization (WHO)
URL: http://www.who.int/en
E-mail: info@who.int
Phone: (41 22) 791 2111
Avenue Appia 20
CH-1211 Geneva 27
Switzerland
Global tobacco use is one of the major health concerns addressed by the WHO, which distributes information about the harm of tobacco use and sponsors the Tobacco Free Initiative.

World Lung Foundation
URL: http://www.worldlung
foundation.org
Phone: (212) 315-8765
61 Broadway
6th Floor
New York, NY 10006
The foundation supports organizations around the world that are working to improve lung health by funding research, pilot projects, training, and programs to promote freedom from smoking.

STATE AND LOCAL ADVOCACY GROUPS

California Tobacco Control Alliance
URL: http://www.tobaccofree
alliance.org
E-mail: admin@tobaccofree
alliance.org
Phone: (916) 554-0390
909 12th Street
Suite 116
Sacramento, CA 95814
This statewide organization works to reduce the use of tobacco in California by uniting government, nonprofit, health, corporate, academic, and business organizations behind a comprehensive statewide tobacco control strategy.

California Tobacco Control Program
URL: http://www.cdph.ca.gov/
programs/Tobacco/Pages
E-mail: partners.webmaster@
cdph.ca.gov
Phone: (916) 449-5500
MS 7206
P.O. Box 997377
Sacramento, CA 95899-7377
To improve the health of all Californians by reducing illness and

241

premature death attributable to the use of tobacco products, the section of the California Department of Public Health helps statewide and local health agencies advocate for a tobacco-free environment.

Capital District Tobacco-Free Coalition
URL: http://www.smokefree capital.org
E-mail: contact@smokefree capital.org
Phone: (518) 233-1106
849 2nd Avenue
Troy, NY 12182
Composed of local organizations and individuals in the Albany area, this coalition works at the local level to reduce adolescent and adult use of tobacco with cooperative programs for prevention, cessation, advocacy, and community education.

Denver Alliance on Tobacco and Health (DATH)
URL: http://www.dath.org
E-mail: info@dath.org
Phone: (303) 436-7949
605 Bannock Street
MC 2600
Denver, CO 80204
A community tobacco control coalition that represents businesses, agencies, community organizations, and individuals in the Denver area and focuses on reducing tobacco use among minority and low socioeconomic groups.

Florida Tobacco Control Clearinghouse Florida State University (FTCC)
URL: http://www.ftcc.fsu.edu

E-mail: ftcc@mailer.fsu.edu
Phone: (877) 682-3822
2555 Pottsdamer Street
Room 211 BFS
P.O. Box 3062800
Tallahassee, FL 32306-2800
A group that provides the latest, most comprehensive, and most accurate resource materials on tobacco use and its effects to those involved with Florida tobacco control efforts.

Georgia Tobacco Prevention Program
URL: http://health.state.ga.us/ programs/tobacco
E-mail: gasmokefreeair@dhr. state.ga.us
Phone: (404) 657-6611
Division of Public Health
Two Peachtree Street, NW
Atlanta, GA 30303-3186
This program aims to reduce the use of tobacco and the burden it causes from related illness and disease in Georgia by coordinating strategy in tobacco use prevention and control. It also serves as a resource center for tobacco issues and provides technical assistance and training on policy development.

Los Angeles County Tobacco Control and Prevention Program
URL: http://www.lapublichealth. org
E-mail: tob@dhs.co.la.ca.us
Phone: (213) 351-7890
3530 Wilshire Boulevard
Suite 800
Los Angeles, CA 90010
Funded by the California Tobacco Tax Initiative, this organization

works to make the county smoke-free through comprehensive tobacco control programs.

New York State Tobacco Control Program
URL: http://www.health.state.ny.us/prevention/tobacco_control
E-mail: tcp@health.state.ny.us
Phone: (518) 474-1515
Corning Tower
Empire State Plaza
Albany, NY 12237
With the goal of tobacco-free communites for all New Yorkers, this program of the New York Department of Health implements promising evidence-based strategies to prevent and reduce tobacco use.

Oregon Tobacco Prevention and Education Program
URL: http://www.oregon.gov/DHS/ph/tobacco
E-mail: tobacco.ohd@state.or.us
Phone: (971) 673-0984
800 NE Oregon Street
Suite 730
Portland, OR 97232
This agency of the Oregon Public Health Divison leads state efforts to reduce tobacco-related illness and death by reducing exposure of Oregonians to secondhand smoke, countering protobacco influences, and helping people quit.

Partnership for a Tobacco-Free Maine
URL: http://www.tobaccofreemaine.org
E-mail: ptm.dhhs@maine.gov
Phone: (207) 287-4627

Key Bank Plaza
4th Floor
11 State House Station
Augusta, ME 04330-0011
This program responsible for tobacco prevention and control in the state of Maine is funded by the tobacco settlement and the Centers for Disease Control and Prevention.

Smokefree Indiana
URL: http://www.smokefreeindiana.org
E-mail: inquiry@smokefreeindiana.org
Phone: (317) 234-1787
2 North Meridian, 7R
Indianapolis, IN 46204
This group of health-promotion specialists in Indiana works in the community to reduce tobacco use.

Texas Tobacco Prevention and Control
URL: http://www.dshs.state.tx.us/tobacco
E-mail: tobacco.free@dshs.state.tx.us
Phone: (512) 206-5810
909 W. 45th Street
Austin, TX 78751
This agency of the Texas Department of Health Services provides technical assistance and information to community organizations, schools, worksites, health professionals, and law enforcement agencies on tobacco use prevention issues. It also sponsors media campaigns to educate Texans about the dangers of tobacco use and the Texas Tobacco Law.

PART III

APPENDICES

APPENDIX A

EXECUTIVE SUMMARY FROM THE HEALTH CONSEQUENCES OF SMOKING: A REPORT OF THE SURGEON GENERAL (2004)

The 2004 report of the Surgeon General, published 40 years after the first 1964 Surgeon General report on smoking and health, concludes that the harm of smoking is even worse than thought previously. Although earlier reports demonstrated that tobacco use causes lung cancer, chronic bronchitis, and heart disease, this new report concludes that smoking harms nearly every organ in the body. The executive summary presented here highlights the key findings of the report, but the full text of the long report can be found at http://www.surgeongeneral.gov/library/smokingconsequences/.

MAJOR CONCLUSIONS

Forty years after the first Surgeon General's report in 1964, the list of diseases and other adverse effects caused by smoking continues to expand. Epidemiologic studies are providing a comprehensive assessment of the risks faced by smokers who continue to smoke across their life spans. Laboratory research now reveals how smoking causes disease at the molecular and cellular levels. Fortunately for former smokers, studies show that the substantial risks of smoking can be reduced by successfully quitting at any age. The evidence reviewed in this and prior reports of the Surgeon General leads to the following major conclusions:

1. Smoking harms nearly every organ of the body, causing many diseases and reducing the health of smokers in general.

2. Quitting smoking has immediate as well as longterm benefits, reducing risks for diseases caused by smoking and improving health in general.
3. Smoking cigarettes with lower machine-measured yields of tar and nicotine provides no clear benefit to health.
4. The list of diseases caused by smoking has been expanded to include abdominal aortic aneurysm, acute myeloid leukemia, cataract, cervical cancer, kidney cancer, pancreatic cancer, pneumonia, periodontitis, and stomach cancer.

CHAPTER CONCLUSIONS

CHAPTER 2. CANCER

Lung Cancer

1. The evidence is sufficient to infer a causal relationship between smoking and lung cancer.
2. Smoking causes genetic changes in cells of the lung that ultimately lead to the development of lung cancer.
3. Although characteristics of cigarettes have changed during the last 50 years and yields of tar and nicotine have declined substantially, as assessed by the Federal Trade Commission's test protocol, the risk of lung cancer in smokers has not declined.
4. Adenocarcinoma has now become the most common type of lung cancer in smokers. The basis for this shift is unclear but may reflect changes in the carcinogens in cigarette smoke.
5. Even after many years of not smoking, the risk of lung cancer in former smokers remains higher than in persons who have never smoked.
6. Lung cancer incidence and mortality rates in men are now declining, reflecting past patterns of cigarette use, while rates in women are still rising.

Laryngeal Cancer

7. The evidence is sufficient to infer a causal relationship between smoking and cancer of the larynx.
8. Together, smoking and alcohol cause most cases of laryngeal cancer in the United States.

Oral Cavity and Pharyngeal Cancers

9. The evidence is sufficient to infer a causal relationship between smoking and cancers of the oral cavity and pharynx.

Appendix A

Esophageal Cancer

10. The evidence is sufficient to infer a causal relationship between smoking and cancers of the esophagus.
11. The evidence is sufficient to infer a causal relationship between smoking and both squamous cell carcinoma and adenocarcinoma of the esophagus.

Pancreatic Cancer

12. The evidence is sufficient to infer a causal relationship between smoking and pancreatic cancer.

Bladder and Kidney Cancers

13. The evidence is sufficient to infer a causal relationship between smoking and renal cell, renal pelvis, and bladder cancers.

Cervical Cancer

14. The evidence is sufficient to infer a causal relationship between smoking and cervical cancer.

Ovarian Cancer

15. The evidence is inadequate to infer the presence or absence of a causal relationship between smoking and ovarian cancer.

Endometrial Cancer

16. The evidence is sufficient to infer that current smoking reduces the risk of endometrial cancer in postmenopausal women.

Stomach Cancer

17. The evidence is sufficient to infer a causal relationship between smoking and gastric cancers.
18. The evidence is suggestive but not sufficient to infer a causal relationship between smoking and noncardia gastric cancers, in particular by modifying the persistence and/or the pathogenicity of *Helicobacter pylori* infections.

Colorectal Cancer

19. The evidence is suggestive but not sufficient to infer a causal relationship between smoking and colorectal adenomatous polyps and colorectal cancer.

Prostate Cancer

20. The evidence is suggestive of no causal relationship between smoking and risk for prostate cancer.
21. The evidence for mortality, although not consistent across all studies, suggests a higher mortality rate from prostate cancer in smokers than in nonsmokers.

Acute Leukemia

22. The evidence is sufficient to infer a causal relationship between smoking and acute myeloid leukemia.
23. The risk for acute myeloid leukemia increases with the number of cigarettes smoked and with duration of smoking.

Liver Cancer

24. The evidence is suggestive but not sufficient to infer a causal relationship between smoking and liver cancer.

Adult Brain Cancer

25. The evidence is suggestive of no causal relationship between smoking cigarettes and brain cancer in men and women.

Breast Cancer

26. The evidence is suggestive of no causal relationship between active smoking and breast cancer.
27. Subgroups of women cannot yet be reliably identified who are at an increased risk of breast cancer because of smoking, compared with the general population of women.
28. Whether women who are at a very high risk of breast cancer because of mutations in *BRCA1* or *BRCA2* genes can lower their risks by not smoking has not been established.

CHAPTER 3. CARDIOVASCULAR DISEASES

Smoking and Subclinical Atherosclerosis

1. The evidence is sufficient to infer a causal relationship between smoking and subclinical atherosclerosis.
2. The evidence is sufficient to infer a causal relationship between smoking and coronary heart disease.
3. The evidence suggests only a weak relationship between the type of cigarette smoked and coronary heart disease risk.

Appendix A

Smoking and Cerebrovascular Disease

4. The evidence is sufficient to infer a causal relationship between smoking and stroke.

Smoking and Abdominal Aortic Aneurysm

5. The evidence is sufficient to infer a causal relationship between smoking and abdominal aortic aneurysm.

CHAPTER 4. RESPIRATORY DISEASES

Acute Respiratory Illnesses

1. The evidence is sufficient to infer a causal relationship between smoking and acute respiratory illnesses, including pneumonia, in persons without underlying smoking-related chronic obstructive lung disease.
2. The evidence is suggestive but not sufficient to infer a causal relationship between smoking and acute respiratory infections among persons with preexisting chronic obstructive pulmonary disease.
3. In persons with asthma, the evidence is inadequate to infer the presence or absence of a causal relationship between smoking and acute asthma exacerbation.

Chronic Respiratory Diseases

4. The evidence is sufficient to infer a causal relationship between maternal smoking during pregnancy and a reduction of lung function in infants.
5. The evidence is suggestive but not sufficient to infer a causal relationship between maternal smoking during pregnancy and an increase in the frequency of lower respiratory tract illnesses during infancy.
6. The evidence is suggestive but not sufficient to infer a causal relationship between maternal smoking during pregnancy and an increased risk for impaired lung function in childhood and adulthood.
7. Active smoking causes injurious biologic processes (i.e., oxidant stress, inflammation, and a protease-antiprotease imbalance) that result in airway and alveolar injury. This injury, if sustained, ultimately leads to the development of chronic obstructive pulmonary disease.
8. The evidence is sufficient to infer a causal relationship between active smoking and impaired lung growth during childhood and adolescence.

9. The evidence is sufficient to infer a causal relationship between active smoking and the early onset of lung function decline during late adolescence and early adulthood.
10. The evidence is sufficient to infer a causal relationship between active smoking in adulthood and a premature onset of and an accelerated age-related decline in lung function.
11. The evidence is sufficient to infer a causal relationship between sustained cessation from smoking and a return of the rate of decline in pulmonary function to that of persons who had never smoked.
12. The evidence is sufficient to infer a causal relationship between active smoking and respiratory symptoms in children and adolescents, including coughing, phlegm, wheezing, and dyspnea.
13. The evidence is sufficient to infer a causal relationship between active smoking and asthma-related symptoms (i.e., wheezing) in childhood and adolescence.
14. The evidence is inadequate to infer the presence or absence of a causal relationship between active smoking and physician-diagnosed asthma in childhood and adolescence.
15. The evidence is suggestive but not sufficient to infer a causal relationship between active smoking and a poorer prognosis for children and adolescents with asthma.
16. The evidence is sufficient to infer a causal relationship between active smoking and all major respiratory symptoms among adults, including coughing, phlegm, wheezing, and dyspnea.
17. The evidence is inadequate to infer the presence or absence of a causal relationship between active smoking and asthma in adults.
18. The evidence is suggestive but not sufficient to infer a causal relationship between active smoking and increased nonspecific bronchial hyperresponsiveness.
19. The evidence is sufficient to infer a causal relationship between active smoking and poor asthma control.
20. The evidence is sufficient to infer a causal relationship between active smoking and chronic obstructive pulmonary disease morbidity and mortality.
21. The evidence is suggestive but not sufficient to infer a causal relationship between lower machine-measured cigarette tar and a lower risk for cough and mucus hypersecretion.
22. The evidence is inadequate to infer the presence or absence of a causal relationship between a lower cigarette tar content and reductions in forced expiratory volume in one second decline rates.
23. The evidence is inadequate to infer the presence or absence of a causal relationship between a lower cigarette tar content and reductions in chronic obstructive pulmonary disease-related mortality.

24. The evidence is inadequate to infer the presence or absence of a causal relationship between active smoking and idiopathic pulmonary fibrosis.

CHAPTER 5. REPRODUCTIVE EFFECTS

Fertility

1. The evidence is inadequate to infer the presence or absence of a causal relationship between active smoking and sperm quality.
2. The evidence is sufficient to infer a causal relationship between smoking and reduced fertility in women.

Pregnancy and Pregnancy Outcomes

3. The evidence is suggestive but not sufficient to infer a causal relationship between maternal active smoking and ectopic pregnancy.
4. The evidence is suggestive but not sufficient to infer a causal relationship between maternal active smoking and spontaneous abortion.
5. The evidence is sufficient to infer a causal relationship between maternal active smoking and premature rupture of the membranes, placenta previa, and placental abruption.
6. The evidence is sufficient to infer a causal relationship between maternal active smoking and a reduced risk for preeclampsia.
7. The evidence is sufficient to infer a causal relationship between maternal active smoking and preterm delivery and shortened gestation.
8. The evidence is sufficient to infer a causal relationship between maternal active smoking and fetal growth restriction and low birth weight.

Congenital Malformations, Infant Mortality, and Child Physical and Cognitive Development

9. The evidence is inadequate to infer the presence or absence of a causal relationship between maternal smoking and congenital malformations in general.
10. The evidence is suggestive but not sufficient to infer a causal relationship between maternal smoking and oral clefts.
11. The evidence is sufficient to infer a causal relationship between sudden infant death syndrome and maternal smoking during and after pregnancy.

12. The evidence is inadequate to infer the presence or absence of a causal relationship between maternal smoking and physical growth and neurocognitive development of children.

CHAPTER 6. OTHER EFFECTS

Diminished Health Status

1. The evidence is sufficient to infer a causal relationship between smoking and diminished health status that may manifest as increased absenteeism from work and increased use of medical care services.
2. The evidence is sufficient to infer a causal relationship between smoking and increased risks for adverse surgical outcomes related to wound healing and respiratory complications.

Loss of Bone Mass and the Risk of Fractures

3. The evidence is inadequate to infer the presence or absence of a causal relationship between smoking and reduced bone density before menopause in women and in younger men.
4. In postmenopausal women, the evidence is sufficient to infer a causal relationship between smoking and low bone density.
5. In older men, the evidence is suggestive but not sufficient to infer a causal relationship between smoking and low bone density.
6. The evidence is sufficient to infer a causal relationship between smoking and hip fractures.
7. The evidence is inadequate to infer the presence or absence of a causal relationship between smoking and fractures at sites other than the hip.

Dental Diseases

8. The evidence is sufficient to infer a causal relationship between smoking and periodontitis.
9. The evidence is inadequate to infer the presence or absence of a causal relationship between smoking and coronal dental caries.
10. The evidence is suggestive but not sufficient to infer a causal relationship between smoking and root-surface caries.

Erectile Dysfunction

11. The evidence is suggestive but not sufficient to infer a causal relationship between smoking and erectile dysfunction.

Eye Diseases

12. The evidence is sufficient to infer a causal relationship between smoking and nuclear cataract.
13. The evidence is suggestive but not sufficient to infer that smoking cessation reduces the risk of nuclear opacity.
14. The evidence is suggestive but not sufficient to infer a causal relationship between current and past smoking, especially heavy smoking, with risk of exudative (neovascular) age-related macular degeneration.
15. The evidence is suggestive but not sufficient to infer a causal relationship between smoking and atrophic age-related macular degeneration.
16. The evidence is suggestive of no causal relationship between smoking and the onset or progression of retinopathy in persons with diabetes.
17. The evidence is inadequate to infer the presence or absence of a causal relationship between smoking and glaucoma.
18. The evidence is suggestive but not sufficient to infer a causal relationship between ophthalmopathy associated with Graves' disease and smoking.

Peptic Ulcer Disease

19. The evidence is sufficient to infer a causal relationship between smoking and peptic ulcer disease in persons who are *Helicobacter pylori* positive.
20. The evidence is inadequate to infer the presence or absence of a causal relationship between smoking and peptic ulcer disease in nonsteroidal antiinflammatory drug users or in those who are *Helicobacter pylori* negative.
21. The evidence is suggestive but not sufficient to infer a causal relationship between smoking and risk of peptic ulcer complications, although this effect might be restricted to nonusers of nonsteroidal anti-inflammatory drugs.
22. The evidence is inadequate to infer the presence or absence of a causal relationship between smoking and the treatment and recurrence of *Helicobacter pylori*-negative ulcers.

CHAPTER 7. THE IMPACT OF SMOKING ON DISEASE AND THE BENEFITS OF SMOKING REDUCTION

1. There have been more than 12 million premature deaths attributable to smoking since the first published Surgeon General's report on

smoking and health in 1964. Smoking remains the leading preventable cause of premature death in the United States.

2. The burden of smoking-attributable mortality will remain at current levels for several decades. Comprehensive programs that reflect the best available science on tobacco use prevention and smoking cessation have the potential to reduce the adverse impact of smoking on population health.

3. Meeting the *Healthy People 2010* goals for current smoking prevalence reductions to 12 percent among persons aged 18 years and older and to 16 percent among youth aged 14 through 17 years will prevent an additional 7.1 million premature deaths after 2010. Without substantially stronger national and state efforts, it is unlikely that this health goal can be achieved. However, even with more modest reductions in tobacco use, significant additional reductions in premature death can be expected.

4. During 1995–1999, estimated annual smoking attributable economic costs in the United States were $157.7 billion, including $75.5 billion for direct medical care (adults), $81.9 billion for lost productivity, and $366 million for neonatal care. In 2001, states alone spent an estimated $12 billion treating smoking attributable diseases.

Source: United States Department of Health & Human Services, Office of the Surgeon General. Available online. URL: http://www.surgeongeneral. gov/library/smokingconsequences/. Last revised on April 24, 2007.

APPENDIX B

SELECTION FROM WHO FRAMEWORK CONVENTION ON TOBACCO CONTROL (2005)

With the growing use of tobacco in developing nations at the same time usage has declined in developed nations, the World Health Organization (WHO) and public health officials have responded with a worldwide program of tobacco control. The program takes the form of a treaty called the WHO Framework Convention on Tobacco Control, which 168 nations have signed. The text of the treaty describes the ambitious goals and methods to be used in this groundbreaking cooperative effort among nations across the world.

FOREWORD

The WHO Framework Convention on Tobacco Control (WHO FCTC) is the first treaty negotiated under the auspices of the World Health Organization. The WHO FCTC is an evidence-based treaty that reaffirms the right of all people to the highest standard of health.

The WHO FCTC represents a paradigm shift in developing a regulatory strategy to address addictive substances; in contrast to previous drug control treaties, the WHO FCTC asserts the importance of demand reduction strategies as well as supply issues.

The WHO FCTC was developed in response to the globalization of the tobacco epidemic. The spread of the tobacco epidemic is facilitated through a variety of complex factors with cross-border effects, including trade liberalization and direct foreign investment. Other factors such as global marketing, transnational tobacco advertising, promotion and sponsorship, and the international movement of contraband and counterfeit cigarettes have also contributed to the explosive increase in tobacco use.

From the first preambular paragraph, which states that the "Parties to this Convention [are] determined to give priority to their right to protect public health", the WHO FCTC is a global trend-setter.

The core demand reduction provisions in the WHO FCTC are contained in articles 6–14:

- Price and tax measures to reduce the demand for tobacco, and
- Non-price measures to reduce the demand for tobacco, namely:
  ○ Protection from exposure to tobacco smoke;
  ○ Regulation of the contents of tobacco products;
  ○ Regulation of tobacco product disclosures;
  ○ Packaging and labelling of tobacco products;
  ○ Education, communication, training and public awareness;
  ○ Tobacco advertising, promotion and sponsorship; and
  ○ Demand reduction measures concerning tobacco dependence and cessation.

The core supply reduction provisions in the WHO FCTC are contained in articles 15–17:

- Illicit trade in tobacco products;
- Sales to and by minors; and
- Provision of support for economically viable alternative activities.

Another novel feature of the Convention is the inclusion of a provision that addresses liability. Mechanisms for scientific and technical cooperation and exchange of information are set out in Articles 20–22.

The WHO FCTC opened for signature on 16 June to 22 June 2003 in Geneva, and thereafter at the United Nations Headquarters in New York, the Depositary of the treaty, from 30 June 2003 to 29 June 2004. The treaty, which is now closed for signature, has 168 Signatories, including the European Community, which makes it the most widely embraced treaties in UN history. Member States that have signed the Convention indicate that they will strive in good faith to ratify, accept, or approve it, and show political commitment not to undermine the objectives set out in it. Countries wishing to become a Party, but that did not sign the Convention by 29 June 2004, may do so by means of accession, which is a one-step process equivalent to ratification.

The Convention entered into force on 27 February 2005—90 days after it has been acceded to, ratified, accepted, or approved by 40 States. Beginning on that date, the forty Contracting Parties are legally bound by the treaty's provisions. For each State that ratifies, accepts or approves the Convention or accedes thereto after the conditions set out in paragraph 1 of Article 36 for entry into force have been fulfilled, the Convention shall enter into force on the ninetieth day following the date of deposit of its instrument of ratification, acceptance, approval or accession. For regional economic integration organizations, the Convention enters into force on the ninetieth day following the date of deposit of its instrument of formal confirmation or accession.

The global network developed over the period of the negotiations of the WHO FCTC will be important in preparing for the implementation of the Convention at country level. In the words of WHO's Director General, Dr Jong-wook LEE: "The WHO FCTC negotiations have already unleashed a process that has resulted in visible differences at country level. The success of the WHO FCTC as a tool for public health will depend on the energy and political commitment that we devote to implementing it in countries in the coming years. A successful result will be global public health gains for all." For this to materialize, the drive and commitment, which was so evident during the negotiations, will need to spread to national and local levels so that the WHO FCTC becomes a concrete reality where it counts most, in countries.

Preamble

The Parties to this Convention,

Determined to give priority to their right to protect public health,

Recognizing that the spread of the tobacco epidemic is a global problem with serious consequences for public health that calls for the widest possible international cooperation and the participation of all countries in an effective, appropriate and comprehensive international response,

Reflecting the concern of the international community about the devastating worldwide health, social, economic and environmental consequences of tobacco consumption and exposure to tobacco smoke,

Seriously concerned about the increase in the worldwide consumption and production of cigarettes and other tobacco products, particularly in developing countries, as well as about the burden this places on families, on the poor, and on national health systems,

Recognizing that scientific evidence has unequivocally established that tobacco consumption and exposure to tobacco smoke cause death, disease and disability, and that there is a time lag between the exposure to smoking and the other uses of tobacco products and the onset of tobacco-related diseases,

Recognizing also that cigarettes and some other products containing tobacco are highly engineered so as to create and maintain dependence, and that many of the compounds they contain and the smoke they produce are pharmacologically active, toxic, mutagenic and carcinogenic, and that tobacco dependence is separately classified as a disorder in major international classifications of diseases,

Acknowledging that there is clear scientific evidence that prenatal exposure to tobacco smoke causes adverse health and developmental conditions for children,

Deeply concerned about the escalation in smoking and other forms of tobacco consumption by children and adolescents worldwide, particularly smoking at increasingly early ages,

Alarmed by the increase in smoking and other forms of tobacco consumption by women and young girls worldwide and keeping in mind the need for full participation of women at all levels of policy-making and implementation and the need for gender-specific tobacco control strategies,

Deeply concerned about the high levels of smoking and other forms of tobacco consumption by indigenous peoples,

Seriously concerned about the impact of all forms of advertising, promotion and sponsorship aimed at encouraging the use of tobacco products,

Recognizing that cooperative action is necessary to eliminate all forms of illicit trade in cigarettes and other tobacco products, including smuggling, illicit manufacturing and counterfeiting,

Acknowledging that tobacco control at all levels and particularly in developing countries and in countries with economies in transition requires sufficient financial and technical resources commensurate with the current and projected need for tobacco control activities,

Recognizing the need to develop appropriate mechanisms to address the long-term social and economic implications of successful tobacco demand reduction strategies,

Mindful of the social and economic difficulties that tobacco control programmes may engender in the medium and long term in some developing countries and countries with economies in transition, and recognizing their need for technical and financial assistance in the context of nationally developed strategies for sustainable development,

Conscious of the valuable work being conducted by many States on tobacco control and commending the leadership of the World Health Organization as well as the efforts of other organizations and bodies of the United Nations system and other international and regional intergovernmental organizations in developing measures on tobacco control,

Emphasizing the special contribution of nongovernmental organizations and other members of civil society not affiliated with the tobacco industry, including health professional bodies, women's, youth, environmental and consumer groups, and academic and health care institutions, to tobacco control efforts nationally and internationally and the vital importance of their participation in national and international tobacco control efforts,

Recognizing the need to be alert to any efforts by the tobacco industry to undermine or subvert tobacco control efforts and the need to be informed of activities of the tobacco industry that have a negative impact on tobacco control efforts,

Recalling Article 12 of the International Covenant on Economic, Social and Cultural Rights, adopted by the United Nations General Assembly on 16 December 1966, which states that it is the right of everyone to the enjoyment of the highest attainable standard of physical and mental health,

Recalling also the preamble to the Constitution of the World Health Organization, which states that the enjoyment of the highest attainable standard of health is one of the fundamental rights of every human being without distinction of race, religion, political belief, economic or social condition,

Determined to promote measures of tobacco control based on current and relevant scientific, technical and economic considerations,

Recalling that the Convention on the Elimination of All Forms of Discrimination against Women, adopted by the United Nations General Assembly on 18 December 1979, provides that States Parties to that Convention shall take appropriate measures to eliminate discrimination against women in the field of health care,

Recalling further that the Convention on the Rights of the Child, adopted by the United Nations General Assembly on 20 November 1989, provides that States Parties to that Convention recognize the right of the child to the enjoyment of the highest attainable standard of health,

Have agreed, as follows:

PART I: INTRODUCTION

Article 1

Use of terms
For the purposes of this Convention:

> (a) "illicit trade" means any practice or conduct prohibited by law and which relates to production, shipment, receipt, possession, distribution,

sale or purchase including any practice or conduct intended to facilitate such activity;

(b) "regional economic integration organization" means an organization that is composed of several sovereign states, and to which its Member States have transferred competence over a range of matters, including the authority to make decisions binding on its Member States in respect of those matters;

(c) "tobacco advertising and promotion" means any form of commercial communication, recommendation or action with the aim, effect or likely effect of promoting a tobacco product or tobacco use either directly or indirectly;

(d) "tobacco control" means a range of supply, demand and harm reduction strategies that aim to improve the health of a population by eliminating or reducing their consumption of tobacco products and exposure to tobacco smoke;

(e) "tobacco industry" means tobacco manufacturers, wholesale distributors and importers of tobacco products;

(f) "tobacco products" means products entirely or partly made of the leaf tobacco as raw material which are manufactured to be used for smoking, sucking, chewing or snuffing;

(g) "tobacco sponsorship" means any form of contribution to any event, activity or individual with the aim, effect or likely effect of promoting a tobacco product or tobacco use either directly or indirectly;

Where appropriate, national will refer equally to regional economic integration organizations.

Article 2

Relationship between this Convention and other agreements and legal instruments

1. In order to better protect human health, Parties are encouraged to implement measures beyond those required by this Convention and its protocols, and nothing in these instruments shall prevent a Party from imposing stricter requirements that are consistent with their provisions and are in accordance with international law.

2. The provisions of the Convention and its protocols shall in no way affect the right of Parties to enter into bilateral or multilateral agreements, including regional or subregional agreements, on issues relevant or additional to the Convention and its protocols, provided that such agreements are compatible with their obligations under the Convention and its protocols. The Parties concerned shall communicate such agreements to the Conference of the Parties through the Secretariat.

PART II: OBJECTIVE, GUIDING PRINCIPLES AND GENERAL OBLIGATIONS

Article 3

Objective
The objective of this Convention and its protocols is to protect present and future generations from the devastating health, social, environmental and economic consequences of tobacco consumption and exposure to tobacco smoke by providing a framework for tobacco control measures to be implemented by the Parties at the national, regional and international levels in order to reduce continually and substantially the prevalence of tobacco use and exposure to tobacco smoke.

Article 4

Guiding principles
To achieve the objective of this Convention and its protocols and to implement its provisions, the Parties shall be guided, *inter alia*, by the principles set out below:

1. Every person should be informed of the health consequences, addictive nature and mortal threat posed by tobacco consumption and exposure to tobacco smoke and effective legislative, executive, administrative or other measures should be contemplated at the appropriate governmental level to protect all persons from exposure to tobacco smoke.
2. Strong political commitment is necessary to develop and support, at the national, regional and international levels, comprehensive multisectoral measures and coordinated responses, taking into consideration:
    (a) the need to take measures to protect all persons from exposure to tobacco smoke;
    (b) the need to take measures to prevent the initiation, to promote and support cessation, and to decrease the consumption of tobacco products in any form;
    (c) the need to take measures to promote the participation of indigenous individuals and communities in the development, implementation and evaluation of tobacco control programmes that are socially and culturally appropriate to their needs and perspectives; and
    (d) the need to take measures to address gender-specific risks when developing tobacco control strategies.
3. International cooperation, particularly transfer of technology, knowledge and financial assistance and provision of related expertise, to

establish and implement effective tobacco control programmes, taking into consideration local culture, as well as social, economic, political and legal factors, is an important part of the Convention.

4. Comprehensive multisectoral measures and responses to reduce consumption of all tobacco products at the national, regional and international levels are essential so as to prevent, in accordance with public health principles, the incidence of diseases, premature disability and mortality due to tobacco consumption and exposure to tobacco smoke.
5. Issues relating to liability, as determined by each Party within its jurisdiction, are an important part of comprehensive tobacco control.
6. The importance of technical and financial assistance to aid the economic transition of tobacco growers and workers whose livelihoods are seriously affected as a consequence of tobacco control programmes in developing country Parties, as well as Parties with economies in transition, should be recognized and addressed in the context of nationally developed strategies for sustainable development.
7. The participation of civil society is essential in achieving the objective of the Convention and its protocols.

Article 5

General obligations

1. Each Party shall develop, implement, periodically update and review comprehensive multisectoral national tobacco control strategies, plans and programmes in accordance with this Convention and the protocols to which it is a Party.
2. Towards this end, each Party shall, in accordance with its capabilities:
   (a) establish or reinforce and finance a national coordinating mechanism or focal points for tobacco control; and
   (b) adopt and implement effective legislative, executive, administrative and/or other measures and cooperate, as appropriate, with other Parties in developing appropriate policies for preventing and reducing tobacco consumption, nicotine addiction and exposure to tobacco smoke.
3. In setting and implementing their public health policies with respect to tobacco control, Parties shall act to protect these policies from commercial and other vested interests of the tobacco industry in accordance with national law.
4. The Parties shall cooperate in the formulation of proposed measures, procedures and guidelines for the implementation of the Convention and the protocols to which they are Parties.

5. The Parties shall cooperate, as appropriate, with competent international and regional intergovernmental organizations and other bodies to achieve the objectives of the Convention and the protocols to which they are Parties.

6. The Parties shall, within means and resources at their disposal, cooperate to raise financial resources for effective implementation of the Convention through bilateral and multilateral funding mechanisms.

PART III: MEASURES RELATING TO THE REDUCTION OF DEMAND FOR TOBACCO

Article 6

Price and tax measures to reduce the demand for tobacco

1. The Parties recognize that price and tax measures are an effective and important means of reducing tobacco consumption by various segments of the population, in particular young persons.

2. Without prejudice to the sovereign right of the Parties to determine and establish their taxation policies, each Party should take account of its national health objectives concerning tobacco control and adopt or maintain, as appropriate, measures which may include:
   (a) implementing tax policies and, where appropriate, price policies, on tobacco products so as to contribute to the health objectives aimed at reducing tobacco consumption; and
   (b) prohibiting or restricting, as appropriate, sales to and/or importations by international travellers of tax- and duty-free tobacco products.

3. The Parties shall provide rates of taxation for tobacco products and trends in tobacco consumption in their periodic reports to the Conference of the Parties, in accordance with Article 21.

Article 7

Non-price measures to reduce the demand for tobacco
The Parties recognize that comprehensive non-price measures are an effective and important means of reducing tobacco consumption. Each Party shall adopt and implement effective legislative, executive, administrative or other measures necessary to implement its obligations pursuant to Articles 8 to 13 and shall cooperate, as appropriate, with each other directly or through competent international bodies with a view to their implementation.

Tobacco Industry and Smoking

The Conference of the Parties shall propose appropriate guidelines for the implementation of the provisions of these Articles.

Article 8

Protection from exposure to tobacco smoke

1. Parties recognize that scientific evidence has unequivocally established that exposure to tobacco smoke causes death, disease and disability.
2. Each Party shall adopt and implement in areas of existing national jurisdiction as determined by national law and actively promote at other jurisdictional levels the adoption and implementation of effective legislative, executive, administrative and/or other measures, providing for protection from exposure to tobacco smoke in indoor workplaces, public transport, indoor public places and, as appropriate, other public places.

Article 9

Regulation of the contents of tobacco products

The Conference of the Parties, in consultation with competent international bodies, shall propose guidelines for testing and measuring the contents and emissions of tobacco products, and for the regulation of these contents and emissions. Each Party shall, where approved by competent national authorities, adopt and implement effective legislative, executive and administrative or other measures for such testing and measuring, and for such regulation.

Article 10

Regulation of tobacco product disclosures

Each Party shall, in accordance with its national law, adopt and implement effective legislative, executive, administrative or other measures requiring manufacturers and importers of tobacco products to disclose to governmental authorities information about the contents and emissions of tobacco products. Each Party shall further adopt and implement effective measures for public disclosure of information about the toxic constituents of the tobacco products and the emissions that they may produce.

Article 11

Packaging and labelling of tobacco products

1. Each Party shall, within a period of three years after entry into force of this Convention for that Party, adopt and implement, in accordance with its national law, effective measures to ensure that:

Appendix B

(a) tobacco product packaging and labelling do not promote a tobacco product by any means that are false, misleading, deceptive or likely to create an erroneous impression about its characteristics, health effects, hazards or emissions, including any term, descriptor, trademark, figurative or any other sign that directly or indirectly creates the false impression that a particular tobacco product is less harmful than other tobacco products. These may include terms such as "low tar", "light", "ultra-light", or "mild"; and

(b) each unit packet and package of tobacco products and any outside packaging and labelling of such products also carry health warnings describing the harmful effects of tobacco use, and may include other appropriate messages. These warnings and messages:

(i) shall be approved by the competent national authority,
(ii) shall be rotating,
(iii) shall be large, clear, visible and legible,
(iv) should be 50% or more of the principal display areas but shall be no less than 30% of the principal display areas,
(v) may be in the form of or include pictures or pictograms.

2. Each unit packet and package of tobacco products and any outside packaging and labelling of such products shall, in addition to the warnings specified in paragraph 1(b) of this Article, contain information on relevant constituents and emissions of tobacco products as defined by national authorities.

3. Each Party shall require that the warnings and other textual information specified in paragraphs 1(b) and paragraph 2 of this Article will appear on each unit packet and package of tobacco products and any outside packaging and labelling of such products in its principal language or languages.

4. For the purposes of this Article, the term "outside packaging and labelling" in relation to tobacco products applies to any packaging and labelling used in the retail sale of the product.

Article 12

Education, communication, training and public awareness

Each Party shall promote and strengthen public awareness of tobacco control issues, using all available communication tools, as appropriate. Towards this end, each Party shall adopt and implement effective legislative, executive, administrative or other measures to promote:

(a) broad access to effective and comprehensive educational and public awareness programmes on the health risks including the addictive characteristics of tobacco consumption and exposure to tobacco smoke;

(b) public awareness about the health risks of tobacco consumption and exposure to tobacco smoke, and about the benefits of the cessation of tobacco use and tobacco-free lifestyles as specified in Article 14.2;

(c) public access, in accordance with national law, to a wide range of information on the tobacco industry as relevant to the objective of this Convention;

(d) effective and appropriate training or sensitization and awareness programmes on tobacco control addressed to persons such as health workers, community workers, social workers, media professionals, educators, decision-makers, administrators and other concerned persons;

(e) awareness and participation of public and private agencies and nongovernmental organizations not affiliated with the tobacco industry in developing and implementing intersectoral programmes and strategies for tobacco control; and

(f) public awareness of and access to information regarding the adverse health, economic, and environmental consequences of tobacco production and consumption.

Article 13

Tobacco advertising, promotion and sponsorship

1. Parties recognize that a comprehensive ban on advertising, promotion and sponsorship would reduce the consumption of tobacco products.
2. Each Party shall, in accordance with its constitution or constitutional principles, undertake a comprehensive ban of all tobacco advertising, promotion and sponsorship. This shall include, subject to the legal environment and technical means available to that Party, a comprehensive ban on cross-border advertising, promotion and sponsorship originating from its territory. In this respect, within the period of five years after entry into force of this Convention for that Party, each Party shall undertake appropriate legislative, executive, administrative and/or other measures and report accordingly in conformity with Article 21.
3. A Party that is not in a position to undertake a comprehensive ban due to its constitution or constitutional principles shall apply restrictions on all tobacco advertising, promotion and sponsorship. This shall include, subject to the legal environment and technical means available to that Party, restrictions or a comprehensive ban on advertising, promotion and sponsorship originating from its territory with cross-border effects. In this respect, each Party shall undertake appropriate

legislative, executive, administrative and/or other measures and report accordingly in conformity with Article 21.

4. As a minimum, and in accordance with its constitution or constitutional principles, each Party shall:

(a) prohibit all forms of tobacco advertising, promotion and sponsorship that promote a tobacco product by any means that are false, misleading or deceptive or likely to create an erroneous impression about its characteristics, health effects, hazards or emissions;

(b) require that health or other appropriate warnings or messages accompany all tobacco advertising and, as appropriate, promotion and sponsorship;

(c) restrict the use of direct or indirect incentives that encourage the purchase of tobacco products by the public;

(d) require, if it does not have a comprehensive ban, the disclosure to relevant governmental authorities of expenditures by the tobacco industry on advertising, promotion and sponsorship not yet prohibited. Those authorities may decide to make those figures available, subject to national law, to the public and to the Conference of the Parties, pursuant to Article 21;

(e) undertake a comprehensive ban or, in the case of a Party that is not in a position to undertake a comprehensive ban due to its constitution or constitutional principles, restrict tobacco advertising, promotion and sponsorship on radio, television, print media and, as appropriate, other media, such as the internet, within a period of five years; and

(f) prohibit, or in the case of a Party that is not in a position to prohibit due to its constitution or constitutional principles restrict, tobacco sponsorship of international events, activities and/or participants therein.

5. Parties are encouraged to implement measures beyond the obligations set out in paragraph 4.

6. Parties shall cooperate in the development of technologies and other means necessary to facilitate the elimination of cross-border advertising.

7. Parties which have a ban on certain forms of tobacco advertising, promotion and sponsorship have the sovereign right to ban those forms of cross-border tobacco advertising, promotion and sponsorship entering their territory and to impose equal penalties as those applicable to domestic advertising, promotion and sponsorship originating from their territory in accordance with their national law. This paragraph does not endorse or approve of any particular penalty.

8. Parties shall consider the elaboration of a protocol setting out appropriate measures that require international collaboration for a

comprehensive ban on cross-border advertising, promotion and sponsorship.

Article 14

Demand reduction measures concerning tobacco dependence and cessation

1. Each Party shall develop and disseminate appropriate, comprehensive and integrated guidelines based on scientific evidence and best practices, taking into account national circumstances and priorities, and shall take effective measures to promote cessation of tobacco use and adequate treatment for tobacco dependence.
2. Towards this end, each Party shall endeavour to:
   (a) design and implement effective programmes aimed at promoting the cessation of tobacco use, in such locations as educational institutions, health care facilities, workplaces and sporting environments;
   (b) include diagnosis and treatment of tobacco dependence and counselling services on cessation of tobacco use in national health and education programmes, plans and strategies, with the participation of health workers, community workers and social workers as appropriate;
   (c) establish in health care facilities and rehabilitation centres programmes for diagnosing, counselling, preventing and treating tobacco dependence; and
   (d) collaborate with other Parties to facilitate accessibility and affordability for treatment of tobacco dependence including pharmaceutical products pursuant to Article 22. Such products and their constituents may include medicines, products used to administer medicines and diagnostics when appropriate.

PART IV: MEASURES RELATING TO THE REDUCTION OF THE SUPPLY OF TOBACCO

Article 15

Illicit trade in tobacco products

1. The Parties recognize that the elimination of all forms of illicit trade in tobacco products, including smuggling, illicit manufacturing and counterfeiting, and the development and implementation of related national law, in addition to subregional, regional and global agreements, are essential components of tobacco control.
2. Each Party shall adopt and implement effective legislative, executive, administrative or other measures to ensure that all unit packets and

packages of tobacco products and any outside packaging of such products are marked to assist Parties in determining the origin of tobacco products, and in accordance with national law and relevant bilateral or multilateral agreements, assist Parties in determining the point of diversion and monitor, document and control the movement of tobacco products and their legal status. In addition, each Party shall:

(a) require that unit packets and packages of tobacco products for retail and wholesale use that are sold on its domestic market carry the statement: *"Sales only allowed in (insert name of the country, subnational, regional or federal unit)"* or carry any other effective marking indicating the final destination or which would assist authorities in determining whether the product is legally for sale on the domestic market; and

(b) consider, as appropriate, developing a practical tracking and tracing regime that would further secure the distribution system and assist in the investigation of illicit trade.

3. Each Party shall require that the packaging information or marking specified in paragraph 2 of this Article shall be presented in legible form and/or appear in its principal language or languages.

4. With a view to eliminating illicit trade in tobacco products, each Party shall:

(a) monitor and collect data on cross-border trade in tobacco products, including illicit trade, and exchange information among customs, tax and other authorities, as appropriate, and in accordance with national law and relevant applicable bilateral or multilateral agreements;

(b) enact or strengthen legislation, with appropriate penalties and remedies, against illicit trade in tobacco products, including counterfeit and contraband cigarettes;

(c) take appropriate steps to ensure that all confiscated manufacturing equipment, counterfeit and contraband cigarettes and other tobacco products are destroyed, using environmentally-friendly methods where feasible, or disposed of in accordance with national law;

(d) adopt and implement measures to monitor, document and control the storage and distribution of tobacco products held or moving under suspension of taxes or duties within its jurisdiction; and

(e) adopt measures as appropriate to enable the confiscation of proceeds derived from the illicit trade in tobacco products.

5. Information collected pursuant to subparagraphs 4(a) and 4(d) of this Article shall, as appropriate, be provided in aggregate form by the Parties in their periodic reports to the Conference of the Parties, in accordance with Article 21.

6. The Parties shall, as appropriate and in accordance with national law, promote cooperation between national agencies, as well as relevant regional and international intergovernmental organizations as it

relates to investigations, prosecutions and proceedings, with a view to eliminating illicit trade in tobacco products. Special emphasis shall be placed on cooperation at regional and subregional levels to combat illicit trade of tobacco products.

7. Each Party shall endeavour to adopt and implement further measures including licensing, where appropriate, to control or regulate the production and distribution of tobacco products in order to prevent illicit trade.

Article 16

Sales to and by minors

1. Each Party shall adopt and implement effective legislative, executive, administrative or other measures at the appropriate government level to prohibit the sales of tobacco products to persons under the age set by domestic law, national law or eighteen. These measures may include:
(a) requiring that all sellers of tobacco products place a clear and prominent indicator inside their point of sale about the prohibition of tobacco sales to minors and, in case of doubt, request that each tobacco purchaser provide appropriate evidence of having reached full legal age;
(b) banning the sale of tobacco products in any manner by which they are directly accessible, such as store shelves;
(c) prohibiting the manufacture and sale of sweets, snacks, toys or any other objects in the form of tobacco products which appeal to minors; and
(d) ensuring that tobacco vending machines under its jurisdiction are not accessible to minors and do not promote the sale of tobacco products to minors.

2. Each Party shall prohibit or promote the prohibition of the distribution of free tobacco products to the public and especially minors.

3. Each Party shall endeavour to prohibit the sale of cigarettes individually or in small packets which increase the affordability of such products to minors.

4. The Parties recognize that in order to increase their effectiveness, measures to prevent tobacco product sales to minors should, where appropriate, be implemented in conjunction with other provisions contained in this Convention.

5. When signing, ratifying, accepting, approving or acceding to the Convention or at any time thereafter, a Party may, by means of a binding written declaration, indicate its commitment to prohibit the introduction of tobacco vending machines within its jurisdiction

or, as appropriate, to a total ban on tobacco vending machines. The declaration made pursuant to this Article shall be circulated by the Depositary to all Parties to the Convention.

6. Each Party shall adopt and implement effective legislative, executive, administrative or other measures, including penalties against sellers and distributors, in order to ensure compliance with the obligations contained in paragraphs 1-5 of this Article.

7. Each Party should, as appropriate, adopt and implement effective legislative, executive, administrative or other measures to prohibit the sales of tobacco products by persons under the age set by domestic law, national law or eighteen.

Article 17

Provision of support for economically viable alternative activities
Parties shall, in cooperation with each other and with competent international and regional intergovernmental organizations, promote, as appropriate, economically viable alternatives for tobacco workers, growers and, as the case may be, individual sellers.

PART V: PROTECTION OF THE ENVIRONMENT

Article 18

Protection of the environment and the health of persons
In carrying out their obligations under this Convention, the Parties agree to have due regard to the protection of the environment and the health of persons in relation to the environment in respect of tobacco cultivation and manufacture within their respective territories.

PART VI: QUESTIONS RELATED TO LIABILITY

Article 19

Liability

1. For the purpose of tobacco control, the Parties shall consider taking legislative action or promoting their existing laws, where necessary, to deal with criminal and civil liability, including compensation where appropriate.

2. Parties shall cooperate with each other in exchanging information through the Conference of the Parties in accordance with Article 21 including:

(a) information on the health effects of the consumption of tobacco products and exposure to tobacco smoke in accordance with Article 20.3(a); and

(b) information on legislation and regulations in force as well as pertinent jurisprudence.

3. The Parties shall, as appropriate and mutually agreed, within the limits of national legislation, policies, legal practices and applicable existing treaty arrangements, afford one another assistance in legal proceedings relating to civil and criminal liability consistent with this Convention.

4. The Convention shall in no way affect or limit any rights of access of the Parties to each other's courts where such rights exist.

5. The Conference of the Parties may consider, if possible, at an early stage, taking account of the work being done in relevant international fora, issues related to liability including appropriate international approaches to these issues and appropriate means to support, upon request, the Parties in their legislative and other activities in accordance with this Article.

PART VII: SCIENTIFIC AND TECHNICAL COOPERATION AND COMMUNICATION OF INFORMATION

Article 20

Research, surveillance and exchange of information

1. The Parties undertake to develop and promote national research and to coordinate research programmes at the regional and international levels in the field of tobacco control. Towards this end, each Party shall:

(a) initiate and cooperate in, directly or through competent international and regional intergovernmental organizations and other bodies, the conduct of research and scientific assessments, and in so doing promote and encourage research that addresses the determinants and consequences of tobacco consumption and exposure to tobacco smoke as well as research for identification of alternative crops; and

(b) promote and strengthen, with the support of competent international and regional intergovernmental organizations and other bodies, training and support for all those engaged in tobacco control activities, including research, implementation and evaluation.

Appendix B

2. The Parties shall establish, as appropriate, programmes for national, regional and global surveillance of the magnitude, patterns, determinants and consequences of tobacco consumption and exposure to tobacco smoke. Towards this end, the Parties should integrate tobacco surveillance programmes into national, regional and global health surveillance programmes so that data are comparable and can be analysed at the regional and international levels, as appropriate.

3. Parties recognize the importance of financial and technical assistance from international and regional intergovernmental organizations and other bodies. Each Party shall endeavour to:
   (a) establish progressively a national system for the epidemiological surveillance of tobacco consumption and related social, economic and health indicators;
   (b) cooperate with competent international and regional intergovernmental organizations and other bodies, including governmental and nongovernmental agencies, in regional and global tobacco surveillance and exchange of information on the indicators specified in paragraph 3(a) of this Article; and
   (c) cooperate with the World Health Organization in the development of general guidelines or procedures for defining the collection, analysis and dissemination of tobacco-related surveillance data.

4. The Parties shall, subject to national law, promote and facilitate the exchange of publicly available scientific, technical, socioeconomic, commercial and legal information, as well as information regarding practices of the tobacco industry and the cultivation of tobacco, which is relevant to this Convention, and in so doing shall take into account and address the special needs of developing country Parties and Parties with economies in transition. Each Party shall endeavour to:
   (a) progressively establish and maintain an updated database of laws and regulations on tobacco control and, as appropriate, information about their enforcement, as well as pertinent jurisprudence, and cooperate in the development of programmes for regional and global tobacco control;
   (b) progressively establish and maintain updated data from national surveillance programmes in accordance with paragraph 3(a) of this Article; and
   (c) cooperate with competent international organizations to progressively establish and maintain a global system to regularly collect and disseminate information on tobacco production, manufacture and the activities of the tobacco industry which have an impact on the Convention or national tobacco control activities.

5. Parties should cooperate in regional and international intergovernmental organizations and financial and development institutions of which they are members, to promote and encourage provision of

275

technical and financial resources to the Secretariat to assist developing country Parties and Parties with economies in transition to meet their commitments on research, surveillance and exchange of information.

Article 21

Reporting and exchange of information

1. Each Party shall submit to the Conference of the Parties, through the Secretariat, periodic reports on its implementation of this Convention, which should include the following:
   (a) information on legislative, executive, administrative or other measures taken to implement the Convention;
   (b) information, as appropriate, on any constraints or barriers encountered in its implementation of the Convention, and on the measures taken to overcome these barriers;
   (c) information, as appropriate, on financial and technical assistance provided or received for tobacco control activities;
   (d) information on surveillance and research as specified in Article 20; and
   (e) information specified in Articles 6.3, 13.2, 13.3, 13.4(d), 15.5 and 19.2.
2. The frequency and format of such reports by all Parties shall be determined by the Conference of the Parties. Each Party shall make its initial report within two years of the entry into force of the Convention for that Party.
3. The Conference of the Parties, pursuant to Articles 22 and 26, shall consider arrangements to assist developing country Parties and Parties with economies in transition, at their request, in meeting their obligations under this Article.
4. The reporting and exchange of information under the Convention shall be subject to national law regarding confidentiality and privacy. The Parties shall protect, as mutually agreed, any confidential information that is exchanged.

Article 22

Cooperation in the scientific, technical, and legal fields and provision of related expertise

1. The Parties shall cooperate directly or through competent international bodies to strengthen their capacity to fulfill the obligations arising from this Convention, taking into account the needs of developing country

Parties and Parties with economies in transition. Such cooperation shall promote the transfer of technical, scientific and legal expertise and technology, as mutually agreed, to establish and strengthen national tobacco control strategies, plans and programmes aiming at, *inter alia:*
(a) facilitation of the development, transfer and acquisition of technology, knowledge, skills, capacity and expertise related to tobacco control;
(b) provision of technical, scientific, legal and other expertise to establish and strengthen national tobacco control strategies, plans and programmes, aiming at implementation of the Convention through, *inter alia:*

   (i) assisting, upon request, in the development of a strong legislative foundation as well as technical programmes, including those on prevention of initiation, promotion of cessation and protection from exposure to tobacco smoke;

   (ii) assisting, as appropriate, tobacco workers in the development of appropriate economically and legally viable alternative livelihoods in an economically viable manner; and

   (iii) assisting, as appropriate, tobacco growers in shifting agricultural production to alternative crops in an economically viable manner;

(c) support for appropriate training or sensitization programmes for appropriate personnel in accordance with Article 12;
(d) provision, as appropriate, of the necessary material, equipment and supplies, as well as logistical support, for tobacco control strategies, plans and programmes;
(e) identification of methods for tobacco control, including comprehensive treatment of nicotine addiction; and
(f) promotion, as appropriate, of research to increase the affordability of comprehensive treatment of nicotine addiction.

2. The Conference of the Parties shall promote and facilitate transfer of technical, scientific and legal expertise and technology with the financial support secured in accordance with Article 26.

PART VIII: INSTITUTIONAL ARRANGEMENTS AND FINANCIAL RESOURCES

Article 23

Conference of the Parties

1. A Conference of the Parties is hereby established. The first session of the Conference shall be convened by the World Health Organization

not later than one year after the entry into force of this Convention. The Conference will determine the venue and timing of subsequent regular sessions at its first session.

2. Extraordinary sessions of the Conference of the Parties shall be held at such other times as may be deemed necessary by the Conference, or at the written request of any Party, provided that, within six months of the request being communicated to them by the Secretariat of the Convention, it is supported by at least one-third of the Parties.

3. The Conference of the Parties shall adopt by consensus its Rules of Procedure at its first session.

4. The Conference of the Parties shall by consensus adopt financial rules for itself as well as governing the funding of any subsidiary bodies it may establish as well as financial provisions governing the functioning of the Secretariat. At each ordinary session, it shall adopt a budget for the financial period until the next ordinary session.

5. The Conference of the Parties shall keep under regular review the implementation of the Convention and take the decisions necessary to promote its effective implementation and may adopt protocols, annexes and amendments to the Convention, in accordance with Articles 28, 29 and 33. Towards this end, it shall:

(a) promote and facilitate the exchange of information pursuant to Articles 20 and 21;

(b) promote and guide the development and periodic refinement of comparable methodologies for research and the collection of data, in addition to those provided for in Article 20, relevant to the implementation of the Convention;

(c) promote, as appropriate, the development, implementation and evaluation of strategies, plans, and programmes, as well as policies, legislation and other measures;

(d) consider reports submitted by the Parties in accordance with Article 21 and adopt regular reports on the implementation of the Convention;

(e) promote and facilitate the mobilization of financial resources for the implementation of the Convention in accordance with Article 26;

(f) establish such subsidiary bodies as are necessary to achieve the objective of the Convention;

(g) request, where appropriate, the services and cooperation of, and information provided by, competent and relevant organizations and bodies of the United Nations system and other international and regional intergovernmental organizations and nongovernmental organizations and bodies as a means of strengthening the implementation of the Convention; and

(h) consider other action, as appropriate, for the achievement of the objective of the Convention in the light of experience gained in its implementation. 6. The Conference of the Parties shall establish the criteria for the participation of observers at its proceedings.

Article 24

Secretariat

1. The Conference of the Parties shall designate a permanent secretariat and make arrangements for its functioning. The Conference of the Parties shall endeavour to do so at its first session.
2. Until such time as a permanent secretariat is designated and established, secretariat functions under this Convention shall be provided by the World Health Organization. 3. Secretariat functions shall be:
(a) to make arrangements for sessions of the Conference of the Parties and any subsidiary bodies and to provide them with services as required;
(b) to transmit reports received by it pursuant to the Convention;
(c) to provide support to the Parties, particularly developing country Parties and Parties with economies in transition, on request, in the compilation and communication of information required in accordance with the provisions of the Convention;
(d) to prepare reports on its activities under the Convention under the guidance of the Conference of the Parties and submit them to the Conference of the Parties;
(e) to ensure, under the guidance of the Conference of the Parties, the necessary coordination with the competent international and regional intergovernmental organizations and other bodies;
(f) to enter, under the guidance of the Conference of the Parties, into such administrative or contractual arrangements as may be required for the effective discharge of its functions; and
(g) to perform other secretariat functions specified by the Convention and by any of its protocols and such other functions as may be determined by the Conference of the Parties.

Article 25

Relations between the Conference of the Parties and intergovernmental organizations
In order to provide technical and financial cooperation for achieving the objective of this Convention, the Conference of the Parties may request the cooperation of competent international and regional intergovernmental organizations including financial and development institutions.

Article 26

Financial resources

1. The Parties recognize the important role that financial resources play in achieving the objective of this Convention.
2. Each Party shall provide financial support in respect of its national activities intended to achieve the objective of the Convention, in accordance with its national plans, priorities and programmes.
3. Parties shall promote, as appropriate, the utilization of bilateral, regional, subregional and other multilateral channels to provide funding for the development and strengthening of multisectoral comprehensive tobacco control programmes of developing country Parties and Parties with economies in transition. Accordingly, economically viable alternatives to tobacco production, including crop diversification should be addressed and supported in the context of nationally developed strategies of sustainable development.
4. Parties represented in relevant regional and international intergovernmental organizations, and financial and development institutions shall encourage these entities to provide financial assistance for developing country Parties and for Parties with economies in transition to assist them in meeting their obligations under the Convention, without limiting the rights of participation within these organizations.
5. The Parties agree that:
   (a) to assist Parties in meeting their obligations under the Convention, all relevant potential and existing resources, financial, technical, or otherwise, both public and private that are available for tobacco control activities, should be mobilized and utilized for the benefit of all Parties, especially developing countries and countries with economies in transition;
   (b) the Secretariat shall advise developing country Parties and Parties with economies in transition, upon request, on available sources of funding to facilitate the implementation of their obligations under the Convention;
   (c) the Conference of the Parties in its first session shall review existing and potential sources and mechanisms of assistance based on a study conducted by the Secretariat and other relevant information, and consider their adequacy; and
   (d) the results of this review shall be taken into account by the Conference of the Parties in determining the necessity to enhance existing mechanisms or to establish a voluntary global fund or other appropriate financial mechanisms to channel additional financial

resources, as needed, to developing country Parties and Parties with economies in transition to assist them in meeting the objectives of the Convention.

Source: World Health Organization, Programmes and Projects. Available online. URL: http://www.who.int/fctc/en/index.html. Accessed on July 14, 2008.

APPENDIX C

EXECUTIVE SUMMARY FROM CLINICAL PRACTICE GUIDELINES: TREATING TOBACCO USE AND DEPENDENCE: 2008 UPDATE

The executive summary of the much larger book contains information on the most effective methods for smoking cessation. The effort comes from the work of more than two dozen scholars to update scientific findings and give useful advice to clinicians trying to help smokers quit.

CONTEXT

The 1996 Smoking Cessation Clinical Practice Guideline emphasized the dire health consequences of tobacco use and dependence, the existence of effective treatments, and the importance of inducing more smokers to use such treatments. It also called for newer, even more effective tobacco dependence treatments. All of these points still are germane. Nevertheless, heartening progress has been made in tobacco control since that time, and this progress is part of a larger pattern of change that stretches back over the past 40 years. This progress reflects the achievements of clinicians, the public health community, scientists, government agencies, health care organizations, insurers, purchasers, and smokers who have successfully quit. As a result, the current prevalence of tobacco use among adults in the United States (about 20.8 percent) is less than half the rate observed in the 1960s (about 44 percent).

This Guideline concludes that tobacco use presents a rare confluence of circumstances: (1) a highly significant health threat; (2) a disinclination among clinicians to intervene consistently; and (3) the presence of effective interventions. This last point is buttressed by evidence that tobacco dependence interventions, if delivered in a timely and effective manner, significantly reduce the smoker's risk of suffering from smoking-related disease. Indeed, it is difficult to identify any other condition that presents such a mix of lethality, prevalence, and neglect, despite effective and readily available interventions.

Although tobacco use still is an enormous threat, the story of tobacco control efforts during the last half century is one of remarkable progress and promise. In 1965, current smokers outnumbered former smokers three to one. During the past 40 years, the rate of quitting has so outstripped the rate of initiation that, today, there are more former smokers than current smokers. Moreover, 40 years ago smoking was viewed as a habit rather than a chronic disease. No scientifically validated treatments were available for the treatment of tobacco use and dependence, and it had little place in health care delivery. Today, numerous effective treatments exist, and tobacco use assessment and intervention are considered to be requisite duties of clinicians and health care delivery entities. Finally, every state now has a telephone quitline, increasing access to effective treatment.

The scant dozen years following the publication of the first Guideline have ushered in similarly impressive changes. In 1997, only 25 percent of managed health care plans covered any tobacco dependence treatment; this figure approached 90 percent by 2003, although this increased coverage often includes barriers to use. Numerous states added Medicaid coverage for tobacco dependence treatment since the publication of the first Guideline so that, by 2005, 72 percent offered coverage for at least one Guideline-recommended treatment. In 2002, The Joint Commission (formerly JCAHO), which accredits some 15,000 hospitals and health care programs, instituted an accreditation requirement for the delivery of evidence-based tobacco dependence interventions for patients with diagnoses of acute myocardial infarction, congestive heart failure, or pneumonia (www.coreoptions.com/new_site/jcahocore.html; hospital-specific results: www.hospitalcompare.hhs.gov). Finally, Medicare, the Veterans Health Administration, and the United States Military now provide coverage for tobacco dependence treatment. Such policies and systems changes are paying off in terms of increased rates of assessment and treatment of tobacco use.

Data show that the rate at which smokers report being advised to quit smoking has approximately doubled since the early 1990s. Recent data also suggest a substantial increase in the proportion of smokers receiving more intensive cessation interventions. The National Committee for Quality Assurance (NCQA) reports steady increases for both commercial insurers and Medicaid in the discussion of both medications and strategies for smoking cessation. Finally, since the first Guideline was published in 1996, smoking prevalence among adults in the United States has declined from about 25 percent to about 21 percent.

An inspection of the 2008 Guideline update shows that substantial progress also has been made in treatment development and delivery. Telephone quitlines have been shown to be effective in providing wide access to evidence-based cessation counseling. Seven U.S. Food and Drug Administration (FDA)-approved medications for treating tobacco dependence are now available, and new evidence has revealed that particular medications or combinations of medications are especially effective.

This Guideline update also casts into stark relief those areas in which more progress is needed. There is a need for innovative and more effective counseling strategies. In addition, although adolescents appear to benefit from counseling, more consistent and effective interventions and options for use with children, adolescents, and young adults clearly are needed. Smoking prevalence remains discouragingly high in certain populations, such as in those with low socioeconomic status (SES)/low educational attainment, some American Indian populations, and individuals with psychiatric disorders, including substance use disorders. New techniques and treatment delivery strategies may be required before the needs of these groups are adequately addressed. Moreover, although much of the available data come from randomized clinical trials occurring in research settings, it is imperative that new research examine implementation of effective treatments in real-world clinical settings. Finally, new strategies are needed to create consumer demand for effective treatments among tobacco users; there has been little increase in the proportion of smokers who make quit attempts, and too few smokers who do try to quit take advantage of evidence-based treatment that can double or triple their odds of success. New research and communication efforts must impart greater hope, confidence, and increased access to treatments so that tobacco users in ever greater numbers attempt tobacco cessation and achieve abstinence. To succeed, all of these areas require adequate funding.

Thus, this 2008 Guideline update serves as a benchmark of the progress made. It should reassure clinicians, policymakers, funding agencies, and the public that tobacco use is amenable to both scientific analysis and clinical interventions. This history of remarkable progress should encourage renewed efforts by clinicians, policymakers, and researchers to help those who remain dependent on tobacco.

GUIDELINE ORIGINS

This Guideline, *Treating Tobacco Use and Dependence: 2008 Update*, a Public Health Service-sponsored Clinical Practice Guideline, is the product of the Treating Tobacco Use and Dependence Guideline Panel ("the Panel"), government liaisons, consultants, and staff. These individuals were charged with the responsibility of identifying effective, experimentally validated tobacco dependence clinical treatments and practices. This Guideline update is the third Public Health Service Clinical Practice Guideline published on tobacco use. The first Guideline, the 1996 *Smoking Cessation Clinical Practice Guideline No. 18*, was sponsored by the Agency for Healthcare Policy and Research (AHCPR, now the Agency for Healthcare Research and Quality [AHRQ]), U.S. Department of Health and Human Services (HHS). That Guideline reflected scientific literature published between 1975 and 1994. The second Guideline, published in 2000, *Treating Tobacco Use and Dependence*, was sponsored by a consortium of U. S. Public Health Service (PHS) agencies (AHRQ; Centers for Disease Control and Prevention [CDC]; National Cancer Institute [NCI]; National Heart, Lung, and Blood Institute [NHLBI]; National Institute on Drug Abuse [NIDA]) as well as the Robert Wood Johnson Foundation (RWJF) and the University of Wisconsin Center for Tobacco Research and Intervention (UW-CTRI). That Guideline reflected the scientific literature published from 1975 to 1999. The current 2008 update addresses literature published from 1975 to 2007.

The updated Guideline was written in response to new, effective clinical treatments for tobacco dependence that have been identified since 1999. These treatments promise to enhance the rates of successful tobacco cessation. The original 1996 Guideline was based on some 3,000 articles on tobacco treatment published between 1975 and 1994. The 2000 Guideline required the collection and screening of an additional 3,000 articles published between 1995 and 1999. The 2008 Guideline update screened an additional 2,700 articles; thus, the present Guideline update reflects the distillation of a literature base of more than 8,700 research articles. This body of research of course was further reviewed to identify a much smaller group of articles, based on rigorous inclusion criteria, which served as the basis for focused Guideline data analyses and review.

The 2008 updated Guideline was sponsored by a consortium of eight Federal Government and private nonprofit organizations: AHRQ, CDC, NCI, NHLBI, NIDA, American Legacy Foundation, RWJF, and UW-CTRI. All of these organizations have as their mission reducing the human costs of tobacco use. Given the importance of this issue to the health of all Americans, the updated Guideline is published by the PHS, HHS.

GUIDELINE STYLE AND STRUCTURE

This Guideline update was written to be applicable to all tobacco users—those using cigarettes as well as other forms of tobacco. Therefore, the terms "tobacco user" and "tobacco dependence" will be used in preference to "smoker" and "cigarette dependence." In some cases, however, the evidence for a particular recommendation consists entirely of studies using cigarette smokers as participants. In these instances, the recommendation and evidence refers to "smoking" to communicate the parochial nature of the evidence. In most cases, though, Guideline recommendations are relevant to all types of tobacco users. Finally, most data reviewed in this Guideline update are based on adult smokers, although data relevant to adolescent smokers are presented in Chapter 7.

The updated Guideline is divided into seven chapters that integrate prior and updated findings:

Chapter 1, Overview and Methods, provides the clinical practice and scientific context of the Guideline update project and describes the methodology used to generate the Guideline findings.

Chapter 2, Assessment of Tobacco Use, describes how each patient presenting at a health care setting should have his or her tobacco use status determined and how tobacco users should be assessed for willingness to make a quit attempt.

Chapter 3, Clinical Interventions for Tobacco Use and Dependence, summarizes effective brief interventions that can easily be delivered in a primary care setting. In this chapter, separate interventions are described for the patient who is *willing* to try to quit at this time, for the patient who is *not yet willing* to try to quit, and for the patient who has recently quit.

Chapter 4, Intensive Interventions for Tobacco Use and Dependence, outlines a prototype of an intensive tobacco cessation treatment that comprises strategies shown to be effective in this Guideline. Because intensive treatments produce the highest success rates, they are an important element in tobacco intervention strategies.

Chapter 5, Systems Interventions, targets health care administrators, insurers, and purchasers, and offers a blueprint to changes in health care delivery and coverage such that tobacco assessment and intervention become a standard of care in health care delivery.

Chapter 6, Evidence and Recommendations, presents the results of Guideline literature reviews and statistical analyses and the recommendations that emanate from them. Guideline analyses address topics such as the effectiveness of different counseling strategies and medications; the relation between treatment intensities and treatment success; whether screening for tobacco use in the clinic setting enhances tobacco user identification; and whether systems changes can increase provision of effective interventions, quit attempts, and actual cessation rates. The Guideline Panel also made specific recommendations regarding future research needs.

Chapter 7, Specific Populations and Other Topics, evaluates evidence on tobacco intervention strategies and effectiveness with specific populations (e.g., HIV-positive smokers; hospitalized smokers; lesbian/gay/bisexual/transgender smokers; smokers with low SES/limited educational attain-

Appendix C

ment; smokers with medical comorbidities; older smokers; smokers with psychiatric disorders, including substance use disorders; racial and ethnic minorities; women smokers; children and adolescents; light smokers; pregnant smokers; and noncigarette tobacco users). The Guideline Panel made specific recommendations for future research on topics relevant to these populations. This chapter also presents information and recommendations relevant to weight gain after smoking cessation, with specific recommendations regarding future research on this topic.

FINDINGS AND RECOMMENDATIONS

The key recommendations of the updated Guideline, *Treating Tobacco Use and Dependence: 2008 Update*, based on the literature review and expert Panel opinion, are as follows:

Ten Key Guideline Recommendations

The overarching goal of these recommendations is that clinicians strongly recommend the use of effective tobacco dependence counseling and medication treatments to their patients who use tobacco, and that health care systems, insurers, and purchasers assist clinicians in making such effective treatments available.

1. Tobacco dependence is a chronic disease that often requires repeated intervention and multiple attempts to quit. Effective treatments exist, however, that can significantly increase rates of long-term abstinence.
2. It is essential that clinicians and health care delivery systems consistently identify and document tobacco use status and treat every tobacco user seen in a health care setting.
3. Tobacco dependence treatments are effective across a broad range of populations. Clinicians should encourage every patient willing to make a quit attempt to use the counseling treatments and medications recommended in this Guideline.
4. Brief tobacco dependence treatment is effective. Clinicians should offer every patient who uses tobacco at least the brief treatments shown to be effective in this Guideline.
5. Individual, group, and telephone counseling are effective, and their effectiveness increases with treatment intensity. Two components of counseling are especially effective, and clinicians should use these when counseling patients making a quit attempt:
   o Practical counseling (problemsolving/skills training)
   o Social support delivered as part of treatment

6. Numerous effective medications are available for tobacco dependence, and clinicians should encourage their use by all patients attempting to quit smoking—except when medically contraindicated or with specific populations for which there is insufficient evidence of effectiveness (i.e., pregnant women, smokeless tobacco users, light smokers, and adolescents).

   Seven first-line medications (5 nicotine and 2 non-nicotine) reliably increase long-term smoking abstinence rates:
   - Bupropion SR
   - Nicotine gum
   - Nicotine inhaler
   - Nicotine lozenge
   - Nicotine nasal spray
   - Nicotine patch
   - Varenicline

   Clinicians also should consider the use of certain combinations of medications identified as effective in this Guideline.

7. Counseling and medication are effective when used by themselves for treating tobacco dependence. The combination of counseling and medication, however, is more effective than either alone. Thus, clinicians should encourage all individuals making a quit attempt to use both counseling and medication.

8. Telephone quitline counseling is effective with diverse populations and has broad reach. Therefore, clinicians and health care delivery systems should both ensure patient access to quitlines and promote quitline use.

9. If a tobacco user currently is unwilling to make a quit attempt, clinicians should use the motivational treatments shown in this Guideline to be effective in increasing future quit attempts.

10. Tobacco dependence treatments are both clinically effective and highly cost-effective relative to interventions for other clinical disorders. Providing coverage for these treatments increases quit rates. Insurers and purchasers should ensure that all insurance plans include the counseling and medication identified as effective in this Guideline as covered benefits.

GUIDELINE UPDATE: ADVANCES

A comparison of the findings of the 2008 Guideline update with the 2000 Guideline reveals the considerable progress made in tobacco research over the brief period separating these two works. Among many important differences between the two documents, the following deserve special note:

- The updated Guideline has produced even stronger evidence that counseling is an effective tobacco use treatment strategy. Of particular note are findings that counseling adds significantly to the effectiveness of tobacco cessation medications, quitline counseling is an effective intervention with a broad reach, and counseling increases abstinence among adolescent smokers.

- The updated Guideline offers the clinician a greater number of effective medications than were identified in the previous Guideline. Seven different effective first-line smoking cessation medications are now approved by the FDA for treating tobacco use and dependence. In addition, multiple combinations of medications have been shown to be effective. Thus, the clinician and patient have many more medication options than in the past. The Guideline also now provides evidence regarding the effectiveness of medications relative to one another.

- The updated Guideline contains new evidence that health care policies significantly affect the likelihood that smokers will receive effective tobacco dependence treatment and successfully stop tobacco use. For instance, making tobacco dependence a benefit covered by insurance plans increases the likelihood that a tobacco user will receive treatment and quit successfully.

FUTURE PROMISE

The research reviewed for this 2008 Guideline update suggests a bright future for treating tobacco use and dependence. Since the first AHCPR Clinical Practice Guideline was published in 1996, encouraging progress has been made in tobacco dependence treatment. An expanding body of research has produced a marked increase in the number and types of effective treatments and has led to multiple new treatment delivery strategies. These new strategies are enhancing the delivery of tobacco interventions both inside and outside health care delivery systems. This means that an unprecedented number of smokers have access to an unprecedented number of effective treatments.

Although the data reviewed in this Guideline update are encouraging and portend even greater advances through future research, for many smokers, the progress has been an undelivered promissory note. Most smokers attempting to quit today still make unaided quit attempts, although the proportion using evidence-based treatments has increased since the publication of the 1996 AHCPR Guideline. Because of the prevalence of such unaided attempts (those that occur without evidence-based counseling or medication), many smokers have successfully quit through this approach. It is clear from the data presented in this Guideline, however, that smokers are significantly more likely to quit successfully if they use an evidence-based counseling or medication treatment than if they try to quit without such aids. Thus, a future challenge for the field is to ensure that smokers, clinicians, and health systems have accurate information on the effectiveness of clinical interventions for tobacco use, and that the 70 percent of smokers who visit a primary care setting each year have greater access to effective treatments. This is of vital public health importance because the costs of failure are so high. Relapse results in continuing lifetime exposure to tobacco, which leads to increased risk of death and disease. Additional progress must be made in educating clinicians and the public about the effectiveness of clinical treatments for tobacco dependence and in making such treatments available and attractive to smokers.

Continued progress is needed in the treatment of tobacco use and dependence. Treatments should be even more effective and available, new counseling strategies should be developed, and research should focus on the development of effective interventions and delivery strategies for populations that carry a disproportionate burden from tobacco (e.g., adolescents; pregnant smokers; American Indians and Alaska Natives; individuals with low SES/limited educational attainment; individuals with psychiatric disorders, including substance use disorders). The decrease in the prevalence of tobacco use in the United States during the past 40 years, however, has been a seminal public health achievement. Treatment of tobacco use and dependence has played an important role in realizing that outcome.

Source: Health Services/Technology Assessment Text, National Institutes of Health. Available online. URL: http://www.ncbi.nlm.nih.gov/books/bv.fcgi?rid=hstat2.section.28189. Accessed on July 14, 2008.

APPENDIX D

GRAPHS AND FIGURES RELATING TO THE TOBACCO INDUSTRY AND SMOKING

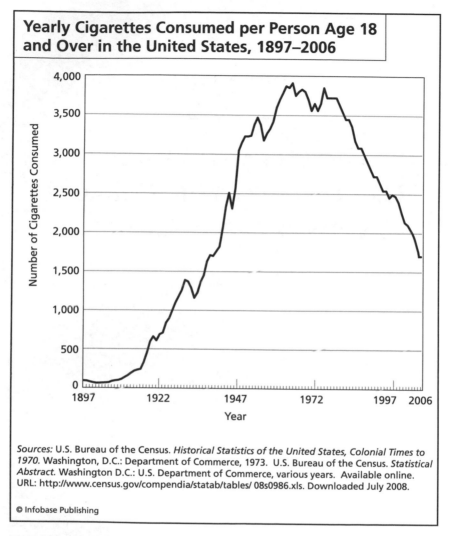

Yearly Cigarettes Consumed per Person Age 18 and Over in the United States, 1897–2006

Sources: U.S. Bureau of the Census. *Historical Statistics of the United States, Colonial Times to 1970.* Washington, D.C.: Department of Commerce, 1973. U.S. Bureau of the Census. *Statistical Abstract.* Washington D.C.: U.S. Department of Commerce, various years. Available online. URL: http://www.census.gov/compendia/statab/tables/ 08s0986.xls. Downloaded July 2008.

© Infobase Publishing

Trends in cigarette consumption show more or less steady growth until a peak in 1963. Consumption declined from the late 1960s and fell to levels not seen since the 1930s. Even so, 1,700 cigarettes consumed per adult in 2006 shows that smoking remains common.

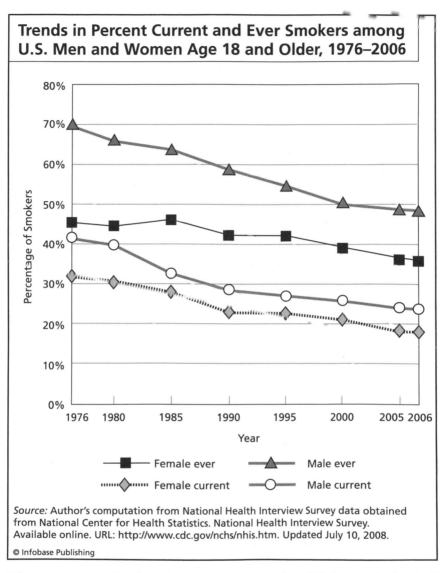

Trends in Percent Current and Ever Smokers among U.S. Men and Women Age 18 and Older, 1976–2006

Female ever
Male ever
Female current
Male current

Source: Author's computation from National Health Interview Survey data obtained from National Center for Health Statistics. National Health Interview Survey. Available online. URL: http://www.cdc.gov/nchs/nhis.htm. Updated July 10, 2008.

© Infobase Publishing

The percentages of male and female current smokers fell during the last half of the 20th century, and the gap between males and females narrowed considerably. Because the percent of ever smokers includes former smokers as well as current smokers, it remains relatively high. Again, however, the gap between men and women narrowed.

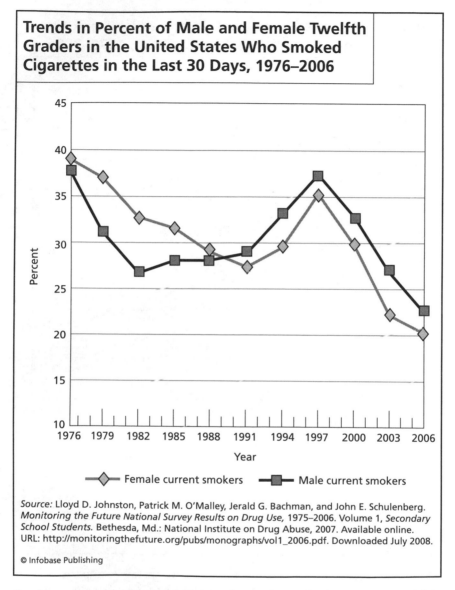

Trends in Percent of Male and Female Twelfth Graders in the United States Who Smoked Cigarettes in the Last 30 Days, 1976–2006

Source: Lloyd D. Johnston, Patrick M. O'Malley, Jerald G. Bachman, and John E. Schulenberg. *Monitoring the Future National Survey Results on Drug Use,* 1975–2006. Volume 1, *Secondary School Students.* Bethesda, Md.: National Institute on Drug Abuse, 2007. Available online. URL: http://monitoringthefuture.org/pubs/monographs/vol1_2006.pdf. Downloaded July 2008.

© Infobase Publishing

Smoking among high school seniors dropped steeply during the 1970s but then declined only slightly during the 1980s and rose during the 1990s. More recently, smoking has again dropped.

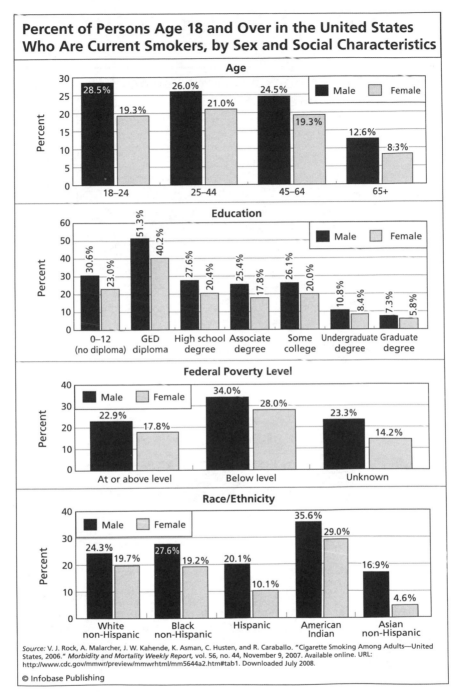

Percent of Persons Age 18 and Over in the United States Who Are Current Smokers, by Sex and Social Characteristics

Age

Male / Female

18–24	25–44	45–64	65+
28.5% (Male) / 19.3% (Female)	26.0% (Male) / 21.0% (Female)	24.5% (Male) / 19.3% (Female)	12.6% (Male) / 8.3% (Female)

Education

Male / Female

0–12 (no diploma)	GED diploma	High school degree	Associate degree	Some college	Undergraduate degree	Graduate degree
30.6% / 23.0%	51.3% / 40.2%	27.6% / 20.4%	25.4% / 17.8%	26.1% / 20.0%	10.8% / 8.4%	7.3% / 5.8%

Federal Poverty Level

Male / Female

At or above level	Below level	Unknown
22.9% / 17.8%	34.0% / 28.0%	23.3% / 14.2%

Race/Ethnicity

Male / Female

White non-Hispanic	Black non-Hispanic	Hispanic	American Indian	Asian non-Hispanic
24.3% / 19.7%	27.6% / 19.2%	20.1% / 10.1%	35.6% / 29.0%	16.9% / 4.6%

Source: V. J. Rock, A. Malarcher, J. W. Kahende, K. Asman, C. Husten, and R. Caraballo. "Cigarette Smoking Among Adults—United States, 2006." *Morbidity and Mortality Weekly Report,* vol. 56, no. 44, November 9, 2007. Available online. URL: http://www.cdc.gov/mmwr/preview/mmwrhtml/mm5644a2.htm#tab1. Downloaded July 2008.

Smoking varies by social characteristics. Men and younger persons smoke more than women and older persons. Those with less education and in poverty smoke more than those with higher education and income. And Hispanics and Asian Americans smoke less than whites, blacks, and Native Americans.

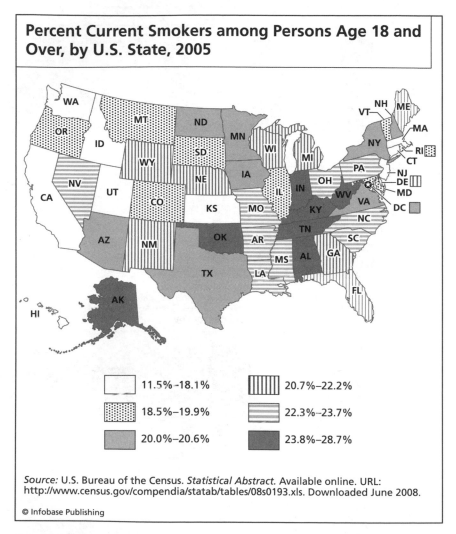

Percent Current Smokers among Persons Age 18 and Over, by U.S. State, 2005

Legend:

- 11.5%–18.1%
- 18.5%–19.9%
- 20.0%–20.6%
- 20.7%–22.2%
- 22.3%–23.7%
- 23.8%–28.7%

Source: U.S. Bureau of the Census. *Statistical Abstract.* Available online. URL: http://www.census.gov/compendia/statab/tables/08s0193.xls. Downloaded June 2008.

© Infobase Publishing

Smoking percentages are highest in midwestern and midsouthern states such as Indiana, Kentucky, Tennessee, and West Virginia. The percentages are lowest in Pacific states, such as California, Washington, and Oregon, and northeastern states, such as Connecticut, Massachusetts, and New Jersey, but Utah stands out as having considerably fewer smokers than all other states.

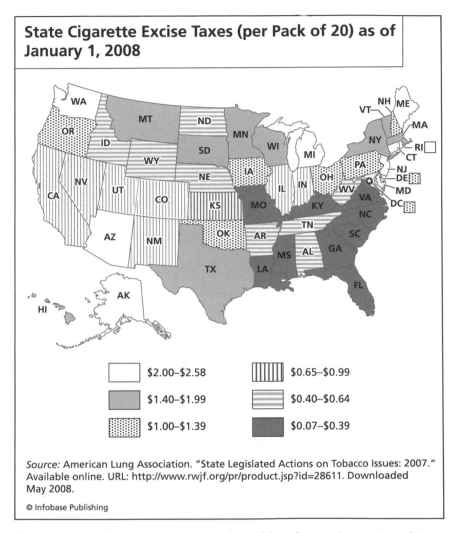

State Cigarette Excise Taxes (per Pack of 20) as of January 1, 2008

$2.00–$2.58

$1.40–$1.99

$1.00–$1.39

$0.65–$0.99

$0.40–$0.64

$0.07–$0.39

Source: American Lung Association. "State Legislated Actions on Tobacco Issues: 2007." Available online. URL: http://www.rwjf.org/pr/product.jsp?id=28611. Downloaded May 2008.

© Infobase Publishing

States vary widely in the excise taxes they add to the purchase price of cigarettes. High taxes represent a form a tobacco control, and state differences in taxes reflect different tobacco control policies.

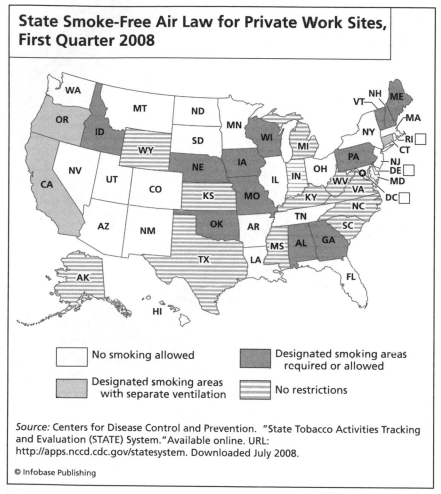

State Smoke-Free Air Law for Private Work Sites, First Quarter 2008

Legend:
- No smoking allowed
- Designated smoking areas required or allowed
- Designated smoking areas with separate ventilation
- No restrictions

Source: Centers for Disease Control and Prevention. "State Tobacco Activities Tracking and Evaluation (STATE) System." Available online. URL: http://apps.nccd.cdc.gov/statesystem. Downloaded July 2008.

© Infobase Publishing

States vary in policies to restrict indoor smoking. Twelve states have no restrictions, but the vast majority limit smoking in workplaces to special areas of buildings or restrict it altogether.

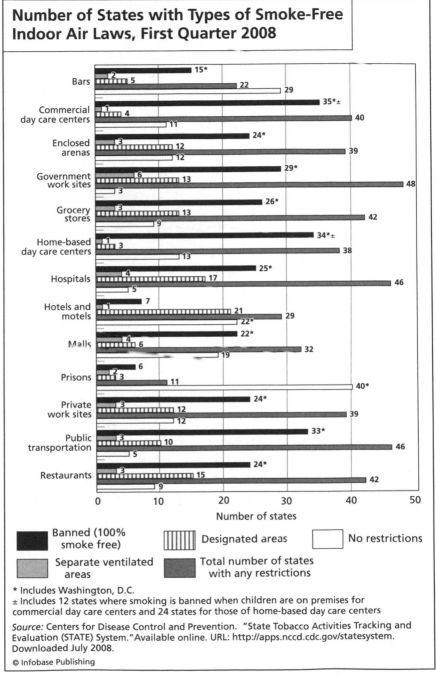

Number of States with Types of Smoke-Free Indoor Air Laws, First Quarter 2008

Bars
- 15*
- 2
- 5
- 22
- 29

Commercial day care centers
- 35*±
- 1
- 4
- 40
- 11

Enclosed arenas
- 24*
- 3
- 12
- 39
- 12

Government work sites
- 29*
- 6
- 13
- 48
- 3

Grocery stores
- 26*
- 3
- 13
- 42
- 9

Home-based day care centers
- 34*±
- 1
- 3
- 38
- 13

Hospitals
- 25*
- 4
- 17
- 46
- 5

Hotels and motels
- 7
- 1
- 21
- 29
- 22*

Malls
- 22*
- 4
- 6
- 32
- 19

Prisons
- 6
- 2
- 3
- 11
- 40*

Private work sites
- 24*
- 3
- 12
- 39
- 12

Public transportation
- 33*
- 3
- 10
- 46
- 5

Restaurants
- 24*
- 3
- 15
- 42
- 9

Number of states: 0 10 20 30 40 50

Legend:
- Banned (100% smoke free)
- Designated areas
- No restrictions
- Separate ventilated areas
- Total number of states with any restrictions

* Includes Washington, D.C.
± Includes 12 states where smoking is banned when children are on premises for commercial day care centers and 24 states for those of home-based day care centers

Source: Centers for Disease Control and Prevention. "State Tobacco Activities Tracking and Evaluation (STATE) System." Available online. URL: http://apps.nccd.cdc.gov/statesystem. Downloaded July 2008.

© Infobase Publishing

The spread of smoke-free indoor air laws across the United States shows in the large number of states that ban smoking altogether in day care centers, hospitals, public transportation, and restaurants. Many other states have partial restrictions on smoking in these places. Full bans on smoking in hotels and prisons remain uncommon but are used in several states.

INDEX

Locators in **boldface** indicate main topics. Locators followed by *c* indicate chronology entries. Locators followed by *b* indicate biographical entries. Locators followed by *g* indicate glossary entries. Locators followed by *t* indicate tables.

A

ACS. *See* American Cancer Society

Action on Smoking and Health (ASH) 130, 140*g*, 237

actors, cigarette use by 114*c*, 119*c*

addiction (term) 140*g*

addictiveness of cigarettes and nicotine 9, **23–26**
  Brown & Williamson's knowledge of 65, 94–96, 122*c*, 139
  Comprehensive Smokeless Tobacco Health Education Act 80
  and continued success of tobacco industry 49–51
  Robert Dole's comments 122*c*, 132
  industry knowledge of 28–29, 91, 122*c*, 135
  and litigation 64, 65
  and persistence of smoking 3–4
  smokers who claim to be addicted 43
  and smoking cessation 56, 57
  Surgeon General's Report (1988) 25, 119*c*
  tobacco executives' denial of 121*c*

additives 45, 80, 84, 100, 121*c*, 140*g*. *See also* flavorings

adolescents. *See* young people

Adolescent Substance Abuse Prevention (ASAP) 234

advertising **16–18**. *See also* antismoking ads; fairness doctrine; *specific ad campaigns, e.g.:* Marlboro Country
  AMA's advocacy of ban on 119*c*
  Brown & Williamson v. FDA 97
  Leo F. Burnett and 131
  California laws 86
  Capital Broadcasting v. Mitchell 117*c*
  for cigars 17
  Comprehensive Smokeless Tobacco Health Education Act 81
  Comprehensive Smoking Education Act 79, 119*c*
  James Duke's cigarette monopoly 11
  Family Smoking Prevention and Tobacco Control Act 84, 127*c*

Federal Cigarette Labeling and Advertising Act 74–76

filter-tip cigarette hearings 115*c*

George Washington Hill and 134

JAMA criticism of 113*c*

late 19th century 8

litigation victories 64

Mangini v. R. J. Reynolds 122*c*

on matchbooks 110*c*

and minors 15, **26–27**, 36, 42, 60

and persistence of smoking 3–4

physicians featured in 17, 19, 29, 113*c*

Public Health Cigarette Smoking Act 77–79, 117*c*

R. J. Reynolds and 124*c*, 137

and racketeering lawsuit settlement 127*c*

radio/television ban 31

regulation limits 124*c*

and smokers' rights 69

smoking prevention campaigns *vs.* 55

by TI 30

300

Index

Index

Index